Wound Healing and Skin Integrity

Wound Healing and Skin Integrity
Principles and Practice

Edited by

Madeleine Flanagan
MSc (Dist), BSc (Hons), Cert Ed (FE), RN

Principal Lecturer
School of Life and Medical Sciences
Postgraduate Medicine
University of Hertfordshire, UK

⟨W⟩ WILEY-BLACKWELL

A John Wiley & Sons, Ltd., Publication

This edition first published 2013
© 2013 by John Wiley & Sons, Ltd

Registered office: John Wiley & Sons, Ltd, The Atrium, Southern Gate, Chichester, West Sussex, PO19 8SQ, UK

Editorial offices: 9600 Garsington Road, Oxford, OX4 2DQ, UK
The Atrium, Southern Gate, Chichester, West Sussex, PO19 8SQ, UK
111 River Street, Hoboken, NJ 07030-5774, USA

For details of our global editorial offices, for customer services and for information about how to apply for permission to reuse the copyright material in this book please see our website at www.wiley.com/wiley-blackwell.

Library of Congress Cataloging-in-Publication Data

Wound healing and skin integrity : principles and practice / edited by Madeleine Flanagan, MSc (Dist), BSc (Hons), Cert Ed (FE), RN, principal lecturer, School of Life and Medical Sciences, Postgraduate Medicine, University of Hertfordshire, UK.
        pages cm
    Includes bibliographical references and index.
    ISBN 978-0-470-65977-9 (pbk. : alk. paper) – ISBN 978-1-118-44181-7 (mobi) – ISBN 978-1-118-44202-9 (ebook/epdf) – ISBN 978-1-118-44206-7 (epub)   1. Wounds and injuries–Treatment.   2. Skin–Wounds and injuries–Treatment.   I. Flanagan, Madeleine.
    RD95.W68 2013
    617.4′77044–dc23

                                                                                2012039436

A catalogue record for this book is available from the British Library.

Wiley also publishes its books in a variety of electronic formats. Some content that appears in print may not be available in electronic books.

Cover images courtesy of Julia Schofield (main image of varicose eczema), Ann Marie Brown (skin tear), Shiu-Ling Briggs (infected leg ulcer) and Madeleine Flanagan (pressure ulcer)
Cover design by Andy Meaden

Set in 9.5/11.5 pt Palatino by Aptara® Inc., New Delhi, India
Printed and bound in Malaysia by Vivar Printing Sdn Bhd

3   2014

Contents

List of Contributors

Jan Apelqvist MD, PhD, Department of Endocrinology, University Hospital of Skåne, Division for Clinical Sciences, University of Lund, Malmö, Sweden

Janice Bianchi MSc, BSc, RGN, RMN, PGcert TLHE, Medical Education Specialist and Honorary Lecturer at Glasgow University, Nursing and Healthcare School, University of Glasgow, Scotland, UK

Annemarie Brown MSc, BSc (Hons), RN, Tissue Viability Solutions, Castle Point and Rochford Primary Care Trust, Southend Primary Care Trust, Southend-on-Sea, Essex, UK

Keryln Carville RN, STN (Cred), PhD, Assoc Professor Domiciliary Nursing Silver Chain Nursing Association & Curtin University of Technology, Osborn Park, Perth, Western Australia

Kim Deroo RN, MN, NP(c), Wound and Chronic Disease Management, Nursing Practice Solutions, Inc, Toronto, Ontario, Canada

Valerie Edwards-Jones PhD, FIBMS, FRSM, School of Research, Enterprise, and Innovation, Faculty of Science and Engineering, Manchester Metropolitan University, Manchester, UK

Madeleine Flanagan MSc (Dist), BSc Hons, Cert Ed (FE), RN, School of Life and Medical Sciences, Postgraduate Medicine, University of Hertfordshire, Hatfield, Hertfordshire, UK

Keith Harding MB, FRCGP, FRCP, FRCS, Director Wound Healing Research Unit, Director TIME Institute, Medical School Cardiff University, Cardiff, Wales, UK

Theresa Hurd MSN, Med, Wound and Chronic Disease Management, Nursing Practice Solutions, Inc., Toronto, Ontario, Canada

David Keast BSc, Aging Rehabilitation and Geriatric Care Research Centre, Lawson Health Research Institute, St Joseph's Parkwood Hospital, London, Ontario, Canada

Arne Langøen RN, Asc. Professor, Stord/ Haugesund University College, Department of Health, Klingenbergvegen, Norway

Mary Martin D4 Consultancy, Dublin, Ireland

Jeanette Muldoon RN, Head of Clinical Services, Activa Healthcare, Burton-on Trent, Staffordshire, UK

Wayne Naylor BSc (Hons), PG Cert (Palliative Care), Nat Cert (Official Statistics), Palliative Care Council of New Zealand, Wellington, New Zealand

Patricia Price PhD, BA (Hons), CPsychol, AFBPsS, FHEA, School of Healthcare Studies, Cardiff University, Cardiff, Wales, UK

Douglas Queen BSc, PhD, MBA, Honorary Research Fellow, Wound Healing Research Unit Medical School, Cardiff University, Cardiff, Wales, UK

Lesley Robertson-Laxton MSN, NP, Wound and Chronic Disease Management, Nursing Practice Solutions, Inc, Toronto, Ontario, Canada

Sabina Sabo RN, MN, Wound, Skin and Ostomy Consultant, Nursing Practice Solutions, Inc., Toronto, Canada

Arlene A. Sardo NP-Adult, MS/ACNP, ENC(C), CCN(C), Wound and Chronic Disease Management, Nursing Practice Solutions, Inc., Toronto, Ontario, Canada; Faculty of Health Sciences, School of Nursing, McMaster University, Hamilton, Ontario, Canada

Julia Schofield MB, Department of Dermatology, Lincoln County Hospital, United Lincolnshire Hospitals NHS Trust, Lincoln, Lincolnshire, UK, School of Life and Medical Sciences, University of Hertfordshire, Hatfield, Hertfordshire, UK

Carolina Weller PhD, MEd (Research), GCHE, BN, RM, RN, School of Public Health and Preventive Medicine, Monash University, Melbourne, Australia

Alan Widgerow MD, MBBCh, FCS (Plast), MMed (Wits), FACS, Laboratory for Tissue Engineering & Regenerative Medicine, Aesthetic & Plastic Surgery Institute, University of California, Irvine, CA, USA

Preface

Wounds are everywhere, occurring in the young and elderly, in hospital and at home, and affect patients in every clinical speciality around the world. Skin breakdown impacts on a significant proportion of the global population each year and has a major effect on sufferers, relatives, and their carers. Many wounds and skin integrity problems are self managed as those affected may lack access to specialist services and professional expertise. As a result, clinicians who manage wounds work in a diverse range of healthcare environments and their work involves addressing the prevention, treatment, care needs, and long-term support of people with skin damage. Even though skin and wound problems are one of the commonest reasons that people present to their doctors, relatively few are referred for specialist advice.

There has always been common ground between wound management and other clinical specialities including dermatology and vascular medicine. But in recent years, the overlap between clinical specialities concerned with the prevention and maintenance of skin integrity has become more apparent as integrated pathways of care have become widely accepted as a way of improving continuity and collaboration among multidisciplinary teams which until now has not been a feature of traditional wound care services. In recent years, an emphasis on service integration has brought the specialities of wound mangement and dermatology much

closer, together as it makes sound economic sense for health providers to develop services which cross traditional boundaries, promoting integrated working, development of extended role practitioners, and improvements in patient care.

This book aims to reflect these trends by cutting across the traditional service boundaries and is designed to be of practical help to any clinician responsible for managing wounds and skin integrity problems in hospitals or community settings including nurses, doctors, podiatrists, pharmacists, and physiotherapists. It has been written with the needs of clinicians with a special interest in the promotion and maintenance of skin integrity in mind and provides the opportunity to develop wound management, skin integrity, and dermatology expertise by integrating relevant aspects of these related disciplines into one comprehensive resource. Thus, the primary goal for this book is to help clinicians acquire and develop advanced knowledge and skills to effectively promote and maintain skin integrity in patients of all ages based on the best available evidence. This supports the global health agenda by building and supporting a skilled workforce with the aim of maintaining and improving health within a knowledge-based, patient-centred healthcare system.

Section 1 covers *Principles of Best Practice* for all wound types beginning with a review of how to effectively make evidence-based clinical decisions to improve quality of everyday practice and continues with applied physiology of skin barrier integrity and wound healing, and chapters focusing on the generic principles of wound management, wound infection, and the psychological impact of skin breakdown.

Section 2, *Challenging Wounds*, considers specific types of nonhealing wounds such as pressure ulcers, leg ulcers, diabetic foot wounds, surgical and malignant wounds as well as lymphoedema and dermatological conditions associated with skin breakdown. Section 3, Improving Skin Integrity Services examines the importance of reducing healthcare costs from a clinical perspective and the need to demonstrate the value of skin integrity service provision to key stakeholders. It concludes with an analysis of the impact that advanced wound technologies have had on the healing revolution and predicts the evolution of wound management in the future. The expert practitioners who have contributed to this book have willingly drawn upon their wealth of personal experience, knowledge, and skills to share practical tips and advice previously not published in a single resource.

Each chapter begins by providing an overview of key issues and summarises the specific principles of wound management by wound type to provide a practical guide that is accessible to clinicians regardless of professional background, and acknowledges that in different healthcare settings a variety of health professionals may assume the lead role for wound management and may do so with limited resources. The book is written from a broad international perspective avoiding nationally specific terms and agendas and addresses the need of clinicians to access evidence-based information for a broad range of wound types and is extensively referenced throughout.

Each chapter concludes with a section on provision of specialist services and "further information" which lists selected, free internet resources that have been carefully chosen because they represent best practice, are evidence based, well written, and relevant to an international audience. Where possible, examples of current, consensus clinical practice guidelines are provided to support clinical decision making.

Chapter 15, *Neglected Wounds*, provides a quick, practical guide to the types of wound sometimes mismanaged due to lack of clinical experience and is written using a concise, easy-to-read style. It provides key details about those wounds that are difficult to heal but less commonly encountered in everyday practice and includes essential information about factors delaying healing, complications, tips for practical wound management, and criteria for specialist referral, and is intended to offer practical, no-nonsense help for busy clinicians.

This book will be useful for anyone with a responsibility for teaching clinicians, students, and patients to manage wounds and skin integrity problems as well as practitioners studying wound healing, skin integrity, pressure ulcer prevention, dermatology, and palliative care as part of science degrees for doctors and health professionals allied to medicine, and those with a research interest in skin integrity and wounds.

The global wound care community is a tight-knit group of dedicated and enthusiastic health professionals who are keen to share their knowledge and experience to improve the life of patients with compromised skin integrity. I am pleased to observe that this community is growing year on year as practitioners researchers, and healthcare industry gain knowledge and push the boundaries about what is possible to improve the lives of patients with nonhealing wounds. If this book helps one clinician heal a single patient's wound, then the effort involved will have been well worth it.

Madeleine Flanagan

Acknowledgements

My thanks go to all the health professionals and patients I have had the privilege to meet during my career who have stimulated my interest in chronic wounds, to my students for asking difficult questions and giving me the impetus to capture current thinking in a book, and to my contributors who were handpicked for their specialist knowledge and practical expertise. But most of all, special thanks goes to Ed and Max who have lived through the writing, editing, and proof reading of this book – without whose unfailing support, I just couldn't have done it.

This book is dedicated to Maxwell Coupland who is a very special little boy.

Section 1

Principles of Best Practice

1 Evidence and Clinical Decision-making

Carolina Weller

School of Public Health and Preventive Medicine, Monash University, Melbourne, Australia

Overview

- Evidence-based practice integrates the best available research evidence with information about patient preferences, clinician skills and available resources to make decisions about patient care.
- Barriers to the use of research-based evidence can occur when time, access to the literature, search skills, critical appraisal skills and implementation skills are lacking.
- Evidence-based clinical decision-making requires comparison of all relevant sources. In the absence of randomised controlled trials involving a direct comparison of treatments of interest, indirect treatment comparisons and systematic reviews provide useful evidence.
- Clinical guidelines appear to be one of the most effective methods of applying evidence to improve quality of care but little is known about the best way to implement them into everyday practice.
- Selective reading of high-quality evidence is one of the most effective strategies to improve research dissemination and changes in practice. There are now good sources of evidence-based information available on the Internet that help identify, appraise and apply research findings to clinical practice.

Introduction: what is effective clinical decision-making?

Clinical decision-making is an essential part of effective wound management and is based on clinical judgement which consists of professional performance and human judgement. Health care providers increasingly recognise the importance of making decisions based on the best possible evidence. Making decisions that will impact on the healing outcome of individuals in the clinical workplace take place every day but reliability of clinical judgement is often variable as many different factors will influence decisions; these include the type of clinical setting, interpersonal relationships, available diagnostic data, scope of practice and individual skill (DiCenso et al., 2010). The process of clinical decision-making should ideally include use of

Wound Healing and Skin Integrity: Principles and Practice, First Edition. Edited by Madeleine Flanagan.
© 2013 John Wiley & Sons, Ltd. Published 2013 by John Wiley & Sons, Ltd.

research findings, clinical guidelines, and evidence-based treatment algorithms (Rose, 2011). Improving the implementation of evidence-based practice (EBP) and public health depends on behaviour change. Health care outcomes such as choice of type of compression to encourage patient adherence to compression therapy are often based on decisions made within an organisation, which adds another layer of complexity to clinical decision-making. Clinical decisions that impact directly on patient safety and quality of care are made by health professionals based on previous knowledge and experience. The care received by patients in relation to wound care is often dependent on factors that are related to characteristics of individual health professionals, such as education and training in wound care as well as behaviour of people in the workplace (Grol, 2002). For patients to benefit from treatment, clinicians must have a mastery of skills, including history-taking and physical examination, although effective clinical decision-making does not begin or end there, continuous, self-directed lifelong learning is paramount to advance wound management and improve quality of care.

What is evidence-based health care?

Best practice research evidence refers to methodologically sound, clinically relevant research about the effectiveness and safety of interventions, the accuracy and precision of assessment measures, the power of prognostic indicators, the strength of causal relationships, the cost-effectiveness of interventions and the meaning of illness or patient experiences (Sackett et al., 1996).

Over 10 years ago, the Cochrane systematic reviews (Cullum et al., 2000; O'Meara et al., 2009) reported the importance of multi-component compression bandages to heal people with venous leg ulcers (VLUs) and the importance of Ankle Brachial Pressure Index (ABPI) assessment to exclude arterial disease prior to compression application. This type of evidence should guide clinical practice, but what if the clinician does not have access to a hand-held Doppler and is unable to refer to a vascular laboratory or specialist wound clinic due to geographical or cost factors? Even if a Doppler is available the clinician may not have the confidence to assess the patients and measure the ABPI as found

in a recent cross-sectional survey of practice nurses (PNs) working in Australian general practice clinics. This study identified that knowledge of VLU management was sub-optimal and current practice did not comply with evidence-based VLU management guidelines (Weller and Evans, 2012). Despite recognition by PNs that specialist wound clinics provide a valuable resource, more than 40% did not refer patients for treatment and a third retained patients for over 3 months before referring them for specialist assessment. In the United Kingdom, PNs typically have sole responsibility for determining the patient's treatment plan (Ertl, 1992; McGuckin and Kerstein, 1998). Despite 70% of PNs having some responsibility for determining VLU management, less than 20% stated that they used best practice guidelines to direct treatment (Weller and Evans, 2012).

Despite availability of evidence to support leg ulcer management, studies have identified deficiencies in general practice management of leg ulceration, specifically the under-use of ABPI measurements, over-reliance on dressings and lack of understanding of compression therapy (McGuckin and Kerstein, 1998; Graham et al., 2003; Sadler et al., 2006).

Research evidence alone is never sufficient to make a clinical decision. Clinicians often weigh up the benefits and risks, inconvenience and costs associated with alternative management strategies, and in doing so consider the patient's values. Patient values and preferences refer to the underlying assumptions and beliefs that are involved when clinicians, together with patients, weigh what they will gain making a clinical management decision such as choosing a compression system that is easy for the nurse to apply, is less expensive and is more comfortable for the patient. Healing time can be improved simply by addressing the issue of nurse application, patient adherence and cost-effectiveness (Weller et al., 2010b, 2010c). EBP involves the incorporation of research evidence, clinical expertise and client values in clinical decision-making (Sackett et al., 1996). Application of high-quality evidence to clinical decision-making requires knowledge of how to access evidence in the first place; includes an understanding of literature searching and application of critical appraisal skills to differentiate lower- from higher-quality clinical studies (Weller, 2009).

Common misperceptions about evidence-based practice

- Clinicians believe they already 'do' EBP;
- EBP is a passing trend;
- EBP leads to 'cook book' medicine;
- EBP is expensive and time-consuming;
- EBP is a restriction of clinical freedom;
- 'I have always done it this way, so I know it works'.

How does evidence fit into clinical decision-making in clinical practice?

The skills necessary to provide an evidence-based solution to a clinical problem includes several aspects such as defining the problem, conducting an efficient search to locate the best evidence, critically appraising the evidence and considering that evidence and its implications in the context of patients' circumstances and values (Box 1.1).

Clinicians report that the major barrier to using current research evidence is time, effort and skills needed to access the right information (Cabana et al., 1999). A high proportion of new research articles are peer reviewed and published, although the addition of systematically combining results in context of other similar studies is still lacking. Ideally, clinicians could access updated well-conducted systematic reviews for all clinical questions, however only about 10% of randomised controlled trials (RCTs) are incorporated in Cochrane reviews (Mallett and Clarke, 2003) and at least 90% of reviews recommended further research (El Dib et al., 2007). Despite these limitations, systematic reviews can improve decision-making (Box 1.2).

EBP integrates the best available research evidence with information about patient preferences, clinician skill level and available resources to make decisions about patient care (Sackett et al., 1996). Attaining these skills requires knowledge, motivation and application (Guyatt et al., 2000). Clinicians often have questions about the care of their patients, but many go unanswered (Dawes and Sampson, 2003). Barriers to the use of research-based evidence can occur when time, access to journal articles, search skills, critical appraisal skills and understanding of the language used in research are lacking.

The aim of evidence-based health care is to provide the appropriate means for making effective clinical decisions, not only for avoiding habitual practice but also for enhancing clinical performance. An EBP culture connects research evidence, patient preferences, the available resources and clinical expertise, to include these factors in the decision-making process. Clinical judgement provides health professionals with a methodology for comparing decisions between practitioners with different training and experience, and improving decision-making. Keeping up to date with wound care research is a mammoth task and is a challenge for busy clinicians. Evidence-based health care requires clinicians to engage with research evidence in decision-making at the workplace. But is it unrealistic to assume that research results will be implemented in clinical practice as translational research can be hindered by two main aspects: how the evidence is generated, and how the evidence is implemented? When generating evidence, one major barrier to uptake of research into clinical practice is that the 'practice' described in clinical trials or research environments may not be generalisable from the setting (hospital community), circumstances (number of clinicians with wound management knowledge), patient groups (chronic, acute wounds) and resources (Doppler ultrasound, wound dressings, compression bandages) available in daily practice of many clinicians.

For evidence to be translated to clinical practice the clinician needs to be aware of the evidence, and accept and adhere to findings. Although it is broadly accepted that effective health care decisions require the integration of research evidence and individual preferences, it is not unusual to find that evidence generated by researchers does not always get implemented in a timely and dependable way and may not take into account patient input (Cabana et al., 1999). One could question whether practitioners and patients benefit from current best practice and whether EBP affects treatment outcomes in a positive way when research that should change practice is often ignored for years, for example pressure ulcer risk assessment and prevention, moist wound healing principles (Winter, 1995, 1962, 2006; Cullum et al., 2000) and compression for treatment of venous ulcers (Fletcher et al., 1997; Cullum et al., 2001; O'Meara et al., 2009).

Box 1.1   Steps for appraising the literature

1. Ask an answerable question from a clinical issue

PICOT is one technique that can used to develop clinical research questions. PICOT is an acronym for the five different areas the technique considers: patient/population, intervention or issue, comparison with another intervention or issue, outcome and timeframe; e.g. *Which interventions help people adhere to compression therapies for venous leg ulceration?*

2. Search for valid external evidence

Quick access to pre-appraised information is available at

- The Cochrane Library
- PubMed Clinical Queries
- ACP Journal Club
- Evidence-based Medicine

3. Critically appraise the evidence for relevance and validity

Methods

Consider

- Study design, e.g. randomised controlled trial, cohort study, survey;
- Clinical setting, e.g. hospital, community;
- Patient population, e.g. sample size, inclusion/exclusion criteria;
- Describe intervention group and control group;
- Blinding (if applicable), e.g. double blind, single blind;
- Statistical analysis, e.g. suitability of tests;
- Relevance of outcome measures, e.g. time to complete healing;
- Follow-up, e.g. duration, all patients accounted for.

Results

Consider

- Relevance of outcomes, e.g. number needed to treat, sensitivity, specificity;
- Time points of reporting;
- Compliance with intervention/therapy/medications;
- Adverse effects.

4. Apply the results back to the patient

There is low-quality evidence that leg ulcer clinical care may not improve adherence to compression therapy or healing rates or prevent recurrence when compared to home care. Because of the lack of reliable evidence, it is not possible to recommend nurse clinical care interventions. There is a need to improve and increase interaction with patients emphasising the adherence in future compression trials (Field, 1994).

5. Record the information for the future

Audit your clinical practice by checking your everyday practice against published EBP on a regular basis.

Although EBP has an increasingly broad-based support in health care, it remains difficult to get health care professionals to engage and practice it (Thompson et al., 2005). Across most domains in wound care, practice has lagged behind research and knowledge by at least several years and often longer (Bates et al., 2003). There are many impediments to introducing evidence and clinical

---

Box 1.2 Summary of systematic review: compression for venous leg ulcers (O'Meara et al., 2009)

Objectives: To undertake a systematic review of all RCTs of the clinical effectiveness of compression bandage or stocking systems in the treatment of venous leg ulceration.
   Specific questions addressed by the review are

- Does the application of compression bandages or stockings aid venous ulcer healing?
- Which compression bandage or stocking system is the most effective?

   Search strategy: For this update the Cochrane Wounds Group Specialised Register (14/10/08) was searched; the Cochrane Central Register of Controlled Trials (CENTRAL) (The Cochrane Library Issue 4 2008); Ovid MEDLINE (1950 to October Week 1 2008); Ovid EMBASE (1980 to 2008 Week 41); and Ovid CINAHL (1982 to October Week 1 2008). No date or language restrictions were applied.
   Selection criteria: RCTs recruiting people with venous leg ulceration that evaluated any type of compression bandage system or compression hosiery were eligible for inclusion. Comparators included no compression (e.g. primary dressing alone, non-compressive bandage) or an alternative type of compression. Trials had to report an objective measure of ulcer healing in order to be included (primary outcome for the review). Secondary outcomes of the review included ulcer recurrence, costs, quality of life, pain, adverse events and withdrawals. There was no restriction on date, language or publication status of trials.
   Data collection and analysis: Details of eligible studies were extracted and summarised using a data extraction table. Data extraction was performed by one review author and verified independently by a second review author.
   Main results: Overall, 39 RCTs reporting 47 comparisons were included. Review question 1: there was reasonable evidence from seven RCTs that venous ulcers heal more rapidly with compression than without. Review question 2: findings from six trials of single-component compression suggested that this strategy was less effective than multi-component compression.
   Authors' conclusions: Compression increases ulcer healing rates compared with no compression. Multi-component systems are more effective than single-component systems. Multi-component systems containing an elastic bandage appear more effective than those composed mainly of inelastic constituents.

---

guidelines into routine daily practice (Grol and Grimshaw, 2003).

One aspect that researchers need to consider when designing a clinical trial is that the population, measurement tools and interventions will be relevant to the clinical patient group. Some have argued that RCTs are too limited (Gottrup, 2010; Gottrup and Apelqvist, 2010) but others disagree and argue that wound care research needs high-level evidence reported in a transparent way so clinicians and health policymakers can improve wound care with the best available evidence to guide practice (Barton, 2000; Weller et al., 2010d; Weller and McNeil, 2010). For implementing evidence, clinical guidelines appear to be one of the most promising and effective tool for improving the quality of care but little is known about the optimal implementation strategy. There are many good examples of internationally agreed clinical guidelines in wound management that define best practice and are easy to implement to guide local practice (SIGN, 2010; Australian Wound Management Association Inc. and New Zealand Wound Care Society Inc., 2011).

Challenges to changing practice

Even when most clinicians are aware of evidence, there may be little impact on quality of care due to the many complexities involved in changing practice. Change within organisation structures may be hindered by many factors, and barriers to transforming clinical competence into clinical performance can arise due to varied reasons (Thompson et al., 2005). For example, the patient or health care system may not be able to afford effective best practice treatments. Practitioners may experience excessive workloads, inadequate practice organisation, financial pressures and lack of time they are able to spend with each patient which may result in less than optimal care. To introduce evidence into clinical practice it is appropriate to identify the groups affected by the proposed change/s in practice. It is paramount to assess the preparedness of the group to change and identify likely enabling factors, including resources, skills and knowledge.

In addition, the practice of 'traditional habits', e.g. failing to apply compression bandage routinely in people with venous ulcers (omission) or inappropriate use of 'new' dressing (commission) can impact negatively on healing outcomes and quality of life for people with chronic wounds. Although individual clinical practice environments will vary for each health professional, aspects such as professional discipline, availability of information and current resources in the workplace need to be considered when considering change to health service environment. The amount, structure and type of clinical information available are often out of date, not evidence based, variable across clinical domains and not centrally organised on information which leads to uncertainty associated with clinical decision-making. However, the first hurdle to overcome is the awareness and ability to identify high-quality evidence.

Health professionals work in different settings/institutions with differing levels of expertise and may handle similar decisions very differently. Clinical organisations limit or shape choices associated with clinical decisions. Some solutions developed in one place may not be directly transferable or applicable to another health care environment or patient group. Although there are many RCTs and published systematic reviews in wound care providing information on decisions about compression therapy as the best practice treatment for people with VLUs, there are still examples of lack of compression application by some communities and PNs (Annells et al., 2008; Newall et al., 2009). Evidence-based health care decision-making requires comparison of all relevant competing interventions. In the absence of RCTs involving a direct comparison of all treatments of interest, indirect treatment comparisons and network meta-analysis provide useful evidence for judiciously selecting the best treatment(s) (Hoaglin et al., 2011). To implement an intervention requires both access and knowledge. For compression, this is challenging enough; becoming familiar with the many different types of bandages, contraindications of application, adverse effects and monitoring require improved education and better specific training in wound care to lead to better wound care outcomes for patients (Gottrup, 2004). Patients must also contend with competing claims and advice from clinicians, adverse effects; or the fear of, and sometimes the lack of funding to pay for compression treatments.

EBP implementation remains limited in clinical practice. There are practical problems of implementation, which include training, access to research, and development of and access to tools to display evidence and support for decision-making. There may also be practical difficulties of implementation due to the disease burden of the patient group, funding models and workforce shortages which have been reported to have hindered successful adoption of evidence-based strategy that was known to improve health outcomes in a wound care group. A supportive professional environment can greatly influence the use of research-based evidence to inform clinical decisions of an individual (Spring, 2008).

Factors influencing clinical judgement

Clinical decision-making is the ability to sift and synthesise information, make decisions and appropriately implement them. Clinical decision-making is a complex process whereby practitioners determine the type of information they collect, recognise problems according to the cues identified during information collection, e.g. wound assessment, and then decide upon appropriate interventions to address those problems (Sox et al., 2010).

Although many factors influence the decision-making process, there are a myriad of other factors that serve as barriers to this process. Even when clinicians know and accept what to do, it is possible that with workloads they forget or neglect to do it (Glasziou and Haynes, 2005). To achieve effective clinical decision-making, health professionals need to be encouraged to make decisions and assume responsibility for their decisions. Evidence from successful health service change projects suggests that an environment that is genuinely collaborative, cooperative, democratic and involves all stakeholder groups including the patient is imperative for success (Atallah, 1999; Adderley and Thompson, 2007; Grol et al., 2007; Avorn and Fischer, 2010). Factors affecting decision-making must be identified and aspects such as adequate time, technical support and sufficient resources to implement the proposed change must be evaluated to encourage shared decision-making. These factors must be understood, the barriers be identified and strategies to minimise these barriers be developed and implemented (Griffin et al., 2011). Habits do not change easily, despite best intentions. Omissions are particularly easy for preventive measures such as compression hosiery when the venous ulcer has healed, as these aspects are not the pressing focus of the management visit.

Patient safety and quality of care will benefit from clarification of decision-making strategies, in the development of guidelines and care pathways. Clinical decision support may include a variety of tools (printed and electronic) that make knowledge and information available to the clinician to access important information (Kawamoto et al., 2005). Much has been written about effecting organisational change within health care (Oxman et al., 1995; Walter et al., 2003; Davies et al., 2008; Wilkinson et al., 2011) and more recently in wound health care (Gottrup et al., 2010), though the need to further promote knowledge and evidence to already busy health professionals can be improved. Groups such as the Cochrane Collaboration, national health and research organisations such as the National Health Scheme, National Health and Medical Research Council, National Institute of Clinical Studies Joanna Briggs Centre and high-quality wound journals that provide high-quality appraisal of research findings and existing evidence can help the clinician to take up the information offered. Some resources available include, but are not limited to, the NHS Evidence Base, American College of Physicians (ACP) database/journal updates journal clubs, online services, BMJ clinical, EBM/Practice Databases, EBM clinical decision support, DYNAMED clinical, Database of Abstracts of Reviews of Effectiveness Centre, Centre for Evidence-Based Medicine, McMaster University Evidence Based Medicine.

Even when high-quality syntheses of evidence is presented to clinicians, the information presented will be shaped by the clinician's previous knowledge (Davies et al., 2008). Clinician's experience is then connected to the context and culture where individuals work, as well as to their role and position in the organisation to shape effective use and implementation of evidence in practice. One aspect that has been successful in part is the initiation of wound care champions (McNees and Kueven, 2011) who take on the responsibility of promoting effective change using research evidence to improve quality of care for people with compromised skin integrity.

Personal contact with respected wound care and dermatology colleagues can bring about change, although it is imperative that these key leaders are competent in identifying and critically appraising the best available evidence and take responsibility for designing and implementing research that is robust. This mechanism may not work if the professional practice of these distinguished and respected wound care experts includes traditional unproven ways of doing things and may in turn be highly resistant to effective implementation of evidence-based care. To achieve EBP in wound care, clinical decision-making should be scientifically based. Future research should focus on which interventions are most effective in optimising wound healing, as well as investigating cost-effectiveness of treatment (Cowan and Stechmiller, 2009).

Evidence-based practice: hierarchy of evidence

Hierarchies of evidence refer to a method of grading the 'best' sources of evidence to support clinical decision-making. These hierarchies of evidence are often depicted as a pyramid with three, four or five levels and although consensus does not exist, one of the most widely accepted is illustrated in Figure 1.1. Research that can be generalised (applied to whole populations), such as Systematic Reviews and RCTs, is positioned at the apex of the

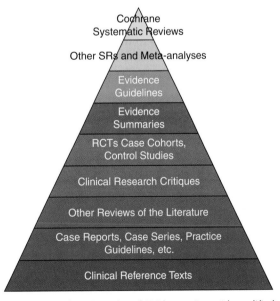

Figure 1.1 The Hierarchy of Evidence. Pyramid modified from *Navigating the Maze*, University of Virginia, Health Sciences Library (2009).

pyramid and evidence where it is not appropriate to generalise, such as data obtained from qualitative research and expert opinion, is usually found at the bottom of these hierarchies. The hierarchy indicates the relative importance that can be given to a particular study design. The higher a methodology is ranked, the stronger it is assumed to be. At the top is the systematic review/meta-analysis which integrates results of a number of similar trials to produce findings of higher statistical power. At the bottom is the opinions of respected authorities, e.g. consensus clinical guidelines thought to provide the weakest level of evidence.

Systematic reviews

A systematic review is a way of summarising the results of multiple research studies in a format that gives a critical assessment of the efficacy and safety of the specific intervention under review. The main objective of a systematic review is to provide summary information to help clinicians make decisions about health care interventions based on best evidence available (Box 1.2).

Systematic reviews are a very efficient way to access the body of research as they save time for busy clinicians who can read a critical synopsis of current research evidence in one document. Searches are undertaken on multiple electronic databases such as CENTRAL and include MEDLINE, EMBASE and other specialist databases (e.g. TRoPHI, CINAHL, LILACS), which ensure a comprehensive search. The search strategy often includes grey literature, trials registers citations, references and may include contacting experts in the field and are not limited by language, year, location and publication status. A systematic review of the literature differs from a literature review, being based on a scientific design, which aims to reduce *bias* and increase reliability and provide a comprehensive picture of all of the available evidence. The information available in a systematic review includes critical appraisal, interpretation of results and reliable basis for decision-making for health care, policy and future research.

Cochrane systematic reviews (Cochrane Wound Group) aim to bring together the body of evidence to inform decision-making. Cochrane reviews are peer reviewed, updated regularly and are free of conflicted funding. Protocols are published prior to review and outline the question definition, eligibil-

ity criteria and outcome measures to reduce impact of bias and are published in The Cochrane Library. Cochrane reviews can be accessed via the Cochrane Library: www.thecochranelibrary.com

A systematic review is comprised of

- clearly stated objectives;
- pre-defined eligibility criteria;
- explicit, reproducible methodology;
- a systematic search;
- assessment of validity of included studies;
- systematic synthesis and presentation of findings.

Other sources of systematic reviews include

- Agency for Healthcare Research and Quality: www.ahrq.gov;
- Joanna Briggs Institute: www.joannabriggs.edu.au;
- BMJ Clinical Evidence: www.clinicalevidence.com;
- Bandolier: www.medicine.ox.ac.uk/bandolier.

Randomised controlled trials

The RCT is considered the best research design to determine the effectiveness of health care interventions. Study participants are randomly assigned to receive a new intervention (experimental group) or standard intervention or no intervention (control group). Randomisation should ensure that chance determines the allocation of participants to one group or other so that the only difference between the two groups should be the intervention. Participants progress is monitored over a specified time period (follow up) and then specific outcomes are evaluated. The random allocation of participants is used to ensure that the intervention and control groups are similar in all respects (which is difficult in chronic conditions) with the exception of the therapeutic or preventative measure being tested (Weller et al., 2010a, 2010c).

Practice point

Is the RCT the best way to provide the evidence base to support wound management decisions?

Originally in medicine RCTs were perceived as the 'gold standard' in terms of levels of evidence and research. In contrast, social science approaches used to explore aspects of patient experience have traditionally been undervalued and seen as unscientific. However, in 1995, Gyatt et al. recognised the greater value of systematic reviews and meta-analyses as they form a comparative analysis of research. Since then, concerns have been raised about the ranking of evidence in relation to which is the most relevant to clinical practice.

The hierarchy is not fixed and there is debate about the relative positions of different research methodologies. Although the RCT is traditionally considered as being an objective method of removing bias, its design is expensive, slow and produces results that may not reflect everyday practice. Methodologies that are lower in ranking are not always inferior, for example a well-conducted observational study may provide more convincing evidence about a treatment than a poorly conducted RCT. Although randomised studies are considered more robust, it would be unethical to perform an RCT which exposed patients to a risk of skin integrity breakdown, for example a study evaluating the effect of no intervention in patients at high risk of pressure ulceration.

Finally, the evidence hierarchy focuses on quantitative research methodologies; however, it is important to choose the most appropriate study design to answer the research question. For example, it is usually not possible to identify individual's feelings and personal experience of living with a chronic wound such as a leg ulcer without using qualitative techniques.

It is therefore important for health care professionals to develop skills to critically evaluate a range of sources of evidence and to raise awareness of the value of evaluating a balanced portfolio of credible evidence when suggesting changes to practice.

Evidence-informed decisions

As stated by Sackett, almost 15 years ago, external clinical evidence can inform, but can never replace, individual clinical expertise, and it is this expertise that decides whether the external evidence applies to the individual patient at all and, if so, how it should be integrated into a clinical decision. Similarly, any external guideline must be integrated with individual clinical expertise in deciding whether and how it matches the patient's clinical state, predicament and preferences, and thus whether it should be applied (Sackett et al., 1996).

A busy clinician will look for the result overview. Aspects such as the type of study, the type of participants and the outcome measures are important as these should be evaluated in their own context

of clinical practice. Some questions that will help when weighing up the relevance of evidence are

(1) Are the participants described similar to my patient group?
(2) Is the intervention something that is used in my practice?
(3) Is the setting similar to my clinical practice environment?
(4) Are the resources used in the study available in my clinical practice for my patient group?

If the answers to these questions are yes, clinicians can make a judgement about the overall quality of evidence based on the criteria as follows:

- risk of bias;
- heterogeneity;
- precision;
- reporting bias;
- generalisability;
- quality (level) of evidence.

The Grading of Recommendations Assessment, Development and Evaluation (GRADE) Working Group has developed a commonsense and transparent approach to grading quality of evidence and strength of recommendations. Many international organizations endorse this approach including the World Health Organisation and the Cochrane Collaboration.

Critical appraisal frameworks

Critical appraisal of research includes both qualitative and quantitative methods, though concentrates on the analysis of the approaches taken to data analysis. Applying a framework of questions to critique a paper allows the reader to critically appraise published work, identify its strengths and limitations and give opportunities to make informed judgements about the study (Box 1.3). The critical appraisal of published research can inform the development of research questions, hypothesis and methodological approaches, or confirm that the body of knowledge that exists is sufficiently robust. Appraising any publication requires three main elements:

(1) What are the results?
(2) Are the results of the study valid?
(3) Are the results applicable to my patients?

Box 1.3   Assessing validity: checklist for various study designs

RCT

- Was the randomisation method outlined adequately?
- Was the randomisation method concealed?
- Were treatment and control groups similar in characteristics (age, gender, etc.) at baseline?
- Were patients and clinicians blinded to treatment?
- Were outcomes assessed objectively?
- Were all patients starting trial accounted for at conclusion?
- Were patients analysed in the groups to which they were randomised, e.g. analysed by intention to treat?

Cohort

- Is the study prospective or retrospective?
- Were the control and study group similar in characteristics at baseline (except for exposure)?
- Were all patients starting the trial accounted for at conclusion?
- Were researchers conducting assessment of outcome blind to exposure status?
- Were the main potential confounders identified and taken into account in the analysis?

Case–control

- Were the cases clearly defined?
- Were cases and controls taken from comparable populations?
- What percentage of cases and controls participated in the study?
- Were study measures identical for cases and controls?
- Were study measures objective or subjective and is recall bias likely if they were subjective?
- Were the main potential confounders identified and taken into account in the analysis?

Cross-sectional study

- Was the study sample clearly defined?
- Was a representative sample achieved?
- Were all relevant exposures, potential confounding factors and outcomes measured accurately?
- Were patients with a wide range of severity of disease assessed?

Case study

- Were cases identified prospectively or retrospectively?
- Are the cases a representative sample?
- Were all relevant exposures, potential confounding factors and outcomes measured accurately?

Other considerations

- Discuss strengths and weaknesses of study (internal and external validity, see above).
- Discuss the study in context of other available literature and/or current standard of care.
- What is the best study design for investigating the research question?
- Can the study outcomes be generalised to your patients?
- What are the clinical implications of this study?

Specific frameworks such as the Consolidated Standards of Reporting Trials (CONSORT) statement (Moher et al., 2010) provides guidance on how to conduct a rigorous RCT for researchers but it can also be used by clinicians as a framework when appraising the results. The CONSORT statement has the potential to play a crucial role in influencing the quality of research and clinical practice and to improve wound care. Implementation of the CONSORT statement can clarify to the reader what exactly was done in the RCT, to whom and when, so that practitioners and health care providers can determine study validity and relevance to their patient group. RCTs are one methodological approach to add to the body of evidence which can inform clinical practice. There are many other quantitative and qualitative approaches that can also inform clinical practice.

Clinical guidelines

Clinical guidelines are 'systematically developed statements to assist clinician and patient decisions about appropriate healthcare for specific circumstances' (Field, 1994). The main purpose of clinical guidelines is to help clinicians provide quality care and to aid in the evaluation of that care with best practice. The development and implementation of (evidence-based) clinical practice guidelines is one of the promising and effective tools for improving the quality of care (Barker and Weller, 2010). However, many guidelines are not used after dissemination. Implementation activities frequently produce only moderate improvement in patient management (Grol and Buchan, 2006; Grol, 2010). Clinical wound care practice guidelines, including specific guidelines for VLUs, skin tears, diabetic foot, pressure ulcers, are now available in many countries (SIGN, 2010) and most take time and resources to collate and distribute.

Practice point

There are many clinical guidelines available for wound and skin care; almost every country has its own version of clinical practice guidelines. Clinicians are faced with the dilemma of choosing from an abundance of guidelines of variable quality or developing new guidelines of their own.

Clinical guidelines should be critically evaluated to ensure that they

- focus on aspects of care delivery that are concerned with difficult decisions or choices to make clinical management easier;
- are based on current scientific evidence drawn from well-designed clinical trials or meta-analyses and clear arguments based on clinical skills and experience;
- contain clear practice recommendations that provide a clear description of desired performance and specific advice about what to do in which situation and which factors should be taken into account;
- are compatible with existing norms and values of clinicians and are not too controversial.

(Burgers et al., 2003)

As users of clinical practice guidelines, health care professionals need to know how much confidence they can place in the practice recommendations made. Systematic methods of making judgements can reduce errors and improve communication, although some guidelines contradict other publications. A system for grading the quality of evidence and the strength of recommendations that can be applied across a wide range of interventions and contexts has been developed (Brouwers et al., 2010). Clinical judgements about the strength of a recommendation require consideration of the balance between benefits and harms, the quality of the evidence and translation of the evidence into specific circumstances. Understanding of EBP is a useful resource when making such judgements. Resource utilisation or how cost-effective the intervention is often lacking in published study results. Good evidence for the cost-effectiveness of many treatments aimed at improving skin integrity are lacking (Grimshaw et al., 2004).

Summary

There is an international effort to improve evidence-based, cost-effective and accountable clinical practice. In Australia, the National Health and Hospitals Reform Commission has a strong focus on continuous learning and evidence-based improvements to health care delivery (Bennett, 2009). In the United States, the Institute of Medicine is building the concept of a value and science-driven learning health care system that is effective and efficient; and in the

United Kingdom, guidance from the National Institute for Health and Clinical Excellence, combined with quality and outcome frameworks that include financial incentives, seeks to align clinical practice with best available evidence (Scott, 2009; Scott and Glasziou, 2012).

Evidence-based guideline development reflects one approach to improving patient care: it assumes health professionals are rational decision-makers who will act on convincing information. A belief that developing and disseminating systematic reviews and guidelines will improve patient outcomes ignores the complexity of change in health care. Guidelines do not implement themselves, they need to be developed, well executed and sustained in implementation programs and even then such programmes usually have only a moderate effect on performance in terms of improvements in patient care (Solberg et al., 2000). Many factors play crucial roles in hindering changes in health care. These factors are related not only to professional decision-making but also to patient behaviour, interaction with colleagues, team functioning and organisational conditions for change, resources and economic or legal conditions (Grol and Buchan, 2006). Challenges can arise when clinical guidelines are introduced into routine daily practice as clinicians find it difficult to be aware of all the relevant valid evidence due to the volume of published research. Plans for change in practice should be based on characteristics of the evidence or guideline itself and barriers and facilitators to change (Grol and Grimshaw, 2003). Some barriers to adoption of evidence may be information overload as it is not uncommon that clinicians find it difficult to be aware of all published evidence as there are so many journals to consider. Even if evidence is accepted, clinicians and guidelines may not target correct groups. To carry out a clinical intervention requires both access and knowledge.

Evidence-based research provides information on which to base clinical decisions and a support for decision-making by providing best outcome data. Comparative effectiveness research using systematic review analysis to compare similar treatments or procedures in maximising the choice of the most effective cost/benefit option within the context of best evidence is a valuable adjunct to protect patients from ineffective or harmful treatments (Lean et al., 2008).

Translational research is the process evolving from EBP that translates the results of clinical trials into sustainable changes in practice (Lean et al., 2008). It has become a useful tool in improving decision-making in the clinical setting and was developed to be a foundation between researchers, clinicians and patients. Translational research using evidence-based and comparative effectiveness research will continue to evolve, and may prove to be a useful tool to improve decision-making in the clinical setting (Bauer and Chiappelli, 2010). EBP that integrates best available research evidence with information about patient preferences, clinician skills and available resources can improve clinical decisions in wound care.

Useful resources

Canadian resources

http://ktclearinghouse.ca – The KT Clearinghouse website is funded by the Canadian Institute of Health Research (CIHR) and is a comprehensive resource incorporating the Centre for Evidence Based Medicine in Toronto.
McMaster University.

European resources

www.thecochranelibrary.com – *Cochrane Systematic Reviews* covers all areas of clinical practice including the Cochrane Skin Group and the Cochrane Wound Group.
www.cks.nhs.uk – It provides summary of evidence-based clinical guidelines (UK).
www.evidence.nhs.uk – National Health Service (UK) approved evidence website.

International resource

The GRADE system to evaluate the quality (level) of evidence and strength of recommendations. Available at: www.gradeworkinggroup.org.

Useful critical appraisal frameworks

CONSORT (Consolidated Standards of Reporting Trials) Transparent Reporting of Trails. Available at: http://www.consort-statement.org/home/

Registered Nurses Association of Ontario. Available at: www.rnao.org/bestpractices

NHS National Institute for Health and Clinical Studies. Available at: www.guidance.nice.org.au

Critical Appraisal Skill Program (CASP). Available at: www.phru.nhs.uk/casp/critical_appraisal_tools.htm

Further reading

Gottrup, F., Apelquvist, J., Price, P. (2010) Outcomes in controlled and comparative studies on nonhealing wounds. *Journal of Wound Care*, 19(6), 237–268.

Greenhalgh, T. (2001) *How to Read a Paper: The Basics of Evidence Based Medicine*. London: BMJ.

Guyatt, G., Rennie, D., Meade, M., Cook, D. (2008) *Users' Guides to the Medical Literature: A Manual for Evidence-Based Clinical Practice*. 2nd ed. Chicago, IL: McGraw-Hill Medical.

References

Adderley, U., Thompson, C. (2007) A study of the factors influencing how frequently district nurses re-apply compression bandaging. *Journal of Wound Care*, 16, 217–221.

Annells, M., O'neill, J., Flowers, C. (2008) Compression bandaging for venous leg ulcers: the essentialness of a willing patient. *Journal of Clinical Nursing*, 17, 350–359.

Atallah, A.N. (1999) The Cochrane Collaboration: shared evidence for improving decision-making in human health. *Sao Paulo Medical Journal*, 117, 183–184.

Australian Wound Management Association Inc., New Zealand Wound Care Society Inc. (2011) *Australia and New Zealand Clinical Practice Guideline for Prevention and Management of Venous Leg Ulcers*. Canberra: Cambridge Publishing.

Avorn, J., Fischer, M. (2010) 'Bench to behavior': translating comparative effectiveness research into improved clinical practice. *Health Affairs*, 29, 1891–900.

Barker, J., Weller, C. (2010) Developing clinical practice guidelines for the prevention and management of venous leg ulcers. *Wound Practice and Research*, 18, 10.

Barton, S. (2000) Which clinical studies provide the best evidence? The best RCT still trumps the best observational study. *British Medical Journal*, 321, 255–256.

Bates, D.W., Kuperman, G.J., Wang, S., et al. (2003) Ten commandments for effective clinical decision support: making the practice of evidence-based medicine a reality. *Journal of the American Medical Informatics Association*, 10, 523–530.

Bauer, J.G., Chiappelli, F. (2010) Transforming scientific evidence into better consumer choices. *Bioinformation*, 5, 297–9.

Bennett, C.C. (2009) A healthier future for all Australians: an overview of the final report of the National Health and Hospitals Reform Commission. *Medical Journal of Australia*, 191, 383–7.

Brouwers, M.C., Kho, M.E., Browman, G.P., et al. (2010) AGREE II: advancing guideline development, reporting and evaluation in health care. *Canadian Medical Association Journal*, 182, E839–E842.

Burgers, J.S., Grol, R.P., Zaat, J.O., et al. (2003) Characteristics of effective clinical guidelines for general practice. *British Journal of General Practice*, 53, 15–19.

Cabana, M.D., Rand, C.S., Powe, N.R., et al. (1999) Why don't physicians follow clinical practice guidelines? A framework for improvement. *The Journal of the American Medical Association*, 282, 1458–1465.

Cowan, L.J., Stechmiller, J. (2009) Prevalence of wet-to-dry dressings in wound care. *Advanced Skin Wound Care*, 22, 567–573.

Cullum, N., Nelson, E.A., Fletcher, A.W., Sheldon, T.A. (2000) Compression for venous leg ulcers. *Cochrane Database of Systematic Reviews*, CD000265.

Cullum, N., Nelson, E.A., Fletcher, A.W., Sheldon, T.A. (2001) Compression for venous leg ulcers. *Cochrane Database of Systematic Reviews*, CD000265.

Davies, H., Nutley, S., Walter, I. (2008) Why 'knowledge transfer' is misconceived for applied social research. *Journal of Health Services Research and Policy*, 13, 188–190.

Dawes, M., Sampson, U. (2003) Knowledge management in clinical practice: a systematic review of information seeking behavior in physicians. *International Journal of Medical Informatics*, 71, 9–15.

Dicenso, A., Bryant-Lukosius, D., Martin-Misener, R., et al. (2010) Factors enabling advanced practice nursing role integration in Canada. *Nursing Leadership (Toronto Ontario)*, 23(2010), 211–238.

El Dib, R.P., Atallah, A.N., Andriolo, R.B. (2007) Mapping the Cochrane evidence for decision making in health care. *Journal of Evaluation in Clinical Practice*, 13, 689–692.

Ertl, P. (1992) How do you make your treatment decision? *Professional Nurse*, 7, 543–552.

Field, M.J. (1994) Practice guidelines and quality of care. *Journal of the National Medical Association*, 86, 255–256.

Fletcher, A.A., Cullum, N.N., Sheldon, T.T. A. (1997) A systematic review of compression treatment for venous leg ulcers. *British Medical Journal*, 315, 576–580.

Glasziou, P., Haynes, B. (2005) The paths from research to improved health outcomes. *ACP Journal Club*, 142, A8–A10.

Gottrup, F. (2004) Optimizing wound treatment through health care structuring and professional education. *Wound Repair and Regeneration*, 12, 129–133.

Gottrup, F. (2010) Controversies in wound healing. *International Journal of Lower Extremity Wounds*, 9, 9.

Gottrup, F., Apelqvist, J. (2010) The challenge of using randomized trials in wound healing. *British Journal of Surgery*, 97, 303–304.

Gottrup, F., Apelqvist, J., Price, P. (2010) Outcomes in controlled and comparative studies on non-healing wounds: recommendations to improve the quality of evidence in wound management. *Journal of Wound Care*, 19, 237–268.

Graham, I.D., Harrison, M.B., Shafey, M., Keast, D. (2003) Knowledge and attitudes regarding care of leg ulcers. Survey of family physicians. *Canadian Family Physician*, 49, 896–902.

Griffin, S.C., Claxton, K.P., Palmer, S.J., Sculpher, M.J. (2011) Dangerous omissions: the consequences of ignoring decision uncertainty. *Health Economics*, 20, 212–224.

Grimshaw, J.M., Thomas, R.E., Maclennan, G., et al. (2004) Effectiveness and efficiency of guideline dissemination and implementation strategies. *Health Technology Assessment*, 8(iii–iv), 1–72.

Grol, R. (2002) Changing physicians' competence and performance: finding the balance between the individual and the organization. *Journal of Continuing Education in the Health Professions*, 22, 244–251.

Grol, R. (2010) Has guideline development gone astray? Yes. *British Medical Journal*, 340, c306.

Grol, R., Buchan, H. (2006) Clinical guidelines: what can we do to increase their use? *Medical Journal of Australia*, 185, 301–302.

Grol, R., Grimshaw, J. (2003) From best evidence to best practice: effective implementation of change in patients' care. *Lancet*, 362, 1225–1230.

Grol, R.P., Bosch, M.C., Hulscher, M.E., Eccles, M.P., Wensing, M. (2007) Planning and studying improvement in patient care: the use of theoretical perspectives. *Milbank Quarterly*, 85, 93–138.

Guyatt, G.H., Meade, M.O., Jaeschke, R.Z., Cook, D.J., Haynes, R.B. (2000) Practitioners of evidence based care. Not all clinicians need to appraise evidence from scratch but all need some skills. *British Medical Journal*, 320, 954–955.

Hoaglin, D.C., Hawkins, N., Jansen, J.P., et al. (2011) Conducting indirect-treatment-comparison and network-meta-analysis studies: report of the ISPOR Task Force on Indirect Treatment Comparisons Good Research Practices: part 2. *Value in Health*, 14, 429–437.

Kawamoto, K., Houlihan, C.A., Balas, E.A., Lobach, D.F. (2005) Improving clinical practice using clinical decision support systems: a systematic review of trials to identify features critical to success. *British Medical Journal*, 330, 765.

Lean, M.E., Mann, J.I., Hoek, J.A., Elliot, R.M., Schofield, G. (2008) Translational research. *British Medical Journal*, 337, a863.

Mallett, S., Clarke, M. (2003) How many Cochrane reviews are needed to cover existing evidence on the effects of health care interventions? *ACP Journal Club*, 139, A11.

Mcguckin, M., Kerstein, M.D. (1998) Venous leg ulcers and the family physician. *Advances in Wound Care*, 11, 344–346.

Mcnees, P., Kueven, J.A. (2011) The bottom line on wound care standardization. *Healthcare Financial Management*, 65, 70–74, 76.

Moher, D., Hopewell, S., Schulz, K.F., et al. (2010) CONSORT 2010 explanation and elaboration: updated guidelines for reporting parallel group randomised trials. *Journal of Clinical Epidemiology*, 63, e1–e37.

Newall, N., Miller, C., Lewin, G., et al. (2009) Nurses' experiences of participating in a randomised controlled trial (RCT) in the community. *Wound Practice and Research*, 17, 24–34.

O'meara, S., Cullum, N.A., Nelson, E.A. (2009) Compression for venous leg ulcers. *Cochrane Database of Systematic Reviews*, CD000265.

Oxman, A.D., Thomson, M.A., Davis, D.A., Haynes, R.B. (1995) No magic bullets: a systematic review of 102 trials of interventions to improve professional practice. *Canadian Medical Association Journal*, 153, 1423–1431.

Rose, L. (2011) Interprofessional collaboration in the ICU: how to define? *Nursing in Critical Care*, 16, 5–10.

Sackett, D.L., Rosenberg, W.M., Gray, J.A., Haynes, R.B., Richardson, W.S. (1996) Evidence based medicine: what it is and what it isn't. *British Medical Journal*, 312, 71–72.

Sadler, G.M., Russell, G.M., Boldy, D.P., Stacey, M.C. (2006) General practitioners' experiences of managing patients with chronic leg ulceration. *Medical Journal of Australia*, 185, 78–81.

Scott, I.A. (2009) The NHHRC final report: view from the hospital sector. *Medical Journal of Australia*, 191, 450–453.

Scott, I.A., Glasziou, P.P. (2012) Improving the effectiveness of clinical medicine: the need for better science. *Medical Journal of Australia*, 196, 304–308.

SIGN (2010) *Scottish Intercollegiate Guidelines Network (SIGN) 120 – National Clinical Guidelines for Management of Chronic Venous Leg Ulcers*. Edinburgh, Scotland: NHS Quality Improvement Scotland.

Solberg, L.I., Brekke, M.L., Fazio, C.J., et al. (2000) Lessons from experienced guideline implementers: attend to many factors and use multiple strategies. *Joint Commission Journal on Quality Improvement*, 26, 171–188.

Sox, H.C., Helfand, M., Grimshaw, J., et al. (2010) Comparative effectiveness research: Challenges for medical journals. *The Cochrane Database of Systematic Reviews*, 8, ED000003.

Spring, B. (2008) Health decision making: lynchpin of evidence-based practice. *Medical Decision Making*, 28, 866–874.

Thompson, C., Mccaughan, D., Cullum, N., Sheldon, T., Raynor, P. (2005) Barriers to evidence-based practice in primary care nursing–why viewing decision-making as context is helpful. *Journal of Advanced Nursing*, 52, 432–444.

Walter, I., Davies, H., Nutley, S. (2003) Increasing research impact through partnerships: evidence from outside health care. *Journal of Health Services Research and Policy*, 8 (Suppl 2), 58–61.

Weller, C., Mcneil, J. (2010) CONSORT 2010 statement: updated guidelines can improve wound care. *Journal of Wound Care*, 19, 347–353.

Weller, C., Mcneil, J., Evans, S., Reid, C. (2010a) Improving venous ulcer healing: designing and reporting randomised controlled trials. *International Wound Journal*, 7, 41–47.

Weller, C.D. (2009) A simple guide to randomised controlled trials in wound care. *European Wound Management Association Journal*, 9, 5–13.

Weller, C.D., Buchbinder, R., Johnston, R. (2010b) Interventions for helping people adhere to compression treatments for venous leg ulceration (Protocol). *Cochrane Database of Systematic Reviews*, 2, 9.

Weller, C.D., Evans, S., Reid, C.M., Wolfe, R., Mcneil, J. (2010c) Protocol for a pilot randomised controlled clinical trial to compare the effectiveness of a graduated three layer straight tubular bandaging system when compared to a standard short stretch compression bandaging system in the management of people with venous ulceration: 3VSS2008. *Trials*, 11, 26.

Weller, C.D., Evans, S.M. (2012) Venous leg ulcer management in general practice: is practice nurse management in accordance with evidence-based guidelines? *Australian Family Physician*. 41, 5, 331–337.

Weller, C.D., Mcneil, J., Evans, S., Reid, C. (2010d) Improving venous ulcer healing: designing and reporting randomised controlled trials. *International Wound Journal*, 7, 41–47.

Wilkinson, J.E., Nutley, S.M., Davies, H.T. (2011) An exploration of the roles of nurse managers in evidence-based practice implementation. *Worldviews Evidence Based Nursing*. 8, 4, 236–246

Winter, G.D. (1962) Formation of the scab and the rate of epithelization of superficial wounds in the skin of the young domestic pig. *Nature*, 193, 293–294.

Winter, G.D. (1995) Formation of the scab and the rate of epithelisation of superficial wounds in the skin of the young domestic pig. 1962. *Journal of Wound Care*, 4, 366–367; discussion 368–371.

Winter, G.D. (2006) Some factors affecting skin and wound healing. *Journal of Tissue Viability*, 16, 20–23.

2 Maintaining Skin Integrity

Arne Langøen[1] and Janice Bianchi[2]

[1]Department of Health, Klingenbergvegen, Norway
[2]Nursing and Healthcare School, University of Glasgow, Glasgow, Scotland, UK

Overview

- Skin health can be threatened by disruption to the epidermis. Conditions such as dry skin, atopic dermatitis and wounds cause skin barrier dysfunction that comprises the ability of the body to protect itself.
- Skin care regimes that include cleansing, hydration and protection are beneficial and help to restore barrier function.
- Skin breakdown is largely preventable with implementation of effective and relatively inexpensive interventions. Yet is often ignored by policymakers and health professionals, resulting in significant impact on quality of life.
- There is a lack of good-quality clinical evidence to guide the use of skin care protocols in clinical practice and further research is urgently required.

Introduction

The most important function of the skin is to provide a semi-permeable barrier to protect the body from the outside world. The outermost layer of the skin is the stratum corneum (SC) that forms the external layer of the epidermis responsible for maintaining skin barrier function and the integrity of healthy skin. Maintaining skin health has been a preoccupation for centuries and is something that individuals often take for granted until damage occurs. Environmental and social factors influence an individual's concerns about their skin: someone living in poverty may be worried about skin infestations or leprosy, someone admitted to hospi-

tal might worry about developing pressure ulcers and a health care professional with the avoidance of hand dermatitis. There is a growing body of evidence to support skin care regimes based on gentle cleansing, moisturisation and application of a skin protectant. This chapter will discuss factors affecting skin integrity and strategies aimed at minimising skin barrier dysfunction.

Clinicians managing chronic wounds encounter patients with a variety of skin-related problems ranging from incontinence-associated dermatitis (IAD) to skin stripping resulting from removal of adhesive dressings. Conditions that affect skin integrity such as eczema or wound breakdown will have a detrimental effect on barrier function.

For example, an inflammatory response in the dermis caused by cellulitis will release chemical mediators such as bradykinin, histamine and serotonin, to increase capillary permeability, oedema and transepidermal water loss (TEWL) causing localised disruption of skin barrier function.

Skin integrity and barrier function

The past decade has provided a better understanding about the skin in general and barrier function in particular (Proksch et al., 2008; Farage et al., 2010). The skin comprises three layers: the thinner epidermis on the outside, the dermis and the supporting subcutaneous tissue. Together they provide the following functions:

- *Protection*: trauma, dehydration, temperature, toxins, ultra-violet (UV) light, micro-organisms;
- *Maintenance of body temperature*: circulatory mechanisms, sweating, insulation;
- *Sensation*: pain, pressure, vibration, temperature;
- *Metabolism*: melanin, vitamin D;
- *Communication*: facial expression, physical appearance, touch.

The epidermis as a physical barrier

The epidermal barrier is a highly specialist, dynamic structure that adapts to environmental conditions (Figure 2.1). As well as providing a physical and chemical barrier to block entry of foreign substances (Figure 2.1), the skin barrier triggers an immunological response against any pathogens that manage to penetrate the barrier. Any breach in the skin barrier must be quickly repaired to prevent infection and maintain normal function and homeostasis.

The barrier function of the skin is situated mostly in the outermost SC which is in direct contact with the external environment. The structure of the epidermis is shown in Figure 2.2. The primary function of the SC is to trap moisture at the surface of the skin to prevent it drying out and protect against the entry of foreign irritants, allergens and microbes (bacteria, fungi and viruses) (Madison, 2003). The epidermis is composed of keratinocytes that are differentiated into layers of specifically structured

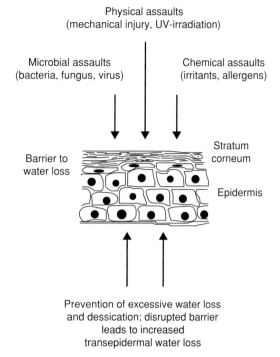

Figure 2.1   The skin barrier (Proksch et al., 2008).

cells that allow it to provide a selectively permeable barrier.

The innermost region of this barrier is the stratum basale, which constantly undergoes cell division. The stratum spinosum is responsible for lipid and protein synthesis which is an integral part of maintaining barrier function. In the stratum granulosum, keratinocytes flatten out to form layers of corneocytes and a protein envelope develops around them lubricated by intra-epidermal lipids consisting mainly of a mix of ceramides (50%), cholesterol (25%) and free fatty acids (15%) (Fluhr and Darlenski, 2009). These lipids are produced from the disintegration of the keratinocytes to form a protective layer around the corneocytes and are crucial to the function of the epidermal permeability barrier. The structure of the healthy epidermal barrier can be seen in Figure 2.3a.

The SC has a brick-and-mortar-like structure where bricks represent flattened, dead keratinocytes that have matured into corneocytes and mortar represents the surrounding inter-cellular lipid membranes (Nemes and Steinert, 1999; Cork and Danby, 2009).

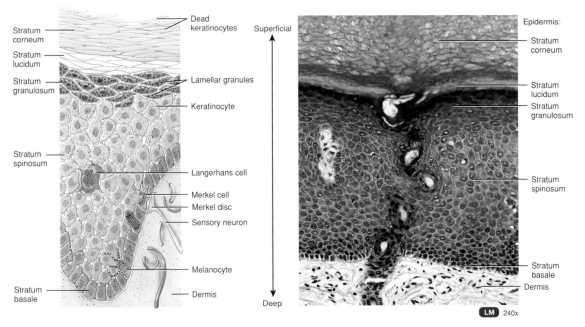

Figure 2.2   The structure of the epidermis. From Tortora and Derrickson (2009). Reproduced with permission from Wiley.

The corneocytes (bricks) are tightly connected by desmosomes in overlapping layers to retain moisture while keeping allergens, pathogens and environmental toxins (such as UV radiation) out. Desmosomes are specialised cell structures that provide cell stability to increase skin resilience (Proksch et al., 2008). They stretch between the cells and anchor them in place, avoiding shearing forces that can easily damage cells (Madison, 2003). The strength and function of desmosomes in the SC are important to maintain the mechanical barrier of the skin by holding the corneocytes tightly together. At the same time, desmosomes have to release corneocytes to shed cells from the skin during the process of desquamation. It takes approximately 24 hours to form one layer of corneocytes in the SC, and in some areas of the epidermis there are up to 15 layers (Egelrud, 2000). The SC is completely renewed about every 15 days. In the SC, a delicate balance between proteases and protease inhibitors is responsible for the release and movement of cells within the extracellular matrix and the regulation of desquamation. Protease inhibitors have an important function to control desquamation to maintain optimal skin barrier function together with intra-epidermal lipids and corneocytes (Proksch et al., 2008).

The extracellular lipids that fill the spaces between the corneocytes (bricks) represent the 'mortar' in the brick and mortar analogy, and form a hydrophobic matrix that waterproofs the epidermis and prevents dehydration. This extracellular matrix provides necessary moisture permeability to the SC.

In healthy skin, the SC is impenetrable to irritants and allergens, and water loss is minimised. However, when the skin dehydrates, the corneocytes shrink, causing cracks to appear between them allowing penetration of external irritants which trigger a local inflammatory response causing discomfort, itching and scratching and further skin damage as seen in Figure 2.3b.

Keratin present in the cells of stratum granulosum (Figure 2.3) forms a matrix protein called filaggrin which is an important epidermal protein that regulates several functions critical to maintain barrier function of the SC such as photoprotection, creation of an anti-bactericidal environment and inhibition of TEWL (Kezic et al., 2008; Brown and McLean, 2012). Filaggrin is destroyed during the maturation of keratinocytes into corneocytes which results in the release of natural moisturising factor (NMF) from the SC and is essential for hydration of the epidermal layer.

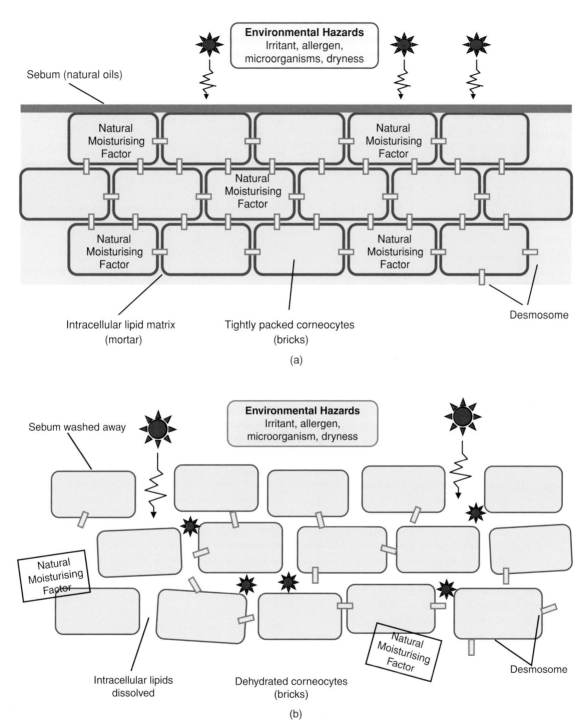

Figure 2.3   (a) Structure of the healthy epidermal barrier. (b) Structure of a damaged epidermal barrier.

NMF is composed of water-soluble compounds that bind water in the epidermis to keep the outermost layers of the SC hydrated and to stop it drying out (Kezic et al., 2008). The lipid layer surrounding the corneocyte helps to prevent loss of NMF but because NMF components are water soluble, they are easily leached from the cells especially when in prolonged contact with moisture which is why repeated contact with water actually makes the skin drier (Robinson et al., 2010). For the same reason, the natural waterproofing function of NMF would be quickly washed off the skin if not protected by intra-epidermal lipids which is why skin cleansing with soap and detergents can be detrimental to barrier function and should be avoided (Thune et al., 1988). If evaporation at the skin's surface is too high or secretion of NMF in the SC is too low, the skin will become dry, flaky and uncomfortable. Dry skin conditions, such as ichtyosis and atopic dermatitis, are partly caused by disruption of intra-epidermal lipids.

The epidermis as a chemical barrier

Maintenance of an effective microbial skin barrier depends on the preservation of resident skin flora and requires the skin pH to be maintained at a physiological level. The surface of the skin is acidic and ranges between a pH of 4.5 and 5 but varies at different sites on the body (Fluhr et al., 2002). The normal skin flora produce free fatty acids from phospholipids to maintain an acidic skin pH which helps to keep the number of transient bacteria and Candida low. A variety of factors including pH, humidity, natural skin cleansing, healthy turnover of cells from the SC contribute to the development of a stable micro-climate of the skin, and helps to maintain barrier function and skin integrity.

Skin pH influences the process of desquamation and the resident bacterial flora of the skin. A permanently raised skin pH will lead to reduced desquamation, with dry and scaly skin and increased levels of bacteria and fungi (Charbonneau et al., 2010). A raised skin pH disturbs the regulation of protease and protease inhibitors that control the rate of desquamation so that the turnover of corneocytes decreases and the skin becomes dry and scaly.

Skin pH is affected by a great number of intrinsic factors such as skin moisture, sweat, sebum, anatomic site, genetic predisposition and age (Fluhr et al., 2002). In addition, extrinsic factors like fre-

quent washing with detergents, skin cleansers and use of occlusive dressings can cause a rise in skin pH (Thune et al., 1988).

The healthy functioning of the SC is dependent on the correct balance of bacteria on the skin surface. These micro-organisms are divided into resident and transient bacteria, transient bacteria do not normally colonise the skin, but are temporarily present as a consequence of surface contamination. Numbers of transient bacteria which are usually found on the surface of the skin are kept to a minimum because of desquamation, whereas resident skin flora can be found in more protected areas such as hair follicles and are more difficult to remove with soaps and skin cleaners (see Chapter 7).

Resident skin flora are important to sustain a healthy micro-climate at the skin's surface to maintain barrier function. The most common species are *Staphylococcus, Micrococcus, Corynebacterium, Rhodococcus, Propionibacterium, Brevibacterium, Dermatobacter* and *Actinobacter* (Charbonneau et al., 2010). But under certain conditions that damage skin barrier function such as increased humidity, protease secretion and use of antibiotics, *Staphylococcus aureus, Streptococcus pyogenes, Candida* spp. and *Actinobacter* may become resident skin flora and cause skin infections. Resident skin flora will try to control transient skin flora by occupying the sites on the skin where transient flora might establish, scavenging the skin's surface to remove nutrients that transient flora need to survive or by producing metabolites that have an anti-microbial effect on transient skin flora. Maintenance of healthy resident skin flora is mainly concerned with regulating numbers of transient and potentially harmful bacteria to such low levels so that they do not damage the skin and penetrate the anti-microbial barrier.

The epidermis as an immunological barrier

The innate immunity of the skin consists of the physical barrier, anti-microbial peptides (AMPs), cytokines and cells containing pattern-recognition receptors or PRRs. To recognise invading micro-organisms, cells such as macrophages, lymphocytes and endothelial cells posses a variety of corresponding receptors called PRRs capable of binding specifically to pathogens (Benedetto et al., 2009). Some PRRs are located on the surface of phagocytes and promote the attachment of micro-organisms to phagocytes leading to their destruction others are found within phagocytes where they have the ability to destroy micro-organisms from within.

AMPs are produced by keratinocytes at the epithelial surface during the inflammatory process and directly kill a wide range of bacteria, fungi, parasites and some virus (Benedetto et al., 2009). AMPs have a central role in resolution of inflammation and infection and can be compared to naturally occurring antibiotics. They induce a variety of responses in host innate immune cells such as monocytes, macrophages, neutrophils and epithelial cells to influence cellular processes such as cytokine release, chemotaxis, angiogenesis and wound healing (Lai and Gallo, 2009). They do this by encouraging leucocyte recruitment to the site of infection and, by influencing cell differentiation and activation. AMP activity results in initiation of adaptive immune responses which protects the body against infection, controls inflammation and promotes wound healing and repair of damaged epithelia (Yang et al., 2004; Lai and Gallo, 2009).

Impaired skin barrier function in the clinical setting

There are many interrelated factors that contribute to failure of skin barrier function and skin breakdown. Effective skin care is an essential element of maintenance of skin integrity and promotion of skin health, but is often taken for granted and given little importance. Many common clinical conditions cause impairment of the barrier function of the skin (Table 2.1). An understanding of these is crucial to preserve and restore skin barrier function in everyday clinical practice.

Effect of age on skin barrier function

The epidermal barrier is influenced by extremes of age: neonates born before 34 weeks gestation and the elderly. There is a strong correlation between gestation age and TEWL, which provides a good indication of the effectiveness of barrier function in neonates. Although babies born at 40 weeks gestation have an average TEWL between 5 and $10 \, g/m^2/h$, children born in the 26th week of gestation have an increased average TEWL of between 70 and $80 \, g/m^2/h$ (Hoath and Maibach, 2003). There are several reasons for the limited barrier function of neonate skin including: the dermal–epidermal junction and corneocytes are not fully developed, and the skin pH is elevated (Behne et al., 2003; Shawayder and Akland, 2005). The overall result is that neonates have fragile, thinner, more immature skin than full-term babies that is prone to trauma from adhesive dressings and tapes, localised pressure from IV lines and tubing, and the risk of extravasation injury.

The terms intrinsic and extrinsic aging are used to describe skin aging. Intrinsic aging refers to the natural degenerative process involving faulty synthesis of collagen and elastin in the dermis and is influenced by physiological factors and occurs in both sun-exposed and non-sun-exposed skin (Fisher et al., 2002). Intrinsic factors such as inherited genes are largely responsible for the rate at which individuals' age. Extrinsic skin aging refers to the cumulative process caused by a variety of environmental factors which include UV radiation, air pollution, nutrition and smoking (Tzellos et al., 2009). The most significant extrinsic skin damage results over time from sun exposure; because of this, extrinsic aging is often referred to as photoaging (Gilchrest, 1989).

Skin changes as a result of ageing were, for many years, only considered to be cosmetic. Intrinsic aging is characterised by dryness, fine wrinkles, skin atrophy and loss of elasticity (Baumann, 2007; Raschke and Elsner 2010). The effects of extrinsic aging include roughness of the skin, coarse wrinkles and uneven pigmentation (Lavker, 1979; Alam and Havey 2010). Skin ageing is now known to be associated with functional changes. The epidermal layer in elderly skin reduces by up to 50% compared with young people, due to flattening and reduced numbers of epidermal cells, and the lipid content is reduced as much as 65% leading to skin drying and reduced water-binding capacity (Farage et al., 2010). Advancing age also decreases epidermal turnover which leads to a reduced ability to repair damage to the epidermis. Numbers of melanocytes and Langerhans cells are also reduced in elderly skin, which lessens the efficacy of the UV barrier and inflammatory response, so older skin is more likely to develop a variety of benign, precancerous and malignant lesions such as seborrheic and actinic keratoses, basal cell carcinoma and squamous cell carcinoma (Cross et al., 1987).

Table 2.1   Clinical conditions affecting skin barrier function

Clinical condition	Factors reducing skin barrier function	Intervention
Neonatal skin problems	Immature skin, risk of skin stripping (due to adhesive tape, dressings, electrodes), absorption of irritants, risk of secondary infection; high environmental temperature	Careful skin assessment, clean skin gently with pH-balanced cleansers; dry skin thoroughly; apply emollient therapy; use skin protectants; minimise risk of additional trauma; control environmental temperature
Dry skin (eczema)	Humidity, dehydration, loss of skin lipids, frequent washing with soap/detergents, contact with irritants, inflammation, secondary infection	Avoid use of very hot water or soap; clean skin gently with pH-balanced cleansers; dry skin thoroughly; avoid skin sensitisers; apply emollient therapy; use moderate—potent topical steroid to control flares; control environmental temperature
Incontinence-associated dermatitis	Prolonged contact with urine, faeces, sweat, proteases (chronic wound fluid), elevated pH, humidity, occlusion, poor skin hygiene, loss of skin lipids, skin occlusion, inflammation, secondary infection	Investigate cause, minimise skin contact with irritants; prevent moisture accumulation; avoid excessive washing/frequent use of soaps/detergents; cleanse skin gently with pH-balanced cleansers; dry skin thoroughly; apply skin protectants
Maceration, intertrigo	Humidity, excess moisture, elevated skin pH, occlusion, skin stripping, inflammation, fungal colonisation/infection	Prevent moisture accumulation; dry skin thoroughly; use skin protectants; treat with anti-fungal agents if indicated; control environmental temperature
Periwound skin problems	Excess moisture, proteases, elevated pH, humidity, occlusion, skin stripping, inflammation, wound infection, fungal colonisation, local tissue hypoxia, ischaemia–reperfusion injury	Prevent moisture accumulation; change absorbent dressings before leakage; consider wound drainage; dry periwound skin thoroughly; apply skin protectants
Wound infection/cellulitis	Elevated bioburden, necrotic tissue, inflammatory response, excess would fluid/proteases, elevated pH, humidity, occlusion, local tissue hypoxia, ischaemia–reperfusion injury	Identify pathogen, treat infection (anti-microbial dressings/antibiotics if indicated), control moisture levels (moisture-retentive dressings); consider use of skin protectants
Pressure damage	Pressure, friction, shear, local tissue hypoxia, ischaemia–reperfusion injury, excess moisture, elevated pH, humidity, occlusion, skin stripping, inflammation, wound infection, fungal colonisation/infection	Systematic risk assessment; prevent moisture accumulation; clean skin gently with pH-balanced cleansers; dry use of appropriate support surfaces, correct positioning.; appropriate management of skin moisture; improve activity levels where possible

The aging process of skin can partly be attributed to intrinsic aging and photoaging which are separate processes. The free radical theory (Harman, 1986) has been proposed to explain skin aging as skin is constantly exposed over time to reactive oxygen species (ROS) from the environment, such as air, solar radiation, or from the normal metabolism. Accumulated ROS have been suggested to play important roles in the intrinsic aging and photoaging of human skin *in vivo* (Kawaguchi et al., 1996). ROS are thought to be responsible for various cutaneous inflammatory disorders and skin cancers (Cross et al., 1987).

Kaya and Saurat (2007) identified the general term 'dermatoporosis' to describe this chronic skin insufficiency/fragility syndrome and suggested that dermatoporosis could be prevented in much the same way as osteoporosis can. The clinical manifestations of dermatoporosis are frequently seen in clinical practice (Figure 2.4) and include actinic purpura and skin atrophy resulting in increased skin fragility and injury from minor trauma such as skin

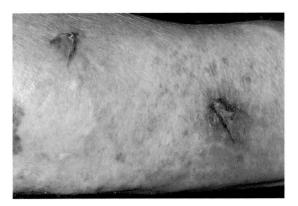

Figure 2.4 Photo of fragile skin in an elderly person showing signs of dermatoporosis. Photo courtesy of Carolyn Wyndam White.

tears, delayed wound healing and in some cases development of subcutaneous bleeding leading to necrosis (Kaya and Saurat, 2007).

Although the epidermis changes quite significantly as a consequence of aging, the barrier function of non-exposed skin is preserved quite well, providing evidence that exposure to the environment especially UVB has a major impact on skin ageing. The ability to recover from injury and restore epidermal barrier function once damaged is greatly reduced in the elderly and takes more time (Ranzer and DiPietro, 2010).

As the skin ages, the microbiological composition of the skin flora changes as some of the transient bacteria become permanent. This is due to several reasons including increased skin pH, reduced skin turnover rate, dryer skin and reduced immune function, which influence the ability to keep the transient skin flora at a non-pathogenic level. *Proteus mirabilis* and *Pseudomonas aeruginosa* have been found to be 25% more common in people over 65 years of age and commonly cause infection in chronic wounds (Charbonneau et al., 2010).

Effect of humidity and moisture on skin barrier function

Skin breakdown related to humidity can occur because of the effect of sweating, incontinence or wound exudate. Periwound skin problems such as maceration and moisture-related skin damage are frequently associated with chronic wounds such as venous leg ulcers, fistula and malignant wounds.

Prolonged exposure of the skin to high levels of moisture causes rehydration of the outer, keratinised layer of epidermal cells which swell and weaken the links between the layers of tissue. Irritant fluids strip away the outer layer of the epidermis to expose the fragile stratum basale layer increasing the risk of secondary infection and further damage. Once the basal layer is exposed to the air, the cells leak serous fluid which dries out quickly to form an eschar leading to progressive tissue damage in deeper layers. These effects significantly alter the ability of the skin to withstand damage from friction in particular, but also sheer and pressure (Mayoritz and Sims, 2001).

Incontinence-associated dermatitis (IAD)

Extensive skin damage can occur when the skin comes into prolonged contact with enzyme-rich fluids, such as urine and faeces, small bowel effluent and chronic wound fluid which strip epidermal tissue rapidly as proteolytic enzymes break down the cell matrix (Ersser et al., 2005; Cooper, 2011). IAD is now the preferred general term to describe this damage as 'erythema and oedema of the surface of the skin, sometimes accompanied by bullae with serous exudate, erosion or secondary cutaneous infection' (Black et al., 2011; Voegeli, 2012). A consensus group in 2005 felt the term IAD more accurately described this type of skin damage than the variety of terms in common use including, diaper dermatitis, perineal dermatitis and moisture lesions (Black et al., 2011; Voegeli, 2012). Recognition is growing that IAD is a distinct form of skin damage that requires further research to understand its aetiology, prevention and treatment.

Fresh soiling from urine and faeces that is cleaned promptly tends not to cause serious skin problems as healthy skin can be exposed to ammonia, a breakdown product of urine, without harming the skin. However, urine, faeces, soap and detergents dissolve the corneocyte linkages in the epidermis increasing the rate of desquamation and epidermal breakdown (Lawton and Langøen, 2009). So if skin cleaning is delayed after soiling, the metabolism of urea by skin flora produces by-products with a high pH which increases the damaging effect of proteases on the skin, leading to an acute inflammatory response in the upper dermis and erythema and

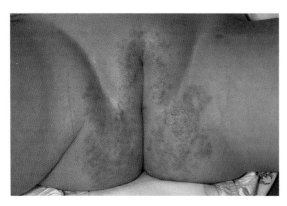

Figure 2.5   Incontinence-associated dermatitis in an infant. Photo courtesy of Madeleine Flanagan.

further damage (Houwing et al., 2007; Zulkowski, 2012).

Once the skin barrier function is breached, damaged skin is very sensitive to ammonia, soap and biliary salts; inflammation intensifies and the surface of the skin erodes further as seen in Figure 2.5. These findings support clinical observation that IAD is a result of top-down skin damage rather than the bottom-up damage due to vascular occlusion in pressure ulcers (Black et al., 2011). Skin excoriation caused by lipase and protease is particularly pronounced in individuals with diarrhoea which can cause sudden and extensive skin breakdown. Within minutes the epidermis can become erythematous and inflamed causing damage to the surface of the epidermis (Buckingham and Berg, 1986; Berg, 1988).

The development of IAD is a complex mechanism that is not fully understood but involves an interaction between urine and faeces on the skin, humidity, mechanical irritants and frequent use of soap and water (Figure 2.6).

Environmental humidity in combination with use of detergents or leaving the skin damp will gradually break down the epidermal mechanical protective barrier. Skin that has been exposed to humid conditions such as between skin folds under the breast, groin, in between the webs of the toes or under occlusive wound dressings will start to break down and gradually turns white. Macerated skin has a higher pH than normal skin, and increases the risk of bacterial and fungal infections.

Some of the same mechanisms that cause incontinence dermatitis, also damage the skin surrounding chronic wounds (Lawton and Langøen, 2009).

If wound dressings or drainage is unable to contain wound exudate, leakage occurs and the skin around the wound becomes soaked in chronic wound fluid which is rich in irritant proteases. Chronic wound fluid in particular due to its high protease content causes maceration and breaks down the SC disrupting barrier function (Trengove et al., 1999). Chronic wounds often contain biofilms, when polymorph nuclear granulocytes try to attack the bacteria present in the biofilm, they are destroyed and release large quantities of destructive matrix metalloproteinase which dissolve the extracellular matrix within the wound, as well as the protein envelope of the corneocytes, damaging epidermal barrier function. This process causes a prolonged inflammatory response in the damaged skin releasing pro-inflammatory cytokines into wound fluid causing additional damage to the SC (Wolcott et al., 2008).

The repeated application and removal of adhesive tapes or dressings to the same site causes stripping of the SC which initiates an inflammatory skin reaction, oedema and soreness (Fluhr et al., 2002; Lawton and Langøen, 2009; Alikhan and Maibach 2010). Skin stripping is influenced by many variables including patient age, skin pathology, properties of the adhesive used and frequency of tape or dressing removal (Fluhr et al., 2002).

In non-healing wounds, the underlying aetiology may contribute to reduction in barrier function. Venous hypertension leads oedema and lipodermatosclerosis, which, in turn, causes varicose eczema. Patients with venous ulcers have an increased tendency to skin sensitivities and allergic reactions (Barbaud et al., 2009), and it can be difficult to differentiate between an irritant wound fluid reaction, varicose eczema or an allergic reaction to topical treatments.

Patients with pressure ulcers are also prone to irritant dermatitis resulting from the combined effects of incontinence, wound secretions, sweat and high humidity which affect the micro-climate of the skin and increase the vulnerability of the soft tissues to pressure, friction and shear (Ersser, 2010; Langøen, 2010). Local pressure will occlude the micro-circulation in the dermis, when this pressure is relived the area is re-perfused causing further inflammation to the tissues (see Chapter 8).

This section has reviewed various conditions that affect the normal physical, chemical and immunological barrier function of the skin. Failed barrier

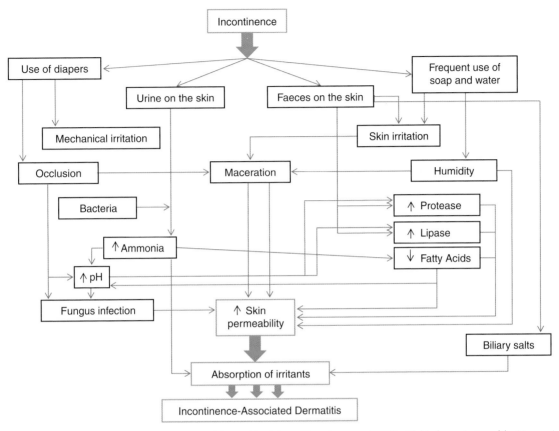

Figure 2.6   Causation of incontinence-associated dermatitis. Adapted from Langøen (1993) with kind permission of the Norwegian Medical Association.

function, whatever the cause, disrupts keratinocytes at the surface of the epidermis allowing irritants to enter and stimulates an inflammatory response in the dermis. Skin barrier dysfunction predisposes to colonisation by micro-organisms and may lead to secondary infection. These cumulative effects cause pruritus and discomfort and initiate the itch–scratch cycle causing further excoriation allowing additional entry of pathogens and irritants setting up a vicious cycle (Figure 2.7).

Management of vulnerable skin

The mainstay of skin health is the maintenance and restoration of barrier function, avoidance of irritants and treatment of inflammation. The most effective way of achieving this is the application of bland (colour and fragrance-free) emollients. The purpose of emollients is to provide occlusion in the form of a greasy film on the surface of the skin to minimise water evaporation and to retain moisture with humectants such as urea and glycerin.

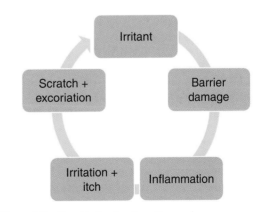

Figure 2.7   The skin barrier disruption cycle.

Moisturisers are commonly used by people with dry skin conditions as well as those with healthy skin. They may be used alone or as an adjuvant to other topical treatments, e.g. topical steroids to reduce eczema flare-ups. There is however, a lack of good-quality clinical data reviewing emollient use in dry skin conditions. Williams and Grindlay (2008) emphasise this lack of evidence does not mean that emollient therapy is not effective in clinical practice and suggests that RCTs should be conducted to evaluate frequency of use of emollients, long-term tolerability and patient preference.

Dry skin

The terms *emollients* and *moisturisers* are often used synonymously to describe topical substances applied to the skin to maintain or repair barrier function. Although both are lipids, emollients primarily work by occluding the epidermis preventing water loss whilst moisturisers add humectant to the skin surface to improve hydration (Voegeli, 2012).

Moisturisers come in many formulations: creams, ointments, gels, sprays, foams and lotions. Choice of emollient is based on a number of factors including personal preference, but also how dry the skin is and what if any sensitivities a person may have. Many people are sensitive to fragrances and preservatives in skin products, lanolin is frequently associated with skin sensitivities and should be avoided (Draelos, 2010). Generally, the more 'greasy' products provide the best emollient effect as they are most effective at trapping moisture in the epidermis. However, individuals may prefer a less oily preparation for daytime use, or for use on exposed areas such as the face.

Complete emollient therapy is the term given to a regime which includes use of soap substitutes, bath additives and moisturisers. There is consensus agreement that soap should be avoided for skin care as it strips the epithelium of natural lipids, alters the protective acidic environment at the surface of the skin and leaves irritant residues (Black et al., 2011; Voegeli, 2012). Bath additives are thought to moisturise the skin by adding a thin layer of oil over the skin. But there is limited evidence to support their effectiveness although some patients find them useful (Drug and Therapeutics Bulletin, 2007).

Principles of emollient use

Emollients are essential to effectively manage dry skin conditions but are often not used appropriately by either patients or health professionals. The following principles for emollient use have been established from best practice guidelines to optimise their effectiveness (Ersser et al., 2009):

- Choice of emollient must be one the patient is willing to use. A trial of a few products, prescribed in small quantities, can help selection. Many individuals find cheaper brands acceptable and effective.
- Emollients should be applied whenever the skin feels dry, to ensure maximum effect. Twice a day is a minimum although three to four times a day is usually more effective. They should be liberally applied after bathing, showering or swimming.
- A detailed explanation of how to use emollients should be provided to encourage concordance and improve effectiveness.
- Generally, less greasy products are more acceptable for use during the day and greasier products for night time. However, choice must be informed by individual preference.
- To be effective, it is important to prescribe the right amount of emollient. For someone with an overall dry skin condition, it is generally accepted that 500 g will last 7–10 days. The prescriber must use their clinical judgement, assessing severity of skin damage, how big the individual is and whether the individual is using the product as both a leave on emollient and soap substitute. As a guide 5 g for full coverage each of the following areas: an arm, thigh, lower leg, chest, abdomen, upper back is a reasonable estimate. As an estimate, one pump from a pump dispenser or a dessert spoonful is equivalent to 1 g (Britton, 2003).
- Emollients should be applied to the skin using a stroking action in the direction of hair growth, avoiding circular or rubbing motions to avoid folliculitis. They should be dotted over the skin and spread to leave a thin film on the skin.
- Complete emollient therapy should be continued once the dry skin condition is controlled as this may help to prevent future exacerbations.

Irritant-associated dermatitis

It is essential that when presented with a patient who is incontinent to take a full history and thorough skin assessment to ensure that causation can be identified and an effective treatment plan implemented. Observation of the distribution of the dermatitis will help clinicians differentiate from other types of tissue damage such as pressure damage and intertrigo (inflamed skin folds caused by exposure to perspiration, friction and bacteria and fungi).

> **Practice point**
>
> Topical anti-fungal or anti-inflammatory products should not routinely be used in patients with AID. Anti-fungals should only be used if a fungal rash is present. If IAD does not improve using barrier products, a weak topical steroid such as 1% hydrocortisone cream or ointment can be applied twice a day to the affected area for 3–5 days. If the skin does not improve then patients should be referred for further evaluation.

The main approach to prevent skin breakdown is by cleansing the skin, applying a moisturiser and the use of skin protectants (Gray et al., 2012). Soap and water should be avoided as soap is made up of a mixture of alkalis and fatty acids. The alkalis in soap are thought to have the potential to raise the pH of the skin damaging the acid mantle which is essential to skin integrity as it aids the natural coexistence of skin flora which has a protective function by acting against pathogenic bacteria (Rippke et al., 2002). The surfactants found in soaps are irritants and are likely to increase skin damage (Voegli, 2008). Skin cleansers are less damaging than soap and water and help to maintain a pH level that minimises skin barrier disruption. They come in different formulations and combine gentle detergents and surfactant ingredients to loosen and remove dirt and irritants. Most are pH balanced and are designed not to be rinsed off the skin as they contain moisturising agents to restore or preserve optimal barrier function so are considered to be the treatment of choice (Gray et al., 2012).

The aim of skin protectants is to prevent skin breakdown by isolating exposed skin from irritants and excess moisture. Liquid barrier films and moisture barrier creams or ointments are frequently used. A study by Hoggarth et al. (2005) demonstrated that petrolatum-based barriers gave protection against irritants and maceration and provided some hydration but that zinc oxide–based products protected against irritants but provided poor skin hydration. The introduction of synthetic barrier products which leave a thin protective polymer layer on the skin have proven useful in recent years to protect skin from high levels of moisture. Skin care systems are available that provide a combination products including moisturising skin cleansers, skin protectant creams and disposable wash clothes which have been shown to maximise carer efficiency and increase adherence with skin care regimes (Warshaw et al., 2002; Hunter et al., 2003).

The management of IAD may require supportive interventions including the use of absorptive products and the use of urinary catheters or stool diversion systems. A Cochrane review on the use of absorbent products for urinary and faecal incontinence concluded that no design was better or worse for maintaining skin health. The reviewers found that individual preference was important and depended on the level of activity of the wearer (Fader et al., 2008). The role of absorptive products and IAD is unclear but appears to be related to occlusion combined with prolonged contact with urine or stool. Although surprisingly, Fader et al. (2003) found that there was no difference in severity of IAD between those who had pads changed frequently or infrequently.

> **Practice point**
>
> What is the most effective way to manage a patient's skin hygiene? Hot water should be avoided as this increases moisture loss from the skin, the use of warm water is preferable. Soaking in a bath for long periods of time is not recommended as the skin can become waterlogged and barrier function is compromised. The use of soap should be avoided and skin cleansers (also known as soap substitutes) should be used. Skin should be gently patted dried taking care to avoid mechanical injury and massage should be avoided as it has the potential to damage the micro-circulation. If skin is left damp, the SC may become macerated and excoriated and will be at increased risk of friction damage (Voegeli, 2012). There is minimal evidence to support specific skin care protocols and most are based on clinical experience and best practice rather than evidence-based practice.

Summary

This chapter has shown that maintenance of skin barrier function is important to prevent loss of skin integrity, which causes discomfort, affects quality of life and may cause deterioration of the patient's general condition. There is now a growing body of evidence to support the use of skin care regimes that focus on cleansing, application of moisturisers and the use of skin protectants. The use of moisturisers should be routinely incorporated into skin care regimes for people with dry skin to promote hydration and reduce the likelihood of skin damage such as IAD and skin tears.

There is a need to raise awareness of the importance of skin health and for wound care practitioners to work more closely with other colleagues who have an interest in skin integrity such as dermatology and continence specialists. Health care facilities should urgently consider adopting a standard skin care protocol that incorporates the principles discussed in this chapter. However, research is urgently required to establish the effectiveness of specific skin care interventions and to validate best practice.

Useful resources

Guidelines

Emollient Best Practice Statement. Available at: www.bdng.org.uk.

Ersser, S.J., Maguire, S., Nicol, N.H., Penzer, R., Peters, J. (2009) Best practice in emollient therapy; a statement for health care professionals. 2nd edn. In: Dermatological Nursing (Supplement), 8(3), pp. 1–22.

Best Practice Statement. Care of the Older Person's Skin. London: Wounds UK, 2012 (Second edition). Available at: www.wounds-uk.com/best-practice-statements/care-of-the-older-persons-skin-best-practice-statement-update

World Union of Wound Healing Societies (WUWHS) (2007) *Principles of Best Practice: Wound Exudate and the Role of Dressings.* London: MEP Ltd. Available at: http://www.woundsinternational.com (accessed 23 November 2011).

Useful websites

www.dermnetnz.org/
www.bdng.org.uk

http://dermatology.cdlib.org/1802/index.html: free dermatology online journal.

References

Alam, M., Havey, J. (2010) Photoaging. In: *Cosmetic Dermatology. Products and Procedures* (ed Z.D. Draelos), pp. 3–13. Oxford: Wiley-Blackwell.

Alikhan, A., Maibach, H.I. (2010) Biology of straum corneum: tape stripping and protein quantification. In: *Textbook of Aging Skin* (eds M.A. Farage, K.W. Miller, H.I. Maibach), pp. 401–407. Berlin: Springer Verlag.

Barbaud, A., Collet, E., Le Coz, C.J., Meaume, S., Gillois, P. (2009) Contact allergy in chronic leg ulcers: results of a multicentre study carried out in 423 patients and proposal for an updated series of patch tests. *Contact Dermatitis*, 60(5), 279–287.

Baumann, L. (2007) Skin ageing and its treatment. *Journal of Pathology*, 211, 241–251.

Behne, M.J., Barry, N.P., Hanson, K.M., et al. (2003) Neonatal development of the stratum corneum pH gradient: localization and mechanisms leading to emergence of optimal barrier function. *Journal of Investigative Dermatology*, 120, 998–1006.

Benedetto, A.D., Agnihothri, R., McGirt, L.Y. (2009) Atopic dermatitis: a disease caused by innate immune defects? *Journal of Investigative Dermatology*, 129, 14–30.

Berg, R.W. (1988) Etiology and pathophysiology of diaper dermatitis. *Advances in Dermatology*, 3, 75–98.

Black, J.M., Gray, M., Bliss, D.Z., et al. (2011) MASD part 2: incontinence-associated dermatitis and intertriginous dermatitis: a consensus. *Journal of Wound, Ostomy and Continence Nursing*, 38, 4, 359–370; quiz 371-372.

Britton, J. (2003) The use of emollients and their correct application. *Journal of Community Nursing*, 17(9), 22–25.

Brown, S.J., McLean, W.H. (2012) One remarkable molecule: filaggrin. *Journal of Investigative Dermatology*, 132, 751–762.

Buckingham, K.W., Berg, R.W. (1986) Etiologic factors in diaper dermatitis: the role of feces. *Pediatric Dermatology*, 3, 107–112.

Charbonneau, D.L., Song, Y.L., Liu, C.X. (2010) Aging skin and microbiology. In: *Textbook of Aging Skin* (eds M.A. Farage, K.W. Miller, H.I. Maibach), pp. 871–881. Berlin: Springer Verlag.

Cross, C.C., Halliwell, B., Borish, E.T., et al. (1987) Davis conference: oxygen radicals and human disease. *Annals of Internal Medicine*, 107, 526–545.

Cooper, P. (2011) Skin care: managing the skin of incontinent patients. *Wound Essentials*, 6, 69–74.

Cork, M.J., Danby, S., Vasilopoulos Y., et al. (2009) Epidermal barrier dysfunction in atopic dermatitis. *Journal of Investigative Dermatology*, 129, 1892–1908.

Draelos, Z.D. (2010) Active agents in common skin care products. *Plastic and Reconstructive Surgery* 125(2), 719–724.

Drug and Therapeutics Bulletin (2007) Bath emollients for atopic eczema: why use them. *Drug and Therapeutics Bulletin*, 45(10), 73–75.

Egelrud, T. (2000) Desquamation in the stratum corneum. *Acta Dermato-Venereologica* (Supp 208), 44–45.

Ersser, S. (2010) Protecting the skin and preventing breakdown. In: *Principles of Skin Care* (eds R. Penzer, S.J. Ersser), pp. 49–69. Oxford: Wiley-Blackwell.

Ersser, S.J., Maguire, S., Nicol, N.H., Penzer, R., Peters, J. (2009). Best practice in emollient therapy; a statement for health care professionals. *Dermatological Nursing (Supplement)*, 8(3), 1–22.

Ersser, S.J., Getliffe, K., Voegeli, D., Regan, S. (2005) A critical review of the inter-relationship between skin vulnerability and urinary incontinence and related nursing intervention. *International Journal of Nursing Stuides*, 42, 823–835.

Fader, M., Cottenden, A.M., Getliffe, K. (2008) Absorbent products for moderate-heavy urinary and/or faecal incontinence in women and men. *Cochrane Database of Systematic Reviews* (4), CD007408.

Fader, M., Clarke-O'Neill, S., Cook, D., et al. (2003) Management of night time urinary incontinence in residential settings for older people: an investigation into the effects of different pad changing regimes on skin health. *Journal of Clinical Nursing*, 12(3), 374–386.

Farage, M.A., Miller, K.W., Maibach, H.I. (2010) Degenerative changes in aging skin. In: *Textbook of Aging Skin* (eds M.A. Farage, K.W. Miller, H.I. Maibach), pp. 25–35. Berlin: Springer Verlag.

Fisher, G.J., Sewon Kang, D., Varani, J., et al. (2002) Mechanisms of photoaging and chronological skin aging. *Archives of Dermatology*, 138, 1462–1470.

Fluhr, J.W., Dickel, H., Kuss, O., Weyher, I., Diepgen, T.L., Berardesca E (2002) Impact of anatomical location on barrier recovery, surface pH, and stratum corneum hydration after acute barrier disruption. *British Journal on Dermatology*, 146(5), 770–776.

Fluhr, J.W., Darlenski, R. (2009) Skin barrier. In: *Life-Threatening Dermatoses and emergencies in Dermatology* (ed J. Revuz), pp. 3–18 Berlin: Springer Verlag.

Gilchrest, B.A. (1989) Skin aging and photoaging: an overview. *Journal of the American Academy of Dermatology*, 21, 610–613.

Harman, D. (1986) Free radical theory of aging: role of free radicals in the origination and evolution of life, aging and disease process. In: *Biology of Aging* (eds J. Johnson, R. Walford, D. Harman, J. Miquel), pp. 3–50. New York: Liss.

Hoath, S.B., Maibach, H.I. (2003) red. *Neonatal Skin*. New York: Marcel Dekker.

Hoggarth, A., Waring, M., Alexander, J., Greenwood, A., Callaghan, T. (2005) A controlled, three-part trial to investigate the barrier function and skin hydration properties of six skin protectants. *Ostomy Wound Manage*, 51(12), 30–42.

Houwing, R.H., Arends, J.W., Canninga-van Dijk, M.R., Koopman, E., Haalboom, J.R. (2007) Is the distinction between superfi cial pressure ulcers and moisture lesions justifiable? A clinical-pathologic study. *Skinmed*, 6(3), 113–117.

Hunter, S., Anderson, J., Hanson, D., Thompson, P., Langemo, D., Klug, M. (2003) Clinical trial of a prevention and treatment protocol for skin breakdown in two nursing homes. *Journal of Wound, Ostomy and Continence Nursing*, 30, 250–258.

Lai, Y., Gallo R.L. (2009) AMPed up immunity: how antimicrobial peptides have multiple roles in immune defense. *Trends in Immunology*, 30(3), 131–141.

Kaya, G., Saurat J.-H. (2007) Dermatoporosis: a chronic cutaneous insufficiency/fragility syndrome. *Dermatology*, 215, 284–294.

Kawaguchi, Y, Tanaka, H, Okada, T, et al. (1996) The effects of ultraviolet A and reactive oxygen species on the mRNA expression of 72-kDa type IV collagenase and its tissue inhibitor in cultured human dermal fibroblasts. *Archives of Dermatological Research*, 288, 39–44.

Kezic, S., Kemperman, P.M., Koster E.S., et al. (2008) Loss-of-function mutations in the filaggrin gene lead to reduced level of natural moisturizing factor in the stratum corneum. *Journal of Investigative Dermatology* 128, 2117–2119.

Lavker, R.M. (1979) Structural alterations in exposed and unexposed aged skin. *Journal of Investigative Dermatology*, 73, 559–566.

Langøen, A., Vik, H., Nyfors, A. (1993) Diaper dermatitis. Classification, occurrence, causes, prevention and treatment. *Tidsskr Nor Laegeforen*, 113(14), 1712–1715.

Langøen, A. (2010) Innovations in care of the skin surrounding pressure ulcers. *Wounds International*, 1(4), 9–12. Available at: http://www.woundsinternational.com/article.php?issueid=326&contentid=122&articleid=9608&page=1.

Lawton, S., Langøen, A. (2009) Dermatological problems and periwound skin. World Wide Wounds, October 2009. Available at: http://www.worldwidewounds.com/2009/October/Lawton-Langoen/vulnerable-skin-2.html.

Madison K. (2003) Barrier function of the skin: "La Raison d'Être" of the epidermis. *Journal of Investigative Dermatology*, 121, 231–241.

Mayoritz, H.N., Sims, N. (2001) Biophysical effects of water and synthetic urine on skin. *Advances in Skin and Wound Care*, 14(6), 302–308.

Nemes, Z., Steinert, P.M. (1999) Brick and mortar of the epidermal barrier. *Experimental and Molecular Medicine*, 31, 5–19.

Proksch E., Brandner J.M., Jensen J.M. (2008) The skin: an indispensable barrier. *Experimental Dermatology*, 17(12), 1063–1072.

Ranzer, M.J., DiPietro, L.A. (2010) Impaired wound repair and delayed angiogenese. In: *Textbook of Aging Skin* (eds M.A. Farage, K.W. Miller, H.I. Maibach), pp. 897–907. Berlin: Springer Verlag.

Raschke, C., Elsner, P. (2010) Skin aging: a brief summary of characteristic changes. In: *Textbook of Aging Skin* (eds M.A. Farage, K.W. Miller, H.I. Maibach), pp. 37–43. Berlin: Springer Verlag.

Rippke, F., Schreiner, V., Schwanitz H.U. (2002) The acid mileu of the horny layer: new findings on the physiology and pathophysiology of the skin pH. *American Journal of Clinical Dermatology*, 3(4), 261–272.

Robinson, M., Visscher, M., Laruffa, A., Wickett, R. (2010) Natural moisturizing factors (NMF) in the stratum corneum (SC). I. Effects of lipid extraction and soaking. *Journal of Cosmetic Science*, 61(1), 13–22.

Shawayder, T., Akland, T. (2005) Neonatal skin barrier: structure, function, and disorders. *Dermatological Therapy*, 18, 87–103.

Tortora, G.J., Derrickson, B.H. (2009) *Principles of Anatomy and Physiology*, 12th edn. New Jersey: Wiley.

Thune, P., Nilsen, T., Hanstad, I.K., Gustavsen T., Lövig Dahl, H. (1988) The water barrier function of the skin in relation to the water content of stratum corneum, pH and skin lipids. The effect of alkaline soap and syndet on dry skin in elderly, non-atopic patients. *Acta Dermato-Venereologica*, 68, 277–283.

Trengove, N.J., Stacey, MC., Macauley, S., et al. (1999) Analysis of the acute and chronic wound environments: the role of proteases and their inhibitors. *Wound Repair and Regeneration*, 7(6), 442–452.

Tzellos, T. G., Klagas, I., Vahtsevanos, K., et al. (2009), Extrinsic ageing in the human skin is associated with alterations in the expression of hyaluronic acid and its metabolizing enzymes. *Experimental Dermatology*, 18, 1028–1035.

Voegeli, D. (2012) Moisture-associated skin damage: aetiology, prevention and treatment. *British Journal of Nursing*, 21, 9, 517–518, 520–521.

Warshaw, E., Nix, D., Kula, J., Markon, C.E. (2002) Clinical and cost effectiveness of a cleanser protectant lotion for treatment of perineal skin breakdown in low-risk patients with incontinence. *Ostomy Wound Manage*, 48, 44–51.

Williams, H.C., Grindlay, D.J.C. (2008) What's new in atopic eczema? An analysis of the clinical significance of systematic reviews on atopic eczema published in 2006 and 2007. *Clinical and Experimental Dermatology*, 33, 685–688.

Wolcott, R.D., Rhoads, D.D., Dowd, S.E. (2008) Biofilms and chronic wound inflammation. *Journal of Wound Care*, 17, 333–341.

Yang, D., Biragyn, A., Hoover, D.M., Lubkowski, J., Oppenheim, J.J. (2004) Multiple roles of antimicrobial defensins, cathelicidins, and eosinophil-derived neurotoxin in host defense *Annual Review of Immunology*, 22, 181–215.

Zulkowski, K. (2012) Diagnosing and treating moisture-associated skin damage. *Advances in Skin and Wound Care*, 25, 5, 231–236; quiz 237-238.

3 Physiology of Wound Healing

Mary Martin

Independent Consultant, D4 Consultancy, Dublin, Ireland

Overview

- The skin is our most accessible organ and is constantly vulnerable to damage and wounds.
- Wounds involving the dermis heal by the complex process of tissue repair which is less efficient than regeneration of the epidermis and results in scar formation.
- The traditional terms 'chronic' and 'acute' wound could be replaced with 'non-healing' and 'healing' as these more accurately reflect the clinical situation.
- The aim of wound management is to facilitate the body's capacity to heal, which relies on an understanding of the physiology of tissue repair, as the goal is to replace injured tissue with regenerated tissue by providing the most favourable conditions and an optimal environment.
- Non-healing wounds are characterised by high levels of exudate that is rich in inflammatory mediators and proteases which impair cell proliferation and growth factor availability causing breakdown of the extracellular matrix (ECM) and skin excoriation.
- Better understanding of the physiology of tissue repair and implementation of best practice currently means that approximately 80% of chronic wounds respond to treatment and go on to heal. Advances in treatment modalities are likely to improve this in the future.

Introduction

Skin is the most visible organ in the body and its observation is often our first point of social contact. Tissue damage is an inevitable consequence of survival in a hostile environment and the human body's capacity to heal is impressive. In recent years, our understanding of the sequence of events, cells involved and molecular signalling required to support this intricate process has increased although the complex relationship between the cell types and processes involved are only just beginning to be fully appreciated. Wound healing is a complex sequence of overlapping events which are often described separately for ease of explanation but in reality form a continuum often referred to as the healing cascade (Diegelmann and Evans, 2004).

Injury refers to a loss of continuity in any body tissue occurring as a result of trauma, infection or pathological process. When the surface of the skin is damaged a wound is created and the body

---

Wound Healing and Skin Integrity: Principles and Practice, First Edition. Edited by Madeleine Flanagan.
© 2013 John Wiley & Sons, Ltd. Published 2013 by John Wiley & Sons, Ltd.

immediately begins to reestablish tissue integrity in an attempt to restore the barrier function of the skin. Wound healing in any tissue follows a predictable sequence of events but wounds have only two mechanisms by which they heal: tissue regeneration and tissue repair (Clark et al., 1998). The epidermis is capable of regeneration of identical cells without loss of function and, in superficial injuries where the basal layer of the dermis remains intact, the epithelial cells will replicate and normal anatomical structure and function is quickly restored (Enoch and Leaper, 2005). Therefore, tissue regeneration is the ideal form of healing giving good cosmetic and functional results. However, in humans, this is only possible in a limited number of cell types such as epithelial and liver cells (Kumar et al., 2010).

If the injury extends deeper into the dermis, damage to its intricate structure including the hair and sweat glands, cells, nerves, blood and lymphatic vessels results in the complex biological process known as tissue repair (Figure 3.1) (Gurtner et al., 2008; Shaw and Martin, 2009). Tissue repair is the mechanism by which all except the most superficial wounds heal. The process of tissue repair replaces damaged or absent tissue and restores skin integrity but the structure and function of the original tissue is lost as even a hair root is too complicated to rebuild (Majno, 1975).

The physiology of wound healing is complex and intricate and involves the related processes of tissue repair and tissue regeneration which the evolution has optimised and are usually very effective (Welt et al., 2009). An understanding of wound-healing

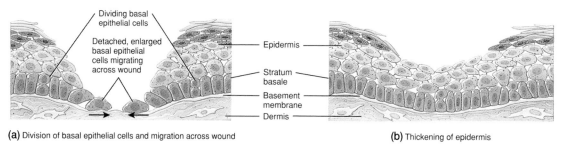

(a) Division of basal epithelial cells and migration across wound

(b) Thickening of epidermis

Epidermal wound healing

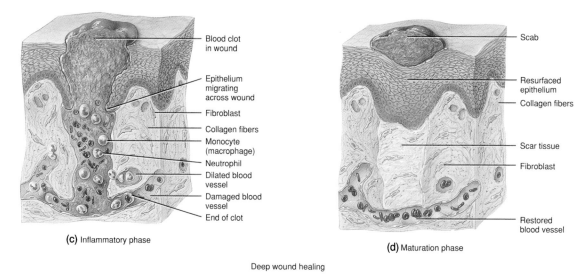

(c) Inflammatory phase

(d) Maturation phase

Deep wound healing

Figure 3.1   Epidermal and deep wound healing. From Tortora and Derrickson (2009). Reproduced with permission from Wiley.

physiology is important because it helps to inform effective clinical management of wounds. In particular, understanding how the body's own immune system responds to tissue injury helps experienced clinicians to interpret the subtle signs and symptoms provided by the wound that may indicate that the progression of healing is delayed.

Types of wound healing

Primary closure

Once skin integrity has been breached, primary closure (sometimes referred to as primary intention) describes the process of wound closure within hours of injury and is possible where the wound edges remain in proximity to each other and there is little or no tissue loss or damage. As long as the wound edges can be mechanically brought together without tension, closure can be achieved using a variety of techniques including adhesive strips, sutures, skin adhesives, staples or clips. Provided there are no factors known to delay healing and complications are treated appropriately, these wounds usually heal quickly. Wounds closed by primary intention typically have the best aesthetic appearance as both wound contraction and scar formation are minimised.

Secondary closure

If primary closure is not possible, wounds should be left open to heal spontaneously by the processes of contraction and reepithelialisation which is known as secondary closure; examples include large traumatic wounds and surgical drainage of abscesses. Secondary closure (alternative term: secondary intention) is associated with wounds where the damage and loss of tissue is caused by an underlying, internal aetiology and pathology, such as venous insufficiency (leg ulcers), unrelieved pressure, shear, or friction (pressure ulceration) and in many cases, healing will be significantly delayed.

Delayed primary closure

Delayed primary closure also known as tertiary wound closure occurs when wound closure is delayed for 3–6 days due to adverse local conditions such as poor vascularity, uncontrolled bleeding or risk of infection (Gottrup, 1999). Once conditions improve, wounds are closed with sutures or other techniques. Delayed primary closure is therefore a compromise between immediate primary closure and allowing local wound conditions to improve prior to delayed closure.

Wound chronicity

One of the most helpful definitions of an acute wound is given by Lazarus et al. (1997), who stated that an acute wound is one that proceeds through an orderly and timely reparative process to establish sustained anatomic and functional integrity. This consensus group described a chronic wound as one that has failed to proceed through an orderly and timely reparative process to produce anatomic and functional integrity or has proceeded through the repair process without establishing a sustained anatomic and functional result. In other words, there are two types of wounds: those that can repair themselves quickly with minimal complications (acute wounds), and those that either heal slowly or heal and recur or never heal at all (chronic wounds).

Enoch and Price (2004) developed this idea further by describing a chronic wound (and its underlying aetiology) as one that does not respond to treatment and/or the demands of treatment are beyond the patient's physical health, tolerance or stamina. Advances in treatment and a better understanding of wound physiology mean that today many chronic wounds will eventually heal although this may take months or even years. One of the defining features of chronic wounds is that they are characterised by alternating patterns of healing and skin breakdown leading to delayed wound healing and frequent recurrence as seen in Figure 3.2.

The conventional approach of describing wounds as either acute or chronic has in recent years been challenged as being over simplistic. Briggs (2010) recommends an alternative viewpoint and suggests wounds could be considered as either 'low risk uncomplicated wounds which are likely to heal' (acute) or 'high risk complicated wounds which are challenging to heal but where healing is possible' (chronic). Others suggest that the terms 'non-healing and healing wounds' are

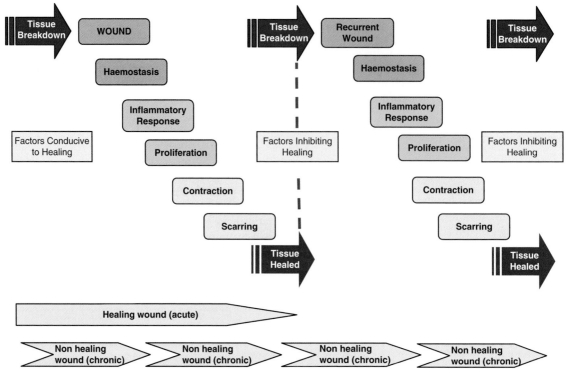

Figure 3.2   Diagrammatic summary of healing and non-healing wounds.

more accurate descriptors and recommend that the traditional term 'chronic' should be replaced with 'non-healing' as this more accurately reflects the clinical situation (Grey et al., 2006; Schultz, 2007; Gottrup et al., 2010). Table 3.1 summarises the most frequently used terms to describe acute and chronic wounds.

Normal wound healing

Uncomplicated, acute wounds are the result of a one-time injury or trauma. They heal in a

Table 3.1   Alternative descriptors for acute and chronic wounds

Acute wounds	Chronic wounds
Low risk	High risk
Uncomplicated wounds	Complicated wounds
Likely to heal	Challenging to heal but possible
Healing wounds	Non-healing wounds
Normal wound healing	Delayed wound healing

microenvironment where cellular communication is clear, controlled and uninhibited, where the ratio between the processes of cellular destruction and synthesis is in balance and where there is an 'elegant coordination' of the wound-healing process (Majno, 1975). Much of our understanding of acute wound healing is however based on animal studies and research findings which cannot always be extrapolated to humans or to the clinical situation.

The dominant research finding over the past 50 years which is clinically well accepted is George Winter's theory of moist wound healing which now forms the basis of modern wound management and has influenced the commercial development of many innovative types of wound dressings (see Chapter 17). Winter's (1962) original small study used pigs to evaluate the effect of occlusion on wound healing and demonstrated that wounds kept moist by a polyurethane film had faster rates of epithelialisation than those exposed to air and allowed to dry out to form a scab. Accumulating evidence from subsequent studies of acute wounds in animal models, including work from Dyson et al. (1988), Chen et al. (1992) and Kunugiza et al. (2010), has confirmed the benefits of moist wound healing which is now supported by clinical experience spanning 40 years.

Moist wound healing:

- has reduced inflammatory response;
- has increased leucocyte activity;
- has reduced infection rates;
- has reduced fibrosis;
- has increased healing rates;
- has improved scar quality.

However, in these uncomplicated acute wound models there is coordination and cooperation between cells and the wound is typically clean and free from significant bioburden, unlike the chronic wound environment. The validity of applying these findings to human wounds where underlying disease and other factors impact on healing has been questioned (Lawrence, 1995; Nelson, 1995). Although the provision of a moist wound environment through occlusive dressings appears to enhance autolytic debridement and inhibit bacterial growth, Winter's theory of moist wound healing is perhaps most applicable to non-healing chronic wounds in the final stages of healing at the point where the successful migration of epithelial cells becomes a priority (Schultz et al., 2003).

The role of wound exudate

Wound exudate is not an inert fluid, its composition is altered by wound aetiology and biochemical changes in the wound environment, e.g. infection and other pathological processes, and vary at different stages of healing. This means that the composition of exudate from healing and non-healing wounds is different (Wysocki et al., 1993; Trengove et al., 1999).

Exudate directly influences the processes of wound healing and initially helps to control inflammation in healing wounds by recruiting neutrophils and macrophages to the injured site. The function of matrix metalloproteases (MMPs) found in wound fluid at this stage is to initiate a clean-up operation by debriding the wound and removing bacteria and damaged collagen molecules. Wound exudate has an important function in normal wound healing as it provides a moist wound healing environment, aids cell migration, enables diffu-

sion of growth factors, provides nutrients, facilitates autolytic debridement of devitalised tissue and keeps the wound hydrated.

Baker and Leaper (2000) examined the constituents of wound fluid from 50 surgical wound drains and concluded that while cellular activity in uncomplicated, surgical wounds has always been considered to be regulated and balanced, fluid from different surgical wounds showed inconsistent levels of proteases and cytokines on the first postoperative day. Various studies have demonstrated that as wounds heal, protease levels fall which is predictive of healing and the level of wound exudate deceases and as a result the composition of exudate will change (Wysocki et al., 1993; Trengove et al., 1999).

The body's response to healing commences immediately after injury with haemostasis, which triggers an inflammatory response leading to proliferation of granulation tissue, reepithelialisation of the defect and remodelling of the dermis which is coordinated by growth factors and cytokines and which is traditionally divided into distinct, overlapping phases resulting in the full restoration of skin integrity (Harding et al., 2002; Moore, 2005; Schultz et al., 2011). However, an exact timeframe cannot be attributed to each phase of tissue repair as, for example, a wound will remain in the inflammatory phase of healing until bacterial balance has been restored and the wound bed is clear of debris. The progression of healing through each phase of the process is dependent on the preceding stage; the intensity and duration of the inflammatory response will affect proliferation which, in turn, will affect remodelling of new tissue.

Practice point

What is the difference between the terms growth factors and cytokines?

In clinical practice, these terms are often used interchangeably. Cytokines and growth factors are both proteins which are synthesised by cells and released into the ECM where they bind to their target cells, and they are critical regulators of healing. However, technically, growth factors are a subset of cytokines. Cytokines primarily target inflammatory cells attracting those cells to the injured area in order to promote an inflammatory response. Growth factors stimulate proliferation and migration of their target cells which include fibroblasts and keratinocytes (Schultz et al., 2005b).

The process of uncomplicated wound healing is often described as being 'dynamic', because progression through the healing process is stimulated by the wound itself (Trengove et al., 1999; Harding et al., 2002; Enoch and Leaper, 2005). However, if this process ceases to be dynamic and the control is lost then healing is delayed, outcomes become unpredictable and the wound is considered to have become chronic.

Optimising healing: general factors

Menon and Kligman (2009) eloquently describe the skin barrier as a 'flexible mosaic of evolutionary triumph' and its restoration is affected by a number of inhibiting factors, such as wound infection and a number of positive actions, such as wound debridement.

Franz et al. (2008) reviewed factors delaying healing of surgical wounds as either local or systemic and examined the strength of evidence supporting each.

This review demonstrated that factors such as inadequate wound perfusion, presence of non-viable tissue, high bacterial bioburden, smoking, malnutrition and systemic conditions such as diabetes mellitus cause significant delays in healing of acute wounds. The factors with the strongest evidence are seen in Table 3.2 (Franz et al., 2008). Other authors (Leaper and Harding, 2000) discuss the negative effect of drug therapies, the aging process and mechanical factors such as pressure and the inappropriate use of dressings. It is also widely

Table 3.2   Summary of evidence supporting physiological factors delaying healing

Guideline	Factors	Effect on wound healing	Level of evidence
1	**Local factors**		
1.1	Inadequate wound perfusion	Increased risk of infection	Level I
1.2	Presence of non-viable tissue	Increased risk of infection	Level I
1.3	Presence of wound haematomas or seromas	Causes wound ischemia, increases dead space, supplies nutrients for bacteria; increases risk of infection	Level I
1.4	Wound infection	Prolongs the inflammatory response	Level I
1.5	Excess proteases	Degrades extracellular matrix	Level I
2	**Systemic factors**		
2.1	Systemic immune deficiency/ suppression, e.g. immuno-suppressant drugs, HIV, cancer	Inhibition of cellular proliferation and function; nutritional deficiency	Level I
2.2	Systemic conditions, e.g. diabetes mellitus	Hyperglycaemia, increased risk of infection, wound ischaemia	Level II
2.3	Increased age	Impaired immune response	Level II
2.4	Obesity	Increased risk of infection, wound dehiscence, pressure ulceration	Level II
2.5	Malnutrition	Protein loss, increased risk of pressure ulceration	Level I
2.6	Cigarette smoking	Higher incidence of complications	Level I
2.7	Corticosteroids	Detrimental effect on growth factors and collagen deposition	Level II

Source: Data from Franz et al. (2008).

Note: Guideline criteria for levels of evidence are:

Level I: Meta-analysis of multiple RCTs or at least two RCTs supporting the intervention of the guideline or multiple laboratory or animal experiments with at least two clinical studies supporting the laboratory results.

Level II: Less than Level I but at least one RCT and at least two significant clinical series or expert opinion papers with literature analysis, RCT or multiple clinical series.

recognised that stress and anxiety also have a detrimental effect on wound healing (Kiecolt-Glaser et al., 1995; Solowiej et al., 2009).

Poor nutritional status can have direct effects on wound healing. Adequate levels of protein are needed for tissue repair, wound tensile strength and resistance to infection (Stechmiller, 2010). When calories are restricted, the body utilises stored fat and protein for sustenance. Reduction in weight due to nutritional deficiencies causes a change in body structure with less subcutaneous fat deposits, more bony prominences and susceptibility to pressure damage. Additionally, these patients are prone to delayed wound healing and wound infections. Protein levels are particularly important in major traumatic wounds such as burn injuries where catabolic states place major demands on energy sources. Deficiencies in vitamins, minerals and trace elements also may influence wound healing. Collagen synthesis and fibrillogenesis (the development of fine fibrils normally present in collagen fibres of connective tissue) is under direct influence of vitamin C; vitamin B is directly involved in protein synthesis, antibody formation, granulation tissue formation and epithelialisation; vitamin A is important in angiogenesis, chemotaxis and macrophage mobility and is important in counteracting some of the wound-healing retarding effects of radiation. Iron is involved in haemoglobin synthesis and thus oxygenation, and copper and zinc are important for stimulating granulation tissue, encouraging collagen formation and epithelialisation (Stechmiller, 2010).

Optimising healing: local factors

Wound hypoxia

The supply of oxygen to wound tissue is essential to promote healing and to regulate resistance to infection (Gottrup, 2004). Hypoxia is defined as levels of oxygen lower than approximately 30 mmHg and is associated with poor healing, inhibiting fibroblast replication and impairing collagen production (Burns et al., 2003). Oxygen plays a dual role in angiogenesis. The initial growth of new vessels is stimulated by hypoxia; however, the later stages of angiogenesis are stimulated by hyperoxia and wounds may not proceed to healing without higher oxygen levels (Knighton et al., 1983; Chambers and

Leaper, 2011). Oxygen supplementation may be beneficial; however, further research is needed to fully determine its benefits (Chambers and Leaper, 2011).

Bioburden

The wound environment provides the ideal conditions for bacterial growth. Hypoxia in chronic wounds produces devitalised tissue, hematoma and slough which provide an abundant food supply for bacteria. Chronicity in wounds is known to begin when levels of bacteria in the tissues are persistently high (Bjarnsholt et al., 2008). Endotoxins secreted by the proliferating bacteria quickly lead to an elevation in pro-inflammatory cytokines which elevates circulating MMPs and results in decreased production of growth factors (Bucknall, 1980; Dowd et al., 2008). This prolonged inflammatory response is detrimental to normal wound healing and must be resolved if the wound is to heal, indeed studies have shown that as wounds heal, bacterial numbers start to fall (Trengove et al., 1999). It is becoming clear that the development of a biofilm, which is prevalent in non-healing wounds supports this persistent inflammatory state and is thought to be one of the principal causes of chronicity (James et al., 2008; Wolcott et al., 2010; Thomson, 2011) (see Chapter 6).

Wound pH

The pH of the wound bed is also an important factor in promoting optimal healing. A pH value of 7 represents neutral with a pH above 7 representing alkaline and a pH below 7 representing acidic environment (Gethin, 2007). The environment of a non-healing wound is alkaline with a pH value in the range of 7.15–8.9 (Schreml et al., 2010; Tsukada et al., 1992). As healing progresses, the pH range moves from neutral to acidic (Tsukada et al., 1992). Since the mechanism of action of proteases is pH dependent, adjusting wound pH by topical therapies and dressings may control protease activity and help to reestablish a healing environment (Greener et al., 2005; Schultz et al., 2005a).

Wound temperature

All cellular activities in the body occur at an optimal rate at normal core body temperature. Tissue repair occurs when the body surface temperature is above 33°C and below 42°C (McGuinness et al., 2004). Maintaining a normothermic wound temperature helps increase tissue perfusion, increase oxygen tension and improve wound tensile strength (Mac-Fie et al., 2005). The avoidance of tissue ischaemia by the use of intraoperative warming during major surgery has been shown to reduce the risk of pressure sores by half (Scott et al., 2006) and it is now recognised that intraoperative hypothermia leads to increased postoperative wound infections and haematoma formation leading to prolonged recovery times (Scott et al., 2006).

Tissue repair is optimised by effective management of these barriers to healing and Wolcott et al. (2009) suggest that a healthy wound, with minimal biofilm infection, exudate and necrotic tissue, is conducive to preparation of the local wound environment which will progress to healing.

Delayed wound healing

The cause of a wound may not necessarily be the reason for delayed healing, for example, a surgical wound may become infected. Empirical research provides a detailed understanding of the process of normal wound healing but it may be unhelpful to assume the same trajectory is relevant in non-healing wounds (see Figure 3.2). The chronic wound environment is characterised by protease levels which are 30 times higher than that of an uncomplicated healing wound (Trengove et al., 1999) and a deficit in growth factors which is not conducive to healing (Schultz et al., 2003; Schultz, 2007; Moor et al., 2009). In a laboratory study of 14 biopsies from chronic pressure ulcers Diegelmann (2003) found the wound microenvironment to be an area of massive tissue destruction due to an excess of neutrophils which are aggressively contributing to tissue degradation, a finding supported by several other studies (Trengove et al., 1999; Yager and Nwomeh, 1999).

Whatever the causes of delayed healing, the dominant feature of non-healing wounds is that the process of healing is disrupted, disorganised, haphazard and unpredictable as the levels of inflammatory mediators and proteases rise and impair cell proliferation and growth factor availability causing breakdown of the ECM and skin excoriation. As a result, chronic wounds become stuck in the inflammatory phase of healing, resulting in a local microenvironment that is not conducive to tissue repair producing increased levels of exudate rich in inflammatory mediators and proteases, particularly where there are concurrent medical conditions such as chronic heart disease and failure of the lymphatic system. Although secretion of wound fluid is a vital part of healing, it is now evident that exudate produced by non-healing wounds can be an irritant and has a detrimental effect on healing by causing further tissue breakdown and delaying cellular proliferation (Trengove et al., 1999; Schultz et al., 2003; Moor et al., 2009).

In summary, non-healing chronic wounds are disorganised, deficient and delayed and are not able to progress until the balance of the local wound environment has been restored and is able to support cellular communication. The main differences between healing and non-healing wounds are summarised in Table 3.3.

Tissue repair in chronic wounds

The largest component of the dermis is the extracellular matrix (ECM), a gel-like matrix consisting primarily of collagen, a fibrous protein, which gives skin its structure and strength, and elastin which provides suppleness and compressibility (Schultz et al., 2005b). Any injury which penetrates the dermis and the ECM results in blood loss and the need for haemostasis. There is an immediate need for cellular defences, particularly against microbiological invasion, and these are deployed by the body's immune system (Davis, 2008). The immediate response is to limit the flow of blood to the injured area by vasoconstriction. Platelets are immediately released from the damaged blood vessels and leak into the surrounding tissue where they come in contact with collagen at the edge of the damaged blood vessels and, responding to the sudden change in environment, become sticky and adhere together with collagen activating the clotting cascade (Silver, 1994; Moore, 2010). The platelets adhere to the severed ends of damaged blood vessels at the injury site forming a platelet plug which acts as a provisional haemostat and

Table 3.3   Differences between healing and non-healing wounds

Acute	Chronic
Controlled inflammatory response	Prolonged inflammatory response
Normal levels of inflammatory cytokines	Increased levels of pro-inflammatory cytokines
Levels of neutrophils, elastase and MMPs within normal limits	Elevated levels of neutrophils, elastase and activated MMPs
Controlled bioburden	Elevated bioburden
Growth factors freely available	Limited availability of growth factors
Wound fluid supports cell proliferation	Wound fluid inhibits cell proliferation
Fibronectin intact	Fibronectin degraded
Normal remodelling of extracellular matrix	Defective remodelling of extracellular matrix
Wound fluid does not damage peri-wound skin	Wound fluid causes peri-wound skin irritation and excoriation
Heal with minimal complications and no recurrence	Defective healing, complications common and frequently recurrence

Source: Data from Trengove et al. (1999) and Shultz et al. (2011).

reservoir for growth factors (Hart, 2002). A network mesh of fibrin fibres quickly forms a fibrin clot around the plug which holds the damaged tissue together, providing a cover and provisional fibrin matrix which supports the necessary migration of cells (Schultz et al., 2005b; Moore, 2010). If exposed to air, the surface of the clot may dry out and become a scab, forcing the cells required for healing to migrate underneath this physical barrier. Unless there is an underlying clotting disorder, haemostasis will be complete within minutes of injury and the delicate process of tissue repair will begin. While haemostasis is the primary function of platelets, they also release cytokines and growth factors which, in turn, recruit neutrophils and macrophages (Li et al., 2007; Sussman and Bates-Jensen, 2007), thereby playing a critical role in advancing the process of healing.

The inflammatory response

Majno (1975) describes the wound at this point as a 'dreadful mess of spilled blood, dead cells, foreign material and bacteria'. While further blood loss has been prevented by vasoconstriction and clotting, the immediate need is to prevent infection, cleanse the injured area and provide optimum conditions for progression to healing. This is essentially achieved by two responses: a vascular and a cellular response known collectively as the inflammatory response (Li et al., 2007). Inflammation is a normal process resulting from any type of injury,

without which there would be no healing (Hart, 2002). During the inflammatory response the initial brief constriction of blood vessels is reversed by vasodilation. Mast cells, which reside in the connective tissue adjacent to the blood vessels, flood the wound releasing histamine and prostaglandins which cause the vessels to dilate and increasing vascular permeability (Ng, 2010). Approximately 10–15 minutes after injury, the blood supply to the area increases and the classic signs of inflammation may now be evident with the area surrounding the wound appearing red, hot, swollen and feeling uncomfortable (Monaco and Lawrence, 2003; Richardson, 2004). The increased flow and pressure changes in the blood vessels in the vicinity of the wounded area allows fluid to pass through the porous vessel walls increasing the extracellular fluid in the surrounding tissue some of which leaks to the surface of the wound as inflammatory exudate. Chemical messengers are released from the platelets and mast cells, including platelet-derived growth factor (PDGF), which attracts neutrophils to the damaged tissue and signal them to proliferate (Woods et al., 2010). White blood cells, which have previously been rushing through the blood vessels, now slow down and congregate on the endothelial lining of the dilated vessels. The neutrophils squeeze through the porous walls of the blood vessels in a process called diapedesis and migrate into the wound space which has already filled with the fibrin clot (Davis, 2008). Their exit through the barrier of the endothelium is helped by the release of elastase and collagenase which facilitates their

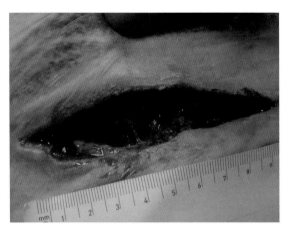

Figure 3.3 Non-healing surgical wound: devitalised tissue and slough evident. Photo courtesy of Nuno Cunha.

movement through the endothelium and enables them to clear the route ahead. Once in the wound environment, neutrophils defend against infection and are responsible for cleaning up the wound by ingesting bacteria and devitalised tissue, in a process known as phagoctyosis. During the inflammatory stage of tissue repair, neutrophils simultaneously release free radicals and proteases into the wounded area as they have a bactericidal effect and promote autolytic debridement to remove damaged cells (Gibson et al., 2009). As they complete their job, neutrophils begin to degenerate and die in a process referred to as apoptosis or programmed cell death (Wolcott et al., 2008). Dead and dying neutophils accumulate on the wound surface and eventually are visible to the naked eye as slough, which is moist, sticky, stringy, devitalised tissue and are typically a creamy yellow colour. Figure 3.3 shows a non-healing surgical wound with devitalised tissue and slough.

Macrophages, derived from blood monocytes, now recognise that these cells are dying and enter the wound to continue the job of phagocytosis (Hart, 2002). Critically, macrophages remove dying neutrophils to prevent them disintegrating into the wound tissue and continuing to release proteases and inflammatory cytokines which prolong the inflammatory process (Wolcott et al., 2008). The wound cannot progress into the proliferative phase of healing until the neutrophils are eliminated by macrophages (Dovi et al., 2004). Li et al. (2007) also consider macrophages as factories for the produc-

tion of the growth factors which recruit fibroblasts and stimulate their proliferation. During the resolution of the inflammatory response, macrophages' dominance over neutrophils increases and the wound environment becomes more able to support new tissue formation (angiogenesis) indicating that the destructive, inflammatory phase of healing is nearing completion (Hart, 2002; Diegelmann and Evans, 2004). The original provisional fibrin matrix is now ready to be replaced by granulation tissue. However, if all is not well at cellular level the point of transition between the inflammatory and proliferative phase of healing may be delayed by a variety of factors, e.g. infection and high protease levels and the wound may be at risk of becoming chronic (Moore, 2003).

The proteases, primarily responsible for the breakdown of the ECM, are the MMPs which play a key destructive role in efficiently removing damaged ECM and bacteria from the wound. However, if not controlled, excessively high levels of proteases have the potential to be in the wrong place at the wrong time resulting in 'off-target' degradation of growth factors inhibiting the cellular messages that stimulate proliferation of cells required for new tissue growth such as fibroblasts and keratinocytes (Gibson et al., 2009). Over the past 20 years, there has been increasing evidence that MMPs are greatly elevated in chronic, non-healing wounds in comparison to healthy healing wounds (Yager et al., 1996; Trengove et al., 1999; Pirila et al., 2007; Moor et al., 2009).

A study comparing wound fluid from acute surgical wounds and non-healing wounds of various aetiologies reported that MMP levels in chronic wound fluid were 30 times higher compared with fluid from acute wounds (Trengove et al., 1999). More recently, investigation into the microenvironment of chronic venous leg ulcers has confirmed the relationship between high levels of MMP9 and delayed healing (Moor et al., 2009). The level and duration of MMP activity in the wound bed are controlled by tissue inhibitors of metalloproteinases (TIMPs) (Percival and Cochrane, 2010). These TIMPs can be overwhelmed by proteases and are known to be present in lower levels in non-healing wounds compared to uncomplicated healing wounds (Gibson et al., 2009). Cullen's circle illustrates the vicious circle of increased inflammatory response and excess protease secretion

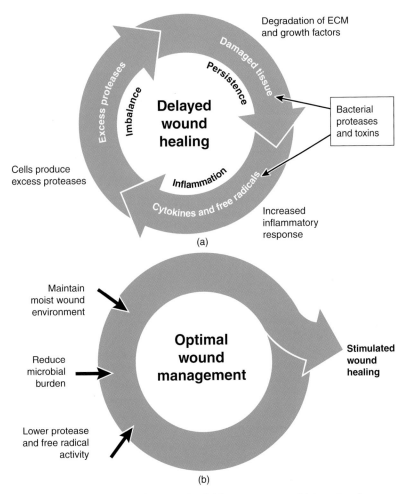

Figure 3.4 (a,b) Cullen's circle. From Gibson et al. (2009). Available at: www.woundsinternational.com

that prolongs healing in Figure 3.4 (Gibson et al., 2009).

Successful progression to healing requires the disruption of this cycle and resolution of the inflammatory response. Since bacteria play a major role in stimulating MMPs and neutrophils, resulting in an overstimulation of the inflammatory response, any concerns regarding increasing levels of bacteria should be addressed (Percival and Cochrane, 2010). Bacteria may remain free-floating or may attach to the wound cells forming biofilm communities (Percival, 2011) which are highly resistant to antibiotics and present challenges for the host immune system (Cooper and Okhiria, 2006).

Proliferation of new tissue

During the proliferative stage of healing the wound needs to develop a new blood supply, a process known as angiogenesis, and create a new matrix to support it. Fibroblasts, the 'fibre makers', respond to growth factors released from platelets and macrophages and migrate to the wound area where they proliferate and produce collagen fibres (Enoch and Leaper, 2005). Fibroblasts crawl over and through the provisional fibrin matrix binding themselves to matrix components. They elongate and find another binding site while the attachment to the original site is broken by MMPs propelling the fibroblast forward so that it can proliferate and lay down collagen to form new ECM (Moore, 2010). Once the original provisional fibrin matrix has performed its function, it is broken down and removed by MMPs. Partially degraded collagen will not bind correctly with newly formed collagen and would result in a weak and disorganised new ECM, so this must also be removed (Schultz et al., 2005b). However, once again the MMPs must be regulated by their tissue inhibitors or the newly formed matrix will be degraded as quickly as it is being built up. The number of times a fibroblast can replicate is limited and they finally lose their ability to divide and multiply becoming senescent and accumulating in the wound (Campisi, 1998). It is now recognised that removing the accumulation of senescent fibroblasts in the wound bed helps to stimulate healing (Falanga, 2004).

The newly formed blood supply in the wound is stimulated by activation of the endothelial cells lining the blood vessels in the wounded area. As the endothelial cells divide, they sprout or bud through the vessel basement membrane into the matrix (Chan, 2009). The tips of these newly formed capillary buds meet, and a cleft develops forming a capillary tube or loop which matures into a new blood vessel (Schultz et al., 2005b; Chan, 2009).

These capillary loops are now embedded in the new matrix and together they comprise granulation tissue which fills the wound from the base up to gradually fill the wound defect. Granulation tissue may initially appear as pale pink, changing to bright red as it proliferates with new blood vessels

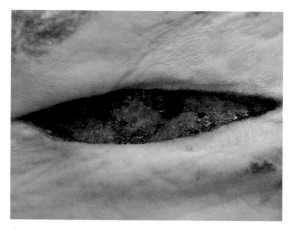

Figure 3.5 Surgical wound healing by secondary intention showing healthy granulation tissue. Note granular appearance of new capillary growth. Photo courtesy of Nuno Cunha.

as seen in Figure 3.5 (Sussman and Bates-Jensen, 2007).

The appearance of granulation tissue is a good indicator of healing. Granulation tissue that appears dark (blackish red) in colour is often a sign that the wound is either poorly perfused or infected. Figure 3.6 shows an arterial leg ulcer with ischemic granulation tissue indicated by its dark red appearance. Table 3.4 summarises the characteristics of healthy and unhealthy granulation tissue.

Since newly formed capillaries and tissue are fragile and have little resistance to mechanical stresses, it is important that the wound is protected against trauma which will cause bleeding and

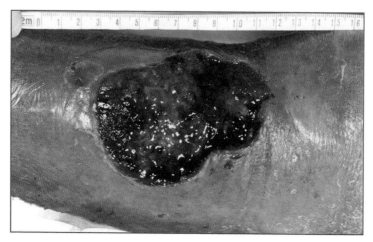

Figure 3.6 Arterial leg ulcer showing unhealthy, fragile granulation tissue. Photo courtesy of Madeleine Flanagan.

Table 3.4 Characteristics of healthy and unhealthy granulation tissue

Healthy granulation tissue	Unhealthy granulation tissue
Bright red or pink	Dark red/bluish discolouration or very pale
Moist	Dehydrated
Shiny surface	Dull surface
Rapid proliferation	Slower growth
Does not bleed easily	Bleeds easily (friable)

restimulate the inflammatory response as this will delay healing and affect scar quality.

Practice point

What is over-granulation and does it delay wound healing?

A complication which may occur at this time is the formation of over-granulation or hypergranulation tissue which is granulation tissue which has grown above the level of the surrounding epithelium causing a barrier to the migrating keratinocytes. Over-granulation is caused by prolonged stimulation of fibroblasts and angiogenesis and appears as mounds of granulation tissue which may bleed easily and leak haemoserous exudate (McGrath, 2011). While the causal trigger is not yet defined, Widgerow and Leak (2010) suggest that possible risk factors may be highly exudating wounds, particularly where moist areas may be subject to repetitive friction or pressure, wounds where a foreign body is present, e.g. a wound drain or orthopaedic pin, wounds which are critically colonised or infected and wounds treated with occlusive dressings. Over-granulation can slow down the rate of healing and increases the risk of infection especially as the tissue is vascular and prone to trauma and bleeds easily. Over-granulation is best treated with simple measures such as application of local pressure to flatten the area and removal of occlusive dressings particularly hydrocolloids. Persistent over-granulation may benefit from the short-term application of self-adhesive polythene tape impregnated with 4 μg/cm^2 fludroxycortide (flurandrenolone) which is a moderately potent corticosteroid.

Wound closure

The surface area and volume of a wound is decreased by the combined processes of granulation, contraction and epithelialisation. At the same time as granulation tissue is being laid down in the wound, keratinocytes (epidermal cells) begin to migrate from the wound margin and intact hair follicles and the wound area will begin to diminish. As long as the local environment is conducive to healing, keratinocytes will creep over the slippery, moist surface of healthy granulation tissue to form a protective layer of epithelium across the wound's surface to repair the epidermal defect.

There are two suggested theories which describe the process of keratinocyte migration: the 'sliding' model where basal keratinocytes at the edge of the wound slide as a moving epithelial sheet (Odland and Ross, 1968; Carter et al., 1990) and the 'rolling' model where the advancing basal keratinocytes stop and the suprabasal keratinocytes leap-frog and tumble over them (Krawczyk, 1971). Usui et al. (2005) propose a model where both basal and suprabasal keratinocytes are activated and suggest that changes to the suprabasal cells are dramatic and that they play the primary role in wound closure. However, the theories are based on *in vitro* remain speculative (Matsumoto and Sugimoto, 2007).

In partial-thickness wounds, keratinocytes also migrate and proliferate from the linings of transected hair follicles, sebaceous glands or sweat ducts which still exist in the damaged tissue. However, in full-thickness wounds, where these dermal appendages are absent, the keratinocyte cells can only proliferate at, and migrate from, the wound margins and it takes longer to provide sufficient cells to cover the wound surface (Moore, 2010). Once the advancing keratinocyte cells make contact with each other, the mechanism of contact inhibition will inhibit further migration and proliferation (Zegers et al., 2003). The wound is now covered by a monolayer of cells which will build upon each other maturing into tough keratinocytes which will quickly reestablish the barrier function of the skin. Clinically, these cells have a white/pink translucent appearance and may appear as small islands of epithelialisation which can be difficult to identify if there is slough or exudate on the wound. It is important to ensure that there is no damage to this newly formed tissue and dressings which are low adherent are an appropriate dressing choice. Moreover, since a moist environment is required for cellular migration, dressings should not allow wound exudate to dry out allowing the formation of a scab which forces the cells to migrate underneath a physical barrier.

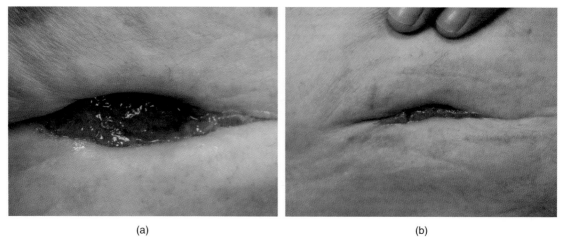

(a)   (b)

Figure 3.7   (a) Contraction of surgical wound (note how granulation tissue has filled in the wound depth). (b) Further contraction of surgical wound (note that the wound defect is completely filled by the combined processes of contraction and granulation. This wound will now epithelialise to close completely). Photos courtesy of Nuno Cunha.

Wound contraction

As the formation of new tissue continues, progress to complete wound closure is helped by wound contraction. Mechanical signals derived from the ECM activate the contractile process that brings the wound edges together and decrease the area requiring coverage by the migrating epithelial cells. This process is particularly relevant in full-thickness wounds where contraction may account for up to a 40% decrease in wound size (Li et al., 2007). There are two opposing theories to describe the mechanisms of wound contraction but physiologists caution against applying findings of *in vitro* studies to complex human wounds (Tejero-Trujeque, 2001; Pellard, 2006; Porter, 2007). One theory supported by Ehrlich (1988) is that the fibroblasts generate uncoordinated traction forces during the remodelling of collagen fibres, thus contracting the wound; the second, supported by Grinnell (1994) and Tomasek et al. (2002) proposes the myofibroblast or cell contraction theory.

Myofibroblasts develop from fibroblasts and are characterised by having components similar to smooth muscle having the ability to extend and retract (Majno, 1975). They connect cell-to-cell and cell-to-matrix and using muscle-like behaviour repeatedly contract and release as the collagen fibres are being laid down thus reducing the area of granulation tissue infill (Ryan et al., 1974; Tomasek

et al., 2002). As the myofibroblasts undergo apoptosis, the granulation tissue will gradually evolve into scar tissue which will continue to be remodelled over time in order for the final scar result to be functionally and cosmetically acceptable (Desmouliere et al., 1995). Stavrou et al. (2009) suggest that both the fibroblast and the myofibroblast appear to play a role in wound contraction; however, this is a process which is not yet completely understood. Figure 3.7a shows the contraction of a surgical wound. Note how granulation tissue has filled in the wound bed providing the right conditions for epithelialisation and final wound closure. Figure 3.7b shows the surgical wound after further contraction. The wound defect is now completely filled by the combined processes of wound contraction and granulation. This wound will now epithelialise quickly to close completely.

Scar maturation and collagen modulation

Inflammation is a necessary component of tissue repair, however, excessive inflammation associated with non-healing wounds result in exaggerated scars of poor quality. Fibroblasts have a central role in wound healing by coordinating the deposition and organisation of the ECM in the wound bed (Blissett et al., 2009). At this stage in the wound-healing process, collagen is continually produced and simultaneously broken down to maintain a balance between the need for tensile strength and remodelling of new tissue. It is this balance which determines the final quality and appearance of scar tissue eventually produced (Roseborough et al., 2004).

Mature collagen type I is the major component of the ECM in most mammalian tissues (Burgeson and Nimni, 1992). As well as providing mechanical strength to the tissue, collagen fibres interact with cells through cell-surface receptors and soluble proteins to support cell proliferation, migration, attachment and differentiation. The formation and assembly of collagen fibres (fibrillogenesis) is a complex process regulated by a variety of collagen-binding proteins (Olaso et al., 2011).

Scar tissue is functionally deficient when compared to uninjured tissue and has no hair follicles, sweat glands or sebaceous glands. As a result it may be associated with lower levels of sensation, chronic itching and hyper pigmentation (Ward, 2007). Collagen maturation goes through phases with collagen type III being present in greater levels in the early scarring phase. As the scar matures, the ratio of type III to type I collagen returns to normal levels so that the quicker the scar matures the lesser the chance of hypertrophy (Widgerow, 2010). Scar tissue may not always produce an ideal aesthetic result; however, it does effectively restore skin barrier function although this may take several months. While scarring is a normal and visible consequence of injury and subsequent tissue repair, it is also a reminder of the inability of dermal tissue to regenerate (Ferguson and O'Kane, 2004).

Practice point

Why do healing wounds often itch?

A healing wound is tissue where many local factors and mechanical conditions are different from normal healthy physiological tissues, so the sources of altered sensation are varied. Itching is the result of an 'intermediate' activation of pain receptors and is a common sensation. There are several theories that explain why healing wounds and scabs itch ranging from the local release of histamines that irritate the skin around the wound to the theory that as the wound heals, the scab becomes more tightly stretched over the rapidly proliferating cells causing the area around the scab to itch. Wound contraction is a physical process that actively draws the wound edges together increasing tension on the nerve fibres within the wound. This shrinkage activates the mechanoreceptive nerves that signal an itch sensation, creating the urge to scratch. Pain neurons have peripheral free nerve terminals which have exposed receptors that come into contact with inflammatory mediators, growth factors and opiates within the wound. These receptors are sensitive and are stimulated by temperature and mechanical stress. As a result they can be activated by a variety of stimuli, typically pressure and touch to produce various sensations such as tickling, itching, tingling and pain. Finally, dehydration exacerbates itching. The sebaceous glands surrounding the injured area may be damaged and not able to lubricate the skin adequately. In reality, the sensation of itching during the final stages of healing is likely to be multifactorial and is a good sign as it is thought to indicate that the wound is healing.

Abnormal scarring

Normal skin has a mature stratum corneum characterised by minimal transepidermal water loss (TEWL). Dehydration of the stratum corneum initiates signalling to keratinocytes to stimulate production of cytokines, which activate dermal fibroblasts to synthesise and release collagen. Excessive collagen production leads to abnormal scarring (Mustoe, 2008). Desmouliere et al. (1995) suggest that the apoptosis of myofibroblasts is the process by which granulation tissue evolves into scar tissue. If myofibroblasts persist and continue the process of remodelling, they can produce excessive amounts of collagen and a hypertrophic scar may occur (Ehrlich et al., 1994). Wounds which are predisposed to hypertrophic scarring include deep burns, wounds with a prolonged inflammatory response due to infection and wounds in areas of high skin tension and movement (Roseborough et al., 2004; Enoch and Leaper, 2005). Hypertrophic scars will regress after approximately 1 year with a reduction in both volume and colour (Teot, 2005).

Keloid scars are often confused with hypertrophic scars (see Chapter 14) but arise from completely different circumstances. Although keloid scars are hypertrophic, they differ by extending beyond the border of the original wound and do not regress over time. Keloid scarring is usually a genetic phenomenon where collagen type I is produced in a tumour-like fashion with uncontrolled growth of scar tissue.

Practice point

How can I tell if an unsightly scar is keloid or hypertrophic?

The patient history of a keloid scar typically involves a wound that has been appropriately managed without infection or complication that could be responsible for its increased size or reactivity. The scar tissue is excessive and overflows the boundary of the wound and is disproportionate to the original injury. It may be painful, sensitive and extremely uncomfortable and previous treatment may be unsatisfactory. In contrast, hypertrophic scarring usually occurs as a natural consequence to normal scarring where exaggeration takes place because either no scar management has been implemented or where suturing technique is lacking or infection has occurred. The hypertropic scar steadily increases its collagen composition and becomes raised and bulky but does not overgrow the wound boundaries. Hypertrophic scars gradually resolve over approximately 1 year and the scar changes colour from pink to white, and flattens into a broad flat scar.

Summary

Wound healing is a complex process performed by cells that are programmed to achieve wound closure. Each cell is capable of multitasking and can perform different functions at different stages of healing depending on the local environment. However, the cells involved in tissue repair need a detailed set of instructions (growth factors) to regulate this process. Critically, these instructions must be delivered to individual cells in the right concentration at the right time. In order to function optimally, the cells responsible for wound healing must be supported by a local environment where conditions are just right. The clinician plays a vital role in supporting the fragile process of tissue repair by understanding the healing trajectory, maintaining the ideal environment to promote healing and observing for signs that it has been delayed.

Although the process of wound healing appears to be simple, advances in molecular science have provided a greater understanding of the complex interactions involved. As understanding of these dynamic physiological processes improves, treatment advances may mean that patients can look forward to scar-less healing; and the routine transplant of tissues engineered from stem cells to improve the outcomes of tissue repair is not too distant future.

Useful resources

Hard-to-heal wounds made easy. (2011) *Wounds International*. 2(4). Available at: http://www.wounds international.com/pdf/content_10140.pdf

MMPs made easy. (2009) *Wounds International*. Available at: http://www.woundsinternational.com

References

Baker, E.A., Leaper, D.J. (2000) Proteinases, their inhibitors, and cytokine profiles in acute wound fluid. *Wound Repair and Regeneration*, 8(5), 392–398.

Bjarnsholt, T., Kirketerp-Møller, K., Jensen, P.Ø., et al. (2008) Why chronic wounds will not heal: a novel hypothesis. *Wound Repair and Regeneration*, 16(1), 2–10.

Blissett, A.R., Garbellini, D., Calomeni, E.P., Mihai, C., Elton, T.S., Agarwal, G. (2009) Regulation of collagen fibrillogenesis by cell-surface expression of kinase dead DDR2. *Journal of Molecular Biology*, 385(3), 902–911.

Briggs, M. (2010) Chronic wounds, non-healing wounds or a possible alternative? *European Wound Management Association Journal*, 10(3), 21–23.

Bucknall, T.E. (1980) The effect of local infection upon wound healing an experimental study. *British Journal of Surgery*, 67, 851–855.

Burgeson, R.E., Nimni, M.E. (1992) Collagen types. Molecular structure and tissue distribution. *Clinical Orthopaedics and Related Research*, 282, 250–272.

Burns, J.L., Mancoll, J.S., Phillips, L.G. (2003) Impairments to wound healing. *Clinics in Plastic Surgery*, 30, 47–56.

Campisi, J. (1998) The role of cellular senescence in skin aging. *Journal of Investigative Dermatology*, 3(1), 1–5.

Carter, W.G., Kaur, P., Gil, S.G., Gahr, P.J., Wayner, E.A. (1990) Distinct functions for integrins alpha 3 beta 1 in focal adhesions and alpha 6 beta 4/bullous pemphigoid antigen in a new stable anchoring contact (SAC) of keratinocytes: relation to hemidesmosomes. *The Journal of Cell Biology*, 111(6 Part 2), 3141–3154. Available at: www.jcb.rupress.org, retrieved on 31 December 2011.

Chan, L.K.W. (2009) Current thoughts on angiogenesis. *Journal of Wound Care*, 18(1), 12–16.

Chambers, A.C., Leaper, D.J. (2011) Role of oxygen in wound healing: a review of evidence. *Journal of Wound Care*, 20(4), 160–164.

Chen, W.Y.J., Rogers, A.A., Lydon, M.J. (1992) Characterization of biologic properties of wound fluid collected during early stages of wound healing. *Journal of Investigative Dermatology*, 99(5), 559–564.

Clark, L.D., Clark, R.K., Heber-Katz, E. (1998) A new murine model for mammalian wound repair and regeneration. *Journal of Clinical Immunology and Immunopathology*, 88(1), 35–45.

Cooper, R., Okhiria, O. (2006) Biofilms, wound infection and the issue of control. *Wounds U.K.*, 2(3), 48–57.

Davis, P. (2008) The immunology of wound healing: the body as a battlefield. *Wounds U.K.*, 4(4), 54–69.

Desmouliere, A., Redard, M., Darby, I., Gabbiani, G. (1995) Apoptosis mediates the decrease in cellularity during the transition between granulation tissue and scar. *American Journal of Pathology*, 146(1), 56–66.

Diegelmann, R.F. (2003) Excessive neutrophils characterize chronic pressure ulcers. *Wound Repair and Regeneration*, 11(6), 490–495.

Diegelmann, R.F., Evans, M.C. (2004) Wound healing: an overview of acute, fibrotic and delayed healing. *Frontiers in Bioscience*, 9, 283–289.

Dowd, S.E., Sun, Y., Secor, P.R., et al. (2008) Survey of bacterial diversity in chronic wounds using pyrosequencing, DGGE, and full ribosome shotgun sequencing. *BMC Microbiol*, 8, 43.

Dovi, J.V., Szpaderska, A.M., DiPietro, L.A. (2004) Neutrophil function in the healing wound: adding insult to injury? *Journal of Thrombosis and Haemostasis*, 92, 275–280.

Dyson, M., Young, S., Pendle, C.L., Webster, D.F., Lang, S.M. (1988) Comparison of the effects of moist and dry conditions on dermal repair. *Journal of Investigative Dermatology*, 91(5), 434–439.

Ehrlich, H.P. (1988) Wound closure: evidence of cooperation between fibroblasts and collagen matrix. *Eye*, 2(2), 149–157.

Ehrlich, H.P., Desmouliere, A., Diegelmann, R.F., et al. (1994) Morphological and immunochemical differences between keloid and hypertrophic scar. *American Journal of Pathology*, 145(1), 105–113.

Enoch, S., Price, P. (2004) Should alternative endpoints be considered to evaluate outcomes in chronic recalcitrant wounds? *World Wide Wounds*. Available at: http://www.worldwidewounds.com/2004/october/Enoch-Part2/Alternative-Enpoints-To-Healing.html, retrieved on 4 April 2011.

Enoch, S., Leaper, D.J. (2005) Basic science of wound healing. *Surgery*, 23(2), 37–42.

Falanga, V. (2004) Wound bed preparation: science applied to practice. In: *Position Document Wound Bed Preparation in Practice*. London: European Wound Management Association (EWMA), MEP Ltd.

Ferguson, M.W.J., O'Kane, S. (2004) Scar-free healing: from embryonic mechanisms to adult therapeutic intervention. *Philosophical Transactions of the Royal Society London*, 359(1445), 839–850.

Franz, M.G., Robson, M.C., Steed, D.L., et al. (2008) Guidelines to aid healing of acute wounds by decreasing impediments of healing. *Wound Repair and Regeneration*, 16, 723–748.

Gethin, G. (2007) The significance of surface pH in chronic wounds. *Wounds U.K.*, 3(3), 52–56.

Gibson, D., Cullen, B., Legerstee, R., Harding, KG., Schults, G. (2009) MMPs made easy. *Wounds International* 1(1). Available at: www.woundsinternational.com, last accessed on 7 November 2012.

Gottrup, F. (1999) Wound closure techniques. *Journal of Wound Care*, 8(8), 397–400.

Gottrup, F. (2004) Oxygen in wound healing and infection. *World Journal of Surgery*, 28(3), 312–315.

Gottrup, F., Apelqvist, J., Price, P. (2010) Outcomes in controlled and comparative studies on non-healing wounds: recommendations to improve the quality of evidence in wound management. EWMA Document. *Journal of Wound Care*, 19(6), 239–268.

Greener, B., Hughes, A.A., Bannister, N.P., Douglass, J. (2005) Proteases and pH in chronic wounds. *Journal of Wound Care*, 14(2), 59–61.

Grey, J.E., Enoch, S., Harding, K.G. (2006) ABC of wound healing: wound assessment. *British Medical Journal*, 332, 285–288.

Grinnell, F. (1994) Mini-review on the cellular mechanisms of disease. Fibroblasts, myofibroblasts, and wound contraction. *The Journal of Cell Biology*, 124(4), 401–404. Available at: www.jcb.rupress.org, retrieved on 5 January 2012.

Gurtner, GC., Werner, S., Barrandon, Y., Longaker, MT. (2008) Wound repair and regeneration. *Nature*, 453, 314–321. Available at: http://www.nature.com/nature/journal/v453/n7193/full/nature07039.html, last accessed on 5 November 2012.

Harding, G.K., Morris, H.L., Patel, G.K. (2002) Science, medicine, and the future: healing chronic wounds. *British Medical Journal*, 324, 160–163.

Hart, J. (2002) Inflammation 1: its role in the healing of acute wounds. *Journal of Wound Care*, 11(6), 205–209.

James, G.A., Swogger, E., Wolcott, R., et al. (2008) Biofilms in chronic wounds. *Wound Repair and Regeneration*, 16(1), 37–44.

Kiecolt- Glaser, J.K., Marucha, P.T., Mercdo, A.M., Malarkey, W.B., Glaser, R. (1995) Slowing of wound healing by psychological stress. *The Lancet*, 346(8984), 1194–1196.

Knighton, D.R., Hunt, T.K., Scheuenstuhl, H., Halliday, B.J., Werb, Z., Banda, M.J. (1983) Oxygen tension regulates the expression of angiogenesis factor by macrophages. *Science*, 221(4617), 1283–1285.

Krawczyk, W.S. (1971) A pattern of epidermal cell migration during wound healing. *The Journal of Cell Biology*, 49, 247–263. Available at: www.jcb.rupress.org, retrieved on 20 December 2011.

Kunugiza, Y., Tomita, T., Moritomo, H., Yoshikawa, H. (2010) A hydrocellular foam dressing versus gauze: effects on the healing of rat excisional wounds. *Journal of Wound Care*, 19(1), 10–14.

Kumar, V., Abbas, A.K., Fausto, N., Aster, J. (2010) *Robbins and Cotran Pathologic Basis of Disease*, 8th edn. pp. 79–110. Philadelphia, PA: Saunders Elsevier.

Lazarus, G.S., Cooper, D.M., Knighton, D.R., et al. (1997) Definitions and guidelines for the assessment of wounds and evaluation of healing. *Archives of Dermatology*, 130, 489–493.

Lawrence, J.C. (1995) Moist wound healing: critique I. *Journal of Wound Care*, 4(8), 369–370.

Leaper, D., Harding, K. (2000) Factors affecting wound healing. In: *An Introduction to Wounds* (eds S. Bale, K. Harding, D. Leaper), pp. 15–22. London: Emap Healthcare Limited.

Li, J., Chen, J., Kirsner, R. (2007) Pathophysiology of acute wound healing. *Clinics in Dermatology*, 25, 9–18.

MacFie, C.C. Melling, A.C., Leaper, D.J. (2005) Effects of warming on healing. *Journal of Wound Care*, 14(3), 133–135.

Majno, G. (1975) *The Healing Hand, Man and Wound in the Ancient World*, pp. 2. Massachusetts: Harvard University Press.

Matsumoto, R., Sugimoto, M. (2007) Dermal matrix proteins initiate re-epithelialization but are not sufficient for coordinated epidermal outgrowth in a new fish skin culture model. *Cell and Tissue Research*, 327, 249–265.

McGuinness, W., Vella, E., Harrison, D. (2004) Influence of dressing changes on wound temperature. *Journal of Wound Care*, 13(9), 383–385.

Menon, G.K., Kligman, A.M. (2009) Barrier functions of human skin: a holistic view. *Skin Pharmacology and Physiology*, 22, 178–189.

Monaco, J.L., Lawrence, W.T. (2003) Acute wound healing an overview. *Clinics in Plastic Surgery*, 30, 1–12.

Moor, A.N., Vachon, D.J., Gouls, L.J. (2009) Proteolytic activity in wound fluids and tissues derived from chronic venous leg ulcers. *Wound Repair and Regeneration*, 17, 832–839.

Moore, K. (2003) Compromised wound healing: a scientific approach to treatment. *British Journal of Community Nursing*, 8(6), 274–278.

Moore, K. (2005) How much science do you need to know? *Wounds U.K.*, 1(3), 50–57.

Moore, K. (2010) Cell biology of normal and impaired healing. In: *Microbiology of Wounds* (eds S.L. Percival, K.F. Cutting), pp. 151–185. Boca Raton, FL: CRC Press.

Mustoe, T. A. (2008) Evolution of silicone therapy and mechanism of action in scar management. *Aesthetic Plastic Surgery*, 32, 82–92.

McGrath, A. (2011) Overcoming the challenge of granulation. *Wounds U.K.*, 7(1), 42–49.

Nelson, E.A. (1995) Moist wound healing: critique II. *Journal of Wound Care*, 4(8), 370–371.

Ng, M.F.Y. (2010) The role of mast cells in wound healing. *International Wound Journal*, 7(1), 55–61.

Odland, G., Ross, R. (1968) Human wound repair I. Epidermal regeneration. *The Journal of Cell Biology*, 39,

135–151. Available at: www.jcb.rupress.org, retrieved on 31 December 2011.

Olaso, E., Lin, H-C., Wang, L-H., Friedman, S.L. (2011) Impaired dermal wound healing in discoidin domain receptor 2-deficient mice associated with defective extracellular matrix remodeling. *Fibrogenesis & Tissue Repair*, 4(1), 5. Available at: http://www.fibrogenesis.com/content/4/1/5, last accessed on 8 November 2012.

Pellard, S. (2006) An overview of the two widely accepted, but contradictory, theories on wound contraction. *Journal of Wound Care*, 15(2), 90–92.

Percival, S.L., Cochrane, C.A. (2010) Wounds, enzymes and proteases. In: *Microbiology of Wounds* (eds S.L. Percival, K.F. Cutting), pp. 249–270. Boca Raton, FL: CRC Press.

Percival, S.L. (2011) Microbiology, biofilms: the future. Biofilms and their management: from concept to reality. *Journal of Wound Care*, 20(5), 220–230.

Pirila, E., Korpi, J.T., Korkiamaki, T., et al. (2007) Collagenase-2 (MMP-8) and matrilysin-2 (MMP-26) expression in human wounds of different etiologies. *Wound Repair and Regeneration*, 15, 47–57.

Porter, S. (2007) The role of the fibroblast in wound contraction and healing. *Wounds U.K.*, 3(1), 33–40.

Richardson, M. (2004) Acute wounds: an overview of the physiological healing process. *Nursing Times*, 100(Suppl. 4), 50–53.

Roseborough, I.E., Grevious, M.A., Lee, R.C. (2004) Prevention and treatment of excessive dermal scarring. *Journal of the National Medical Association*, 96(1), 108–116.

Ryan, G.B., Cliff, W.J., Gabbiani, G., et al. (1974) Myofibroblasts in human granulation tissue. *Human Pathology*, 5(1), 55–67.

Schreml, S., Szeimies, R.M., Karrer, S., Heinlin, J., Landthaler, M., Babilas, P. (2010) The impact of the pH value on skin integrity and cutaneous wound healing. *Journal of the European Academy of Dermatology and Venereology*, 24(4), 373–378. Epub 2009 Aug 23.

Schultz, G.S., Sibbald, R.G., Falanga, V., et al. (2003) Wound bed preparation: a systematic approach to wound management. *Wound Repair and Regeneration*, 11(2), S1–S28.

Schultz, G., Mozingo, D., Romanelli, M., Claxton, K. (2005a) Wound healing and TIME; new concepts and scientific applications. *Wound Repair and Regeneration*, 13(4), S1–S11.

Schultz, G.S., Ladwig, G., Wysocki, A. (2005b) Extracellular matrix: review of its roles in acute and chronic wounds. *World Wide Wounds*, Available at: http://www.worldwidewounds.com/2005/august/Schultz/Extrace-Matric-Acute-Chronic-Wounds.html, retrieved on 21 March 2011.

Schultz, G.S. (2007) The physiology of wound bed preparation. In: *Surgical Wound Healing and Management* (eds M.S. Granick, R.L. Gamelli), pp. 1–16. New York: Informa Healthcare.

Schultz, G.S., Davidson, J.M., Kirsner, R.S., Bornstein, P., Herman, I. (2011) Dynamic reciprocity in the wound microenvironment. *Wound Repair and Regeneration*, 19(2), 134–148.

Scott, E.M., Buckland, R. (2006) A systematic review of intraoperative warming to prevent postoperative complications. *AORN Journal*, 83(5), 1090–1104, 1107.

Shaw, T.J., Martin, P. (2009) Wound repair at a glance. *Journal of Cell Science*, 122(18), 3209–3213. Available at: http://jcs.biologists.org/cgi/content/full/122/18/3209, last accessed on 8 November 2012.

Silver, I.A. (1994) The physiology of wound healing. *Journal of Wound Care*, 3(2), 106–109.

Solowiej, K., Mason, V., Upton, D. (2009) Review of the relationship between stress and wound healing: part 1. *Journal of Wound Care*, 18(9), 357–366.

Stavrou, D., Haik, J., Weissman, O., Millet, E., Winkler, E. (2009) From traction and contraction to wound closure. *Journal of Wound Ostomy and Continence Nursing*, 36(4), 365–366.

Stechmiller, J.K. (2010) Understanding the role of nutrition and wound healing. *Nutrition in Clinical Practice*, 25(1), 61–68.

Sussman, C., Bates-Jensen, B.M. (2007) Wound healing physiology: acute and chronic. In: *Wound Care: A Collaborative Practice Manual for Health Professionals* (eds C. Sussman, B.M. Bates-Jensen), 3rd edn. pp. 21–50. Baltimore, MD: Lippincott Williams & Wilkins.

Tejero-Trujeque, R. (2001) How do fibroblasts interact with the extracellular matrix in wound contraction? *Journal of Wound Care*, 10(6), 237–242.

Teot, L. (2005) Scar evaluation and management: recommendations. *Journal of Tissue Viability*, 15(4), 6–14.

Tomasek, J.J., Gabbiani, G., Hinz, B., Chaponnier, C., Brown, R.A. (2002) Myofibroblasts and mechano-regulation of connective tissue remodeling. *Nature Reviews Molecular Cell Biology* 3(5), 349–363. doi:10.1038/nrm809, last accessed on 8 November 2012.

Thomson, C.H. (2011) Biofilms: do they affect wound healing? *International Wound Journal*, 8, 63–67.

Tortora, G.J., Derrickson, B.H. (2009) *Introduction to the Human Body: Essentials of Anatomy and Physiology*. 8th edn. Hoboken, NJ: John Wiley & Sons, Inc.

Trengove, N.J., Stacey, M.C., Macauley, S., et al. (1999) Analysis of the acute and chronic wound environments: the role of proteases and their inhibitors. *Wound Repair and Regeneration*, 7(6), 442–452.

Tsukada, K., Tokunaga, K., Iwama, T., Mishima, Y. (1992) The pH changes of pressure ulcers related to the healing process of wounds. *Wounds*, 4(1), 16–20.

Usui, M.L., Underwood, R.A., Mansbridge, J.N., Muffley, L.A., Carter, W.G., Olerud, J.E. (2005) Morphological evidence for the role of suprabasal keratinocytes in wound re-epithelialization. *Wound Repair and Regeneration*, 13(5), 468–479.

Ward, R.S. (2007) Management of scar. In: *Wound Care: A Collaborative Practice Manual for Health Professionals* (eds C. Sussman, B.M. Bates-Jensen), pp. 309–318. Baltimore, MD: Lippincott Williams & Wilkins.

Welt, K., Hinrichs, R., Weiss, J.M., Burgdorf, W., Krieg, Th., Scharffetter-Kochanek, K. (2009) Wound healing. In: *European Dermatology Forum White Book Skin Diseases in Europe* (ed P. Fritsch). *European Journal of Dermatology*, 19(4), 413–416. Available at: http://www.john-libbey-eurotext.fr/e-docs/00/04/4C/43/vers_alt/VersionPDF.pdf, last accessed on 28 October 2012.

Widgerow, A.D. (2010) Scar management – marrying the practical with the science. *Wound Healing Southern Africa*, 3(1), 7–10.

Widgerow, A.D., Leak, K. (2010) Hypergranulation tissue: evolution, control and potential elimination. *Wound Healing Southern Africa*, 3(2), 1–3.

Winter, G. (1962) Formation of the scab and the rate of epithelialisation of superficial wounds in the skin of the young domestic pig. *Nature*, 193, 293–294.

Wolcott, R.D., Rhoads, D.D., Dowd, S.E. (2008) Biofilms and chronic wound inflammation. *Journal of Wound Care*, 17(8), 333–341.

Wolcott, R.D., Kennedy, J.P., Dowd, S.E. (2009) Regular debridement is the main tool for maintaining a healthy wound bed in most chronic wounds. *Journal of Wound Care*, 18(2), 54–56.

Wolcott, R.D., Rhoads, D.D., Bennett, M.E., et al. (2010) Chronic wounds and the medical biofilm paradigm. *Journal of Wound Care*, 19(2), 45–53.

Woods, E.J., Davis, P., Barnett, J., Percival, S.L. (2010) Wound healing immunology and biofilms. In: *Microbiology of Wounds* (eds S.L. Percival, K.F Cutting), pp. 271–291. Boca Raton, FL: CRC Press.

Wysocki, A.B., Staiano-Coico, L., Grinnell, F. (1993) Wound fluid from chronic leg ulcers contains elevated levels of metalloproteinases MMP-2 and MMp-9. *Journal of Investigative Dermatology*, 101(1), 64–68.

Yager, D.R., Zhang, L.Y., Liang, H.X., Diegelmann, R.F., Cohen, I.K. (1996) Wound fluids from human pressure ulcers contain elevated matrix metalloproteinase levels and activity compared to surgical wound fluids. *Journal of Investigative Dermatology*, 107(5), 743–748.

Yager, D.R., Nwomeh, B.C. (1999) The proteolytic environment of chronic wounds. *Wound Repair and Regeneration*, 7, 433–441.

Zegers, M.M.P., Forget, M-A., Chernoff, J., Mostov, K.E., ter Beest, M.B.A., Hansen, S.H. (2003) Pak1 and PIX regulate contact inhibition during epithelial wound healing. *Journal of the European Molecular Biology Organization*, 22(16), 4155–4165.

4 Assessing Skin Integrity

Annemarie Brown[1] and Madeleine Flanagan[2]

[1] Tissue Viability Solutions, Essex, UK
[2] School of Life and Medical Sciences, University of Hertfordshire, Hertfordshire, UK

Overview

- Wound assessment is a complex process that helps to determine wound aetiology and the progress of healing over time.
- The patient consultation is the cornerstone of any assessment and is based on effective communication skills that elicit information about the patient's problem and allow the clinician to plan and make appropriate management decisions.
- Wound assessment has three important clinical components: diagnostic, monitoring and legislative.
- Precise wound area measurement can help predict healing rates of some chronic wounds and improve effectiveness of clinical decision-making.
- Wound measurement techniques are only approximate; the use of protocols in clinical practice could help minimise the margin of error.

Introduction

Skin damage is caused by a variety of factors which may result in a break in the surface of the skin, commonly referred to as a wound. Skin breakdown varies in severity, from imperceptible damage that may be invisible to the naked eye to extensive, life-threatening wounds. Assessing skin integrity is a complex, dynamic and continuous process which requires an understanding of the normal structure and function of the skin and underlying tissues and of the factors affecting tissue repair.

Wound assessment should identify potential barriers to healing, prioritise treatment objectives and enable the practitioner to consider possible treatment options, taking into account evidence-based efficacy, cost-effectiveness and availability of local resources (see Chapter 1).

The first step is to take a detailed patient history with examination, as this will provide information which helps determining the cause of skin breakdown and implementation of the most appropriate treatment strategy. There are many assessment frameworks available to guide practitioners through a problem-solving approach in a logical, concise way. This chapter offers a simple but

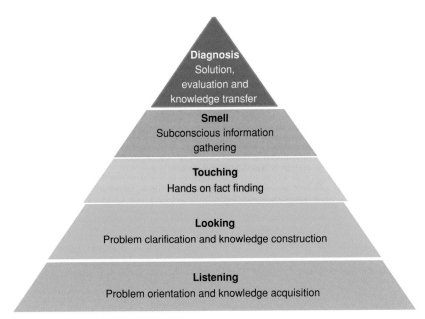

Figure 4.1   Hierarchical approach to skin assessment.

comprehensive approach to assessing skin integrity based on an existing problem-solving model utilising four of the five human senses as seen in Figure 4.1 (Finch, 2003; Salcido, 2005; Cook, 2011).

Assessing skin integrity

A detailed skin and wound assessment is of critical importance to help identify the patient's general physical condition and factors responsible for skin integrity problems so that an appropriate management plan based on these can be implemented.

The key principles of skin integrity assessment are as follows (Naylor, 2002):

- identify cause of skin breakdown;
- identify associated risk factors;
- correct or treat the underlying cause where possible;
- identify appropriate management options;
- control wound-related symptoms;
- prevent further skin/wound deterioration;
- identify patient's expectations and goals of treatment;
- focus on enhancing quality of life if cure is not possible;
- provide psychosocial support;
- promote patient independence.

At initial consultation, a head-to-toe skin assessment should be performed, as it may provide important clues to diagnosis and management of the existing problem. If the practitioner performing the assessment does not have a diagnostic responsibility, then their role is to provide accurate information to assist colleagues who do make appropriate management decisions.

Listening: problem orientation and knowledge

At initial assessment, it is important to gather information about the patient's skin integrity problem by carefully asking the right questions and listening to the patient. Gathering a reliable history is achieved by allowing the patient to tell their story, as this optimises the chance of establishing an accurate history of the presenting problem. An experienced practitioner is able to guide the patient or their carer to provide key information to help determine the cause of the wound or skin problem. A framework of questions to enable clinicians to initiate the consultation and elicit a focused patient history is suggested in Table 4.1. Additional questions may be added, depending on the type of wound or skin condition.

Table 4.1   Prompts to establish a reliable patient history

Prompt	Rationale
What is the problem with your wound or skin and what help do you need?	• Establishes starting point for examination/assessment • Gain understanding of patient's concerns • Identifies patient's expectations
Where is the wound or skin damage?	• Location helps establish diagnosis, e.g. possible pressure damage, leg ulceration, lacerations, stasis eczema • Provides information for treatment
How long have you had the wound or skin damage?	• Duration may be an important indicator of healing potential (Schultz et al., 2005) • Helps to determine wound chronicity
What caused the wound?	• The patient may not always know how the wound initially occurred especially in chronic wounds.
How is your general health?	• Enables identification of potential barriers to healing, e.g. diabetes, peripheral vascular disease, cancer treatment, anaemia, inflammatory or autoimmune diseases
What medications do you take?	• Identifies medications which may adversely affect wound healing, e.g. corticosteroids, chemotherapy, amlodipine, warfarin • Also consider the use of over-the-counter or traditional remedies • Consider potential effect on healing
Tell me about your lifestyle?	• Explore relevant social/environmental and personal factors that may affect healing such as home environment, mobility, family support, occupation, financial status • Identify any negative lifestyle choices – alcohol, tobacco or drug usage, poor nutrition
What makes the wound or your skin better?	• Identify interventions or actions that improve the wound or skin, e.g. resting, using emollients, changing dressings daily • Patients' coping strategies may give further clues as to the cause of skin breakdown, e.g. sitting upright in a chair at night to reduce pain in arterial leg ulceration
What makes the wound or your skin worse?	• Establish any factors which aggravate the wound or skin, causing deterioration.
What is your wound or skin like when it is worse?	• Description of deterioration may help • Note any allergies/skin reactions to topical preparations, dressings, bandages, etc.
Have you had any previous treatment for your wound or skin?	• Establish successful/unsuccessful treatment modalities – these will influence any future treatment plans • Identify what has helped and what has not • Identify patient's likes/dislikes
Is your wound or skin painful?	• Pain descriptors may indicate factors related to wound aetiology, e.g. neuropathic pain is often described as 'sharp shooting pain' (Bunn and Griffiths, 2011)
What is the worst thing about your wound or skin?	• Helps prioritise patient's treatment objectives • Identifies patient's expectations of treatment
How does your wound or skin affect you every day?	• Demonstrates impact on quality of life, self-esteem, occupation • Begins to explore patient's health beliefs

The listening element of the information-gathering process is essential to explore the patient's perspective of the skin/wound problem and assess his or her expectations before moving onto the medical aspect of the consultation. The use of open-ended questions, appropriate verbal prompts and following patients' cues will help the clinician gain insight into the patient's concerns and start to build trust and develop a relationship with the patient before moving onto the physical examination (Kurtz et al., 2005).

History-taking provides a formal structure and leads the clinician onto the physical examination element of the consultation. Effective assessment documentation should be structured to reflect the logical flow of history-taking. A good example of a structured model for a patient consultation is the Calgary-Cambridge Guide to the Medical

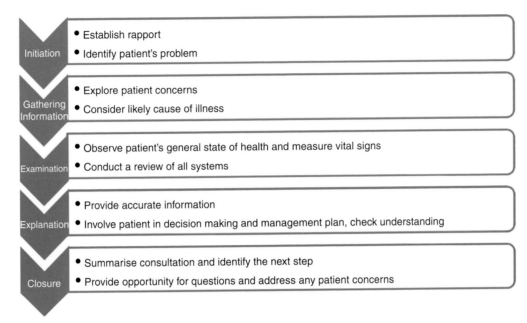

Figure 4.2   Structured patient consultation following the Calgary-Cambridge model. Adapted from Kurtz et al. (2005).

Interview (Kurtz et al., 2005), which clearly demonstrates the interrelationship between the communication process and the physical assessment content of a consultation (Figure 4.2). The five elements of the consultation – understanding the patient's perspective, building a relationship and developing rapport, explaining and planning, and closing the session – provides organisational structure to the consultation using an informal, person-centred approach.

Looking: problem clarification and knowledge construction

Before focusing on the skin integrity issue or wound, it is important to assess the patient's general appearance, including the overall skin condition as this often reflects health status, e.g. looking flushed or pale. Table 4.2 identifies general factors that should be taken into account when assessing a patient.

Once the clinician has conducted this preliminary assessment of the patient, a more detailed examination of the general skin condition should be undertaken. This will involve asking the patient to remove their clothing, where appropriate, so that examination of the skin can be undertaken. This should be performed in a calm, private, warm and well-lit (natural light) environment, ensuring that the patient's dignity is maintained at all times. The following should be noted and carefully recorded on a body plan using the appropriate terminology:

- areas of dry or scaly skin;
- trauma: bruising, petechiae, haemorrhage, skin tears;
- skin colour/pigmentation: jaundice, lipodermatosclerosis;
- oedema: pitting/non-pitting, leakage, location;
- rashes: distribution, characteristics;
- skin perfusion: mottled, pale, shiny, hairless skin, missing digits;
- skin breaks: excoriation, trauma, maceration;
- skin lesions: distribution, character, shape;
- wounds: size, location, duration;
- skin infections: signs/symptoms – bacterial, fungal infections;
- scarring: appearance, quality, hypertrophic, keloid

It is important to use the correct terminology to avoid confusion, particularly when other health professionals are to be involved in the patient's management. Abbreviations and acronyms should also be avoided in documentation, since these may

Table 4.2   Factors to consider when conducting a general patient examination

Considerations	Rationale
General demeanour	• Determine if patient is anxious, confused, depressed or in pain • Good interpersonal and communication skills will elicit why the patient feels this way • Establish source of pain, consider use of pain scales, if appropriate
Age of patient	• Helps to establish likely origin of wound or skin condition • May influence treatment choice • May affect patient concordance
Illness status	• Determine if the patient has any concurrent illness or co-morbidities • Helps determine if patient is immune-compromised, which may delay healing
Mobility	• Level of mobility may influence treatment decisions, e.g. compression systems • Restricted mobility is a risk factor for pressure damage and has a negative outcome on the healing of venous leg ulcers (Franks et al., 1995)
Body weight	• Consider nutritional assessment for patients with extremes of body weight, as this may affect healing • High body weight – consider need for specialist equipment and increased risk of complications, e.g. wound dehiscence • Low body weight – consider increased risk of pressure damage • Identify any manual-handling issues

be misinterpreted if they are not universally recognised.

Developing astute observation skills helps in eliciting additional valuable information from the assessment process to assist diagnosis. However, it is also necessary to examine the skin by touching, to gather additional information about its condition (Lawton, 2001).

Practice point

How to assess pigmented skin

It is important that clinicians are able to recognise early skin damage in patients with pigmented skin to diagnose and treat them effectively. Often, lesions which in Caucasian skin appear red or brown will appear black or purple in pigmented skin, and mild erythema may be masked completely (Bryant and Nix, 2011). The localised area of skin damage may be purplish or bluish (eggplant colour) which is comparable to the erythema or redness seen in persons with lighter skin tones (Bennett, 1995). The general principle is that tissue damage will cause localised skin colour changes which differ from the patient's usual skin colour.

Local inflammation commonly leads to pigmentary skin changes which may be either lighter or darker (depending on the individual), and which may persist for a long time after the initial dermatosis has resolved. Pigmented skin shows more of a pigmentary reaction following trauma or inflammation than non-pigmented or lightly pigmented skin (Bryant and Nix, 2011). Consequently, postinflammatory hyperpigmentation and hypopigmenta-

tion pose particular problems for black patients. In inflammatory skin diseases such as atopic eczema, acne vulgaris and lichen planus, postinflammatory hyperpigmentation can persist well after the active disease process has subsided and sometimes indefinitely. Hypopigmentation may also be seen with pityriasis alba, sarcoidosis, leprosy, pityriasis versicolor and may also occur as a result of damage caused by eczema, herpes zoster, cryotherapy and the use of topical steroids.

Touch: hands on fact finding

The use of touch enables the clinician to elicit information that may not always be visually obvious. Physical examination is often neglected to the detriment of a thorough skin assessment. Factors such as skin texture, moisture and temperature can yield important information on which to base a diagnosis, e.g. localised heat may indicate inflammation, induration or infection, and may be the first sign of category 1 pressure damage (nonblanchable erythema) (Bryant and Nix, 2011).

Damaged, intact skin may feel warm when touched due to localised heat (from the inflammatory process) when compared with surrounding skin (Bennett, 1995). Localised oedema may also be felt as induration immediately surrounding the damaged area. The skin looks taut and shiny and may be broken or intact. As tissue becomes

Table 4.3   Information gained from touching the skin

Skin texture	• Induration in the gaiter area of the lower limb may indicate venous disease • Roughness – xerotic skin may be rough and scaly and may be the result of medication or chronic illness • Consistency of tissue, e.g. firm, boggy, normal
Dry skin	• Pathological dry skin. Dry skin is a normal consequence of ageing but may indicate dehydration, malnutrition, eczema, renal failure, liver disease, anaemia, diabetes
Wet, macerated skin	• High moisture levels may cause moisture lesions and fungal nail infections as a result of incontinence, sweat, wound exudate • Presence of moisture may indicate lymphorrhoea as a result of untreated lymphoedema • Fluid loss due to cellulitis, dependency oedema, large exudating wounds sinus or fistula
Oedema	• Pitting/non-pitting, location • 'Spongy', water-logged tissues (fluctuance)
Temperature (warm)	• Reactive hyperaemia • Inflammation – acute lipodermatosclerosis • May indicate category 1 pressure damage – non-blanchable erythema • Presence of infection, e.g. cellulitis, surgical infection, abscess
Temperature (cool)	• Occluded/decreased arterial supply • Indicator of deep tissue pressure damage as tissue death occurs
Pain	• Elevated pain levels may indicate inflammation localised infection or ischemia
Skin sensitivity	• Abnormal sensations on being touched, such as increased levels of pain, numbness or burning (dysaesthesia), or tingling, feeling of electric shock and stabbing (paraesthesia) are associated with sensory neuropathy (Jensen and Baron, 2003)

devitalised the skin may feel cooler to touch when fingers or the back of the hand is used (Bryant and Nix, 2011).

Reactive hyperaemia occurs when there is a transient increase in organ blood flow following a brief period of ischaemia. This may occur following repeated brachial blood pressure readings on the same arm, or when the patient is repositioned following a period of unrelieved pressure. The area will be red and warm to touch initially but will blanch on digital pressure, indicating that the microcirculation is still intact. Erythema may be difficult to observe in darkly pigmented skin and is more easily felt. Table 4.3 identifies information that can be elicited by touching the patient's skin.

Practitioners should also be aware of and document the presence of hyperalgesia, which is an increased sensitivity to pain. Patients may exhibit an increased level of pain when touched in the area of damaged tissue (primary hyperalgesia) or in the surrounding undamaged tissue (secondary hyperalgesia). This may occur in patients with painful chronic conditions and can be associated with long-term opioid use (Chu et al., 2008).

Abnormal sensations on being touched, such as increased levels of pain, numbness or burning (dysaesthesia), or tingling, feelings of electric shock and stabbing (paraesthesia) are associated with sensory neuropathy (Jensen and Baron, 2003) and can be a consequence of many conditions, including herpes zoster and diabetes. Patients with diabetes may suffer from peripheral neuropathy with extreme sensitivity to the lightest touch – for example, the weight of a sheet can be agonizing. On the other hand, numbness or reduced ability to feel pain or change in temperature especially in their feet or toes may lead to muscle weakness, difficulty in walking and serious foot problems, such as ulcers, infections and deformities of the toes/feet (Jensen and Baron, 2003). Gloves should not be worn by practitioners during a skin assessment, as they diminish sensitivity to changes in skin temperature, although meticulous attention should be paid to hand hygiene to avoid cross infection.

Smell: subconscious information gathering

The final human sense that practitioners use subconsciously when assessing a patient is smell. This sense is undervalued during assessment and can provide useful information about the condition of the skin and hygiene status but must be used sensitively as odour is associated with social stigma and causes embarrassment. Smell affects how patients relate to their loved ones and caregivers and can disturb sleep, cause loss of appetite and social isolation.

Skin may produce an unpleasant or distinctive odour for the following reasons:

- *Poor personal hygiene*: can result in skin breakdown, intertrigo due to fungal infections caused by *Candida albicans* in skin folds, e.g. under breasts and in the toe webs.
- *Urine*: a distinctive odour is produced if urine is not cleaned from the skin or left soaked into bandages due to the breakdown of ketones, nitrates and phosphates.
- *Faeces*: sacral wounds and fistulae are particularly susceptible to faecal contamination. The distinctive malodour is produced by skatole (a 3-methylindole crystalline compound) and is designed to repel humans and prevent ingestion (Suarez et al., 1998).
- *Wound infection*: may cause unpleasant odour caused by multiplication of aerobic bacteria such as *Pseudomonas aeruginosa* which is associated with a distinctive sweet, rancid smell produced by a combination of volatile compounds including hydrogen cyanide gas.
- *Exudating wounds*: chronic wounds such as pressure ulcers, diabetic foot ulcers and venous leg ulcers often have a characteristic smell due to a combination of factors including build-up of chronic wound fluid, high bacterial load and presence of devitalised tissue.
- *Necrotic tissue or slough*: in wounds may produce a distinctive odour due to tissue breakdown and colonisation with anaerobic bacteria that produce unstable sulphur compounds and short-chain fatty acids as metabolic end products.
- *Malignant wounds*: are often malodourous due to the presence of putrescine and cadaverine which are volatile fatty acids released as the tumour erodes surrounding tissue (Haughton and Young, 2003; Piggin and Jones, 2007).

Wound odour may be pungent, sweet, musty or faecal depending on the cause. The presence, type and possible cause of the odour must be documented; however, clinicians must be mindful that patients might request to see these records and documentation must be factual and objective.

Assessing wounds

Inexperienced practitioners tend to focus on wound and skin integrity problems in isolation, and fail to consider skin integrity in the wider context of the patient's general condition. As a consequence, meaningful information may be lost. The frameworks above will enable the clinician to assess the wound in the context of the whole person, resulting in an individualised, meaningful and comprehensive assessment. Failure to take an appropriate history and detailed examination may result in valuable information being missed. The Wound Bed Preparation section will discuss the assessment of the wound or skin integrity problem, utilising all four senses previously discussed. Table 4.4 lists the important wound characteristics and the rationale for assessment.

Wound bed preparation

There are several systematic frameworks available to help clinicians conduct a formal structured assessment of a wound to develop an individualised management plan. One of the most popular of these is wound bed preparation (WBP) (Sibbald et al., 2000). WBP was introduced in 2000 and has gained international recognition as a conceptual framework for managing chronic wounds, based on the wound healing processes at cellular level (Sibbald et al., 2000; Moffatt et al., 2004; Sibbald et al., 2007). Schultz and colleagues developed the four core elements of WBP which were later summarised as the acronym TIME to facilitate understanding of the pathogenesis of chronic wounds and to act as a practical decision-making tool to optimise wound care practice (Falanga, 2004; Dowsett, 2009):

T: tissue, non-viable or deficient;
I: inflammation and infection;
M: moisture balance;
E: epithelial (edge) advancement.

The basis of the WBP assessment framework is that each individual component of the TIME model should be considered when assessing wounds and that a systematic plan of care be developed based on findings. This allows clinicians to prioritise and

Table 4.4   Wound characteristics and rationale for assessment

Wound characteristic	Rationale
Duration	• Indicates chronic/acute wound • 4 wk duration may be indicative of stalled healing (Schultz et al., 2003) • May highlight psychological and social issues
Previous treatments	• May indicate appropriate or inappropriate management • Dressings or alternative therapies used • Indicates patient preference/adherence
Location	• May indicate type of wound, e.g. pressure damage, venous leg ulcer • Will influence dressing choice, fixation problems, cosmetic appearance
Size, depth and shape	• Selection of appropriate dressing size and shape to fit wound • Monitor improvement or deterioration of wound in response to treatment
Type of tissue present	• Will indicate phase of wound healing • Will help determine treatment aims • Will influence dressing choice
Amount and type of exudate	• May indicate infection/bleeding • Amount of exudate will decrease as healing occurs; increased levels may indicate infection • Malodour may indicate infection/presence of necrotic tissue
Peri-wound or surrounding skin	• Maceration/excoriation will indicate high wound exudate levels and inadequate fluid-handling properties of dressings. • Skin texture may indicate aetiology of wound, e.g. hyperkeratosis in venous hypertension
Wound edges	• May indicate signs of epithelialisation • Rolled edges may indicate epibole • Can help to differentiate between different types of leg ulceration aetiology

Source: Courtesy of Wayne Naylor.

implement interventions aimed at minimising barriers to healing found within the chronic wound (Figure 4.3).

The original WBP model placed the emphasis on the physiological and molecular barriers to healing at an advanced level. This led to criticism by some (Schultz et al., 2004; WUWHS, 2008; Mulder, 2009) since inexperienced practitioners may have a tendency to focus on the wound in isolation, losing the broader contextual information gained from a general patient assessment. The importance of addressing patient-centred factors such as concordance, lifestyle factors and psychosocial needs was later incorporated into the model (Inlow et al., 2000; Falanga, 2004; Harding et al., 2008; Dowsett, 2009).

It must also be remembered that the WBP was developed primarily for nonhealing, chronic wounds and is not always appropriate for all wound types, for example, for traumatic, or surgical wounds, and for wounds where active intervention may not be appropriate, such as uncomplicated venous ulcers (Moffatt et al., 2004) and diabetic neuroischaemic foot wounds (Edmonds et al., 2004).

Despite these criticisms, the benefits of implementing WBP as a decision-making framework have helped clinicians around the world make more effective clinical decisions, based on assessment of local conditions at the wound bed. The WBP framework is now widely acknowledged to help rationalise implementation of advanced treatment modalities and monitor progression to healing (Moffatt et al., 2004; Dowsett and Newton, 2005; Mulder, 2009; Ousey and McIntosh, 2010). In addition, it has been used successfully to underpin teaching intervention designed to increase nurses' wound care knowledge (Dowsett, 2009).

However, some authors believe that formal wound assessment tools such as WBP are not effectively used in clinical practice as some clinicians fail to see the link between wound assessment and the selection of appropriate dressing products (Cook, 2011). Cook (2011) conducted a survey into competency and current practice in wound assessment

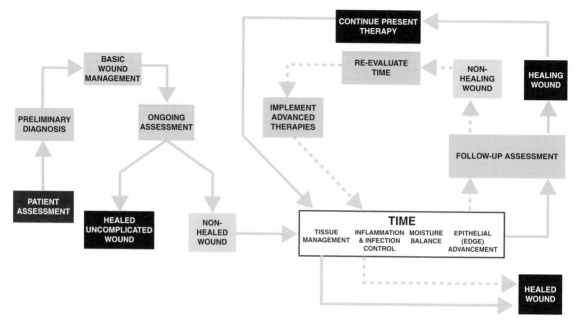

Figure 4.3   Wound bed preparation. From Falanga (2004).

and found that 73% of wound care practitioners did not use any type of assessment tool to aid wound assessment as they found concepts such as WBP difficult to interpret and implement in everyday practice situations.

The need for a standardised wound assessment form has now been recognised and is currently under development (Watret, 2005; Fletcher, 2007; Fletcher, 2010). It is hoped that adoption of this form might help to ensure that adequate data are collected across both primary and secondary healthcare settings to plan appropriate patient care and allow for audit of patient outcomes in the future. A copy of the assessment form can be downloaded from the link given in Useful Resources section at the end of this chapter.

Data collection

The ideal data collection form should allow for the gathering of both qualitative and quantitative information. Qualitative information includes the assessment of the patient's general health and appearance, skin quality, documentation of the wound characteristics or skin integrity problem, including treatment aims and evaluation of interventions, together with a record of any patient-centred concerns.

Quantitative information includes information gathered from risk assessment tools, such as pressure ulcer risk assessment, pain assessment, nutritional status and manual handling, together with the results of specific diagnostic tests, e.g. Doppler results, 10-g monofilament tests. Wound measurements or photography should also be recorded and plotted to assess healing or wound deterioration. Any physiological data, such as blood pressure readings, urinalysis, swab results and blood test results should be recorded on the initial assessment form.

Investigations

Depending on the clinical setting and the type of wound or skin integrity problem, additional investigations may be appropriate. These include routine blood tests such as full blood count, urea and electrolytes, and haemoglobin levels, together with additional tests such as C-reactive protein levels (CRP) and erythrocyte sedimentation rate (ESR), to identify inflammation. Routine tests such as blood pressure, pulse and blood glucose levels will also aid diagnosis. When signs of clinical infection are present, wound swabs for culture and sensitivity should be taken, and actions taken on positive results be recorded. Specific investigations such as Doppler ultrasound or sonography are required to assess particular wound aetiologies and will be discussed in the relevant chapters.

Wound measurement

Wound measurement is an important component of wound assessment and has the potential to provide baseline measurements and monitor healing rates to predict treatment outcomes. Apart from as an outcome measure of clinical trials or within specialist centres, wound measurements over time are not normally documented in everyday clinical practice due to lack of time and resources.

Small changes in wound size are not always visible to the naked eye but there is good evidence that a reduction of 20–40% in wound area after 2–4 weeks of treatment is a reliable predictor of healing at 12 weeks in venous leg ulcers (Kantor and Margolis, 2000), and that a wound area reduction of >50%

by 4 weeks is predictive of healing in diabetic foot ulcers (Sheehan et al., 2003; Lavery et al., 2008; Snyder et al., 2010). This evidence supports the value of regular measurement of wound circumference during the first few weeks of treatment to determine if the wound is responding. However, this is difficult to achieve in clinical practice as wound measurement methods are not standardised, there is no consensus on which wound-healing parameters are the most reliable (Mani, 1999; Schultz et al., 2005) and healing rates vary between different wound aetiologies (Kantor and Margolis, 2000; Phillips, et al., 2000; Keast and Cranney, 2004). Clinicians in some specialised centres record wound measurements over time to plot wound-healing curves and find this a useful visual method of monitoring the healing trajectory of indolent wounds (Figure 4.4). If adopted more widely in other clinical settings, this practice could help justify the use of advanced treatment modalities.

Measurement of wound dimensions is a fundamental element of wound assessment but it

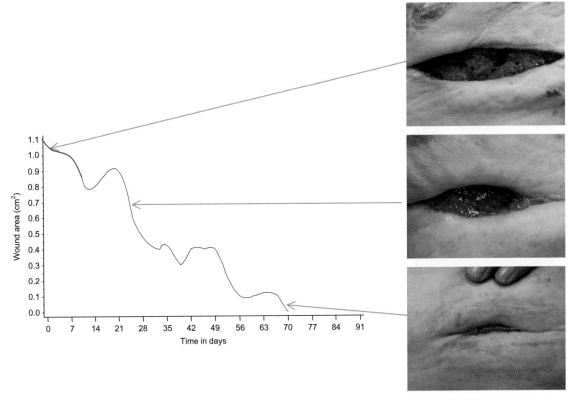

Figure 4.4 Wound healing curve showing decreasing wound measurements as healing occurs in a surgical wound. Photos courtesy of Nuno Cunha.

is not accurate. Length multiplied by width as an isolated measurement falls short of the precision required when monitoring wound progress as wounds change shape over time. These measurements are not representative of overall wound size, as the area of the wound could remain static whilst overall dimensions could change. Length multiplied by width as a method of estimating area is inaccurate especially with irregular-shaped wounds because area is generally overestimated and as such diameter product measurements are only useful as a crude visual indicator of wound dimension (Flanagan, 2003).

It is acknowledged that counting the number of grid squares covering the wound is a time-consuming approximation of surface area which does not facilitate clinical decision-making. Many different procedures have been recommended to improve accuracy of diameter product measurements but precision has not been effectively demonstrated in clinical practice. Measurements of wounds performed on digital photographs using planimetry software have been shown to be more accurate than diameter product measurements, and are simple and convenient (Thawer et al., 2002; Wendelken et al., 2011).

> **Practice point**
>
> The accuracy of measuring wound dimensions, length and width tracings can be improved by implementing the following steps:
>
> - A fine-tip permanent black pen should be used as it can be easy to misinterpret the wound edge when using a thick-tipped pen.
> - Leaning too heavily on the wound margin can distort the wound shape and should be avoided.
> - Ensure, when possible, that the patient is in the same position each time the wound is measured or photographed.
> - Date and label each wound surface area tracing, for records in the patient's notes.

For any measurement to be of value, it must be capable of comparison with other measurements. This can only happen if measurements are made under the same conditions using exactly the same procedures which is challenging in clinical practice. The specification of simple wound measurement protocols could do much to improve accuracy of this aspect of wound assessment.

A protocol should define how to measure the:

- wound margin;
- total wound area;
- areas of tissue type within the wound bed expressed as percentage of total wound area;
- frequency of measurement as a percentage of area reduction in the first 2–4 weeks.

The progress of wound healing should be monitored and treatment aims be evaluated every 2–4 weeks.

Wound photography

Digital photography is a quick, easy and relatively inexpensive method of documenting wound and skin integrity problems and provides visual evidence of skin damage, regardless of whether the epidermis is intact or not, e.g. in bruising, erythema. A series of photographs can help to monitor the progress of healing and can be a useful educational tool. Photography should never be used in isolation from other methods of assessment, as colour reproduction may not be accurate. Always adhere to local policy for information relating to consent, documentation and storage of images.

> **Practice point**
>
> **How can one improve the quality of photographs taken for wound assessment purpose?**
>
> *Consent and documentation*:
>
> - Obtain written consent for each photo and specify if the image is to be used for publication or teaching.
> - Do not assume consent has been given. If patient is unable to give consent, seek advice and follow local protocol.
> - Never photograph patient's face or any other distinguishing features.
>
> *Image quality*:
>
> - Position patient consistently for each photo; ensure patient safety.
> - Do not clean wound before taking photograph.
> - Include a disposable ruler with date, length/width/depth in each photo.
> - Use natural light when possible and try not to use flash facility.
> - Take photograph from a distance of approximately 1 m, or closer if zoom facility used.

- Take the photo from the same angle every time.
- Point camera perpendicular to the wound.
- Avoid blurring by steadying the camera by standing firmly with feet shoulder distance apart and tuck elbows in to avoid shaking.
- Showcase the wound on a solid plain background.
- Avoid clutter in the background.
- If possible, ensure hands are not visible in the photograph.

Frequency:

- Take three photos per wound on each occasion and review.
- Re-take photo if necessary.
- One photo at initial consultation, then weekly thereafter, until wound closure.

Storage:

- As soon as possible, transfer image to a secure, password-protected computer.
- Save as a JPEG file, and record patient's initials and date.
- Do not attempt to manipulate or change the image in any way.
- Store image in patient's medical records in accordance with local protocol.

Effective documentation

Wound assessment is a complex activity that requires collation of much clinical data. Documentation should be user-friendly, concise, comprehensive, and able to withstand legal scrutiny and assist practitioners to make informed treatment choices based on the data collected (Culley, 2001). There is some evidence that well-designed wound assessment forms act as an *aide-memoire* providing cues for clinicians to gather relevant information and provide a structured, systematic approach to assessment (Sterling, 1996). Furthermore, a well-designed assessment form will include prompts to assist clinicians identify barriers to healing (Maylor, 2003).

Accurate documentation is becoming increasingly important in the litigious environment that most health professionals practice in. Clinical negligence cases involving mismanagement of wounds have in recent years resulted in an explosion of legal claims for compensation globally. The simple fact is that determining liability in negligence is dependent upon factual and concise documentation of wound assessment and treatment evaluation.

When to seek specialist help?

Following wound assessment, practitioners sometimes lack confidence in their diagnostic skills or may seek confirmation of the likely cause of skin breakdown. The following criteria indicate when specialist help should be sought:

- wounds of unknown cause – diagnostic uncertainty always requires further investigation before appropriate treatment can be implemented;
- patients with complex co-morbidities, e.g. diabetes, renal failure, rheumatoid arthritis, should be monitored by an appropriately trained specialist;
- wounds that are static or not responding to standard treatment after 4 weeks should be referred for a case review;
- wounds that are rapidly deteriorating are most likely to be due to ischaemia or infection, and should be immediately referred to an appropriately trained specialist;
- unusual lesions or suspicious areas of exuberant granulation tissue which do not respond to treatment should be referred to a dermatologist;
- unconfirmed sinuses/fistulae where the endpoint cannot be determined may need exploration or sinography performed. Referral to a surgical team is necessary
- clinical suspicion of factitious wounds (self-harm) should be referred to the psychiatric team.

This list is not exhaustive, and clinicians should refer to local referral policies for specific guidance. Clinical experience around the world demonstrates that effective wound care cannot ever be managed by one professional group in isolation and benefits from a multidisciplinary team approach. Good communication facilitated by effective reporting mechanisms with organisational support will ensure that patients have access to appropriate specialist skills if required in achieve healing.

Summary

Wound assessment is not always performed as regularly or as accurately as it should be, and can become a routine task. This chapter has highlighted the importance of adopting a structured approach to the assessment of skin breakdown and wounds based on four of the human senses using a problem-solving approach. Practitioners may be tempted to focus on wound and skin integrity problems in isolation, however, by taking a step back and systematically assessing the patient from head to toe, valuable additional information could be gathered, ensuring that the correct assessment is made and timely and appropriate intervention implemented to achieve wound healing.

Development of new therapeutic techniques to measure other parameters of wound healing such as temperature, pH and protease levels currently exist but are not yet widely available. These techniques are already providing additional methods of monitoring progress to healing but are still in their infancy.

Accurate wound assessment ensures that patients receive the most appropriate treatment as soon as possible; that clinicians have confidence that barriers to healing have been identified and progress to healing is being monitored; and that healthcare organisations are assured that governance requirements have been met.

Useful resources

Development of a new wound assessment form. Available at: http://www.wounds-uk.com/pdf/content_9344.pdf

References

Bennett, A.M. (1995) Report of the task force on the implications for darkly pigmented intact skin in the prediction and prevention of pressure ulcers. *Advances in Wound Care: The Journal for Prevention and Healing*, 8(6), 34–35.

Bryant, R., Nix, D. (2011) Developing and maintaining a pressure ulcer program. In: *Acute and Chronic Wounds: Current Management Concepts* (eds R. Bryant, D. Nix), 4th edn. St. Louis, MO: Mosby.

Bunn, R., Griffiths, M. (2011) Understanding breakthrough pain. *Journal of Community Nursing*, 25(3), 24–29.

Chu, L.F., Angst, M.S., Clark, D. (2008) Opioid-induced hyperalgesia in humans: molecular mechanisms and clinical considerations. *Clinical Journal of Pain*, 24(6), 479–496.

Cook, L. (2011) Wound assessment: exploring competency and current practice. *British Journal of Community Nursing*, 16(12 Suppl.), S34–S40.

Culley, F. (2001) The tissue viability nurse and effective documentation. *British Journal of Nursing*, 10(15 Suppl.), S30–S39.

Dowsett, C. (2009) Use of TIME to improve community nurses' wound care knowledge and practice. *Wounds UK*, 5(3), 14–21.

Dowsett, C., Newton, H. (2005) Wound bed preparation: TIME in practice. *Wounds UK*, 1(3), 58–70.

Edmonds, M., Foster, A.V.M., Vowden, P. (2004) Wound bed preparation for diabetic foot ulcers. *Position Document: Wound Bed Preparation in Practice*. London: MEP Ltd.

Falanga, V. (2004) Wound bed preparation: science applied to practice. *Position Document: Wound Bed Preparation in Practice*. London: MEP Ltd.

Finch, M. (2003) Assessing of skin in older people. *Nursing Older People*, 15(2), 29–30.

Flanagan, M. (2003) Wound measurement: can it help us to monitor progression to healing? *Journal of Wound Care*, 12(5), 189–194.

Fletcher, J. (2007) Wound assessment and the TIME framework. *British Journal of Community Nursing*, 16(8), 462–466.

Fletcher J. (2010) Development of a new wound assessment form. *Wounds UK*, 6(1), 92–99.

Franks, P.J., Moffatt, C.J., Connolly, M., et al. (1995) Factors associated with healing leg ulcers with high compression. *Age and Ageing*, 24(5), 407–410.

Harding, K.G., Chadwick, P., Dowsett, C., Findlay, S., Fletcher, J., Gethin, G. (2008) *Best Practice Statement Optimising Wound Care*. Aberdeen: Wounds UK.

Haughton, W., Young, T. (2003) Common problems in wound care: malodorous wounds. *British Journal of Nursing*, 4(16), 959–963.

Inlow, S., Orsted, H., Sibbald, R.G. (2000) Best practices for the prevention, diagnosis and treatment of diabetic foot ulcers. *Ostomy Wound Management*, 46, 55–68.

Jensen, T.S., Baron, R. (2003) Translation of symptoms and signs into mechanisms in neuropathic pain. *Pain*, 102, 1–8.

Kantor, J., Margolis, D.J. (2000) A multicentre study of percentage change in venous leg ulcer area as a prognostic index of healing at 24 weeks. *British Journal of Dermatology*, 142, 960–964.

Keast, D.H., Cranney, G. (2003) Does wound surface area as measured by length and width reflect true area: analysis of a wound data base. In: *Paper given at Ninth Annual Conference, Canadian Association of Wound Care*, Toronto, Canada, 6–9 November.

Kurtz, S., Silverman, J., Draper, J. (2005) *Teaching and Learning Communication Skills in Medicine*, 2nd edn, Oxford: Radcliffe Publishing.

Lavery, L., Seaman, J.W., Barnes, S.A., Armstrong, D.G., Keith, M.S. (2008) Prediction of healing for postoperative diabetic foot wounds based on early wound area progression. *Diabetes Care*, 31(1), 26–29.

Lawton, S. (2001) Assessing the patient with a skin condition. *Journal of Tissue Viability*, 11(3), 113–115.

Mani, R. (1999) Science of measurements in wound healing. *Wound Repair and Regeneration*, 7, 330–334.

Maylor, M.E. (2003) Problems identified in gaining non-expert consensus for a hypothetical Wound Assessment Form. *Journal of Clinical Nursing*, 12, 824–833.

Moffatt, C., Morison, M.J., Pina, E. (2004) Wound bed preparation for venous leg ulcers. In: *European Wound Management Association (EWMA). Position Document: Wound Bed Preparation in Practice*. London: MEP Ltd.

Mulder, M. (2009) The selection of wound care products for wound bed preparation. *Wound Healing Southern Africa*, 2(2), 76–78.

Naylor, W. (2002) Malignant wounds: aetiology and principles of management. *British Journal of Nursing*, 10(20), 33–50.

Ousey, K., McIntosh, C. (2010) Understanding wound bed preparation and wound debridement. *British Journal of Community Nursing*, 15(3 Suppl.), S24–S28.

Phillips, T.J., Machado, F., Trout, R., Porter, J., Olin J., Falanga, V. (2000) Prognostic indicators in venous ulcers. *Journal of the American Academy of Dermatology*, 43, 627–630.

Piggin, C., Jones, V. (2007) Malignant fungating wounds: an analysis of the lived experience. *International Journal of Palliative Nursing*, 13(8), 384–391.

Salcido, R.S. (2005) Using our senses in wound care. *Advances in Skin and Wound Care*, 18(1), 8–11.

Schultz, G.S.S., Sibbald, R.G., Falanga, V. et al. (2003) Wound bed preparation: a systematic approach to wound management. *Wound Repair and Regeneration*, 11, 1–28.

Schultz, G.S., Barillo, D.J., Mozingo, D.W., Chine, G.A. (2004) Wound bed preparation and a brief history of TIME. *International Wound Journal*, 1, 19–32.

Schultz, G., Mozingo, D., Romanelli, M., Claxton, K. (2005) Wound healing and TIME: new concepts and scientific applications. *Wound Repair and Regeneration*, 13 (Suppl.), S1–S11.

Sheehan, P., Jones, P., Caselli D., Giurini, J.M., Veves, A. (2003) Percentage change in wound area of diabetic foot ulcers over a 4-week period is a robust predictor of complete healing by in a 12-week prospective trial. *Diabetes Care*, 26(6), 1879–1882.

Sibbald, R.G., Williamson, D., Orsted, H.L., et al. (2000) Preparing the wound bed – debridement, bacterial balance and moisture balance. *Ostomy/Wound Management*, 46(11), 14–35.

Sibbald, R.G., Woo, K.Y., Queen, D. (2007) Wound bed preparation and oxygen balance – a new component? *International Wound Journal*, 4(Suppl. 3), 9–17.

Snyder, R.J., Cardinal, M., Dauphinee, D.M., Stavosky, J. (2010) A post-hoc analysis of reduction in diabetic foot ulcer size at 4 weeks as a predictor of healing by 12 weeks. *Ostomy Wound Management*, 56(3), 44–50.

Sterling, C. (1996) Methods of wound assessment documentation: a study. *Nursing Standard*, 11(10), 38–41.

Suarez, F.L., Springfield J., Levitt, M.D. (1998) Identification of gases responsible for the odour of human flatus and evaluation of a device purported to reduce this odour. *Gut*, 43, 100–104.

Thawer, H., Houghton, A., Woodbury, E., Keast, G., Campbell, D.A. (2002) Comparison of computer-assisted and manual wound size measurement. *Ostomy Wound Manage*, 48(10), 46–52.

Watret, L. (2005) *Standardised Assessment Tools and the Management of Complex Wounds*. Wound Care Society Educational Leaflet, Wound Care Society, England.

Wendelken, M.E., Berg, W.T., Lichtenstein, P., Markowitz, L., Comfort, C., Alvarez, O.M. (2011) Wounds measured from digital photographs using photo-digital planimetry software: validation and rater reliability. *WOUNDS*, 23(9), 267–275.

World Union of Wound Healing Societies (WUWHS) (2008) Principles of Best Practice: Diagnostics and wounds. A consensus document. London: MEP Ltd.

5 Principles of Wound Management

Madeleine Flanagan

School of Life and Medical Sciences, University of Hertfordshire, Hertfordshire, UK

Overview

- An understanding of the physiological barriers that impair wound healing is required to effectively manage wounds and underpin the principles of chronic wound management: reduce the bacterial and necrotic burden, regulate moisture balance and protect the wound environment.
- Systematic reviews on wound treatments repeatedly highlighted the paucity of high-quality studies using clinically relevant end points to evaluate efficacy of wound therapies.
- Selection of the correct wound dressing is only part of the overall management of chronic wounds. Despite technological advances, dressings optimise local conditions in the wound bed rather than manage the underlying cause and are therefore only an adjunct to wound management.
- Negative pressure wound therapy (NPWT) has emerged as an alternative wound-healing modality to dressings that has transformed the practical management of complex wounds.
- A stepwise approach to use wound management treatments allows more expensive, advanced treatment modalities to be reserved for those patients with more complicated indolent wounds.

Introduction

Chronic wounds are difficult to heal and may persist for months or years or reoccur once healed due to underlying disease processes that can be difficult to manage. Treatment, therefore, requires a comprehensive approach involving the multidisciplinary team so that the underlying pathophysiology can be managed while promoting healing (Atiyeh et al., 2002; Enoch and Harding, 2003). Before a wound can begin to close, the barriers to healing must be eliminated where possible so that the local wound environment can support the delicate physiological process of tissue repair. This may require removal of non-viable tissue, control of bacterial burden, maintenance of moisture balance and provision of an environment to stimulate epithelialisation. This approach is now referred to as wound bed preparation (WBP) (Falanga, 2000; Schultz et al., 2003) and highlights the need to identify treatment aims based on assessment of the patient and their wound (Sibbald et al., 2000).

This chapter will provide an overview of treatment modalities used to manage wounds and

---

Wound Healing and Skin Integrity: Principles and Practice, First Edition. Edited by Madeleine Flanagan.
© 2013 John Wiley & Sons, Ltd. Published 2013 by John Wiley & Sons, Ltd.

describe broad indications for use. The information provided is not intended as a detailed guide and manufacturer's guidelines should be checked to ensure they are up to date.

Principles of wound management

WBP defines the guiding principles of chronic wound management as maintenance of debridement, moisture balance and bacterial balance while taking into account the patient's wider health care needs and allows application of our understanding of the physiology of healing to clinical practice to support appropriate wound management interventions.

The aim of local wound management is to provide optimum conditions to maximise the body's ability to repair injured tissue. This is achieved by:

- controlling haemostasis;
- correcting the underlying cause of tissue breakdown;
- controlling bacterial burden;
- removing the necrotic burden;
- regulating moisture balance;
- protecting the wound and surrounding skin.

The ultimate goal of wound management is to minimise the risk of opportunistic infection while promoting the development of healthy granulation tissue and uneventful healing.

Effective wound management

The majority of wounds will heal without complication using standard treatment. First-line management should aim to implement best practice starting with a thorough patient assessment, identification and treatment of underlying problems such as hyperglycaemia, poor nutrition, restoration of adequate tissue perfusion, etc. First-line interventions would, for example include simple measures such as covering the wound with a moist wound dressing and application of compression therapy in the case of venous leg ulceration. Wounds that fail to respond to standard wound management strategies should then be reassessed and stepped up to intermediate therapies. Figure 5.1 illustrates a stepwise approach to the selection of wound management modalities.

WBP provides a framework for clinical decision-making so that non-healing wounds can be identi-

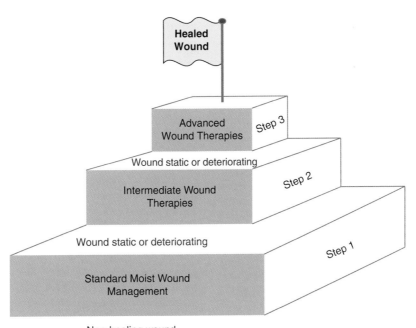

Figure 5.1   A step-wise approach to the selection of wound management modalities. Adapted from World Health Organization (WHO). WHO's Pain Relief Ladder [Illustration] (2005) Available at:www.who.int/cancer/palliative/painladder/en/

fied and more advanced interventions can be implemented (Sibbald et al., 2000). In this way, the use of intermediate therapies such as NPWT and electrical stimulation or advanced therapies such as bioengineered tissue alternatives or stem cell therapy may stimulate healing in indolent wounds. This stepwise approach helps to ensure that more expensive treatments are targeted at the smaller number of people with harder-to-heal wounds who might benefit from them making best use of limited resources. The rationale for choice at each level for therapeutic options is often guided by local wound management policies or protocols and many excellent examples are available on the Internet.

Many standard and advanced wound treatment modalities are thought to demonstrate clinical efficacy in practice and their use is supported by expert opinion. However, it should be recognised that the quality of evidence to support the use of one wound management intervention over another is limited and that the varying conditions found in different types of chronic wounds makes evaluation difficult (Vermeulen et al., 2004; Chaby et al., 2007; MeReC Bulletin, 2010; NICE, 2011).

Controlling bacterial burden: wound cleansing

Open wounds quickly become contaminated with bacteria within 48 hours (Bowler, 2002). The normal host immune response to bacteria invasion is inflammation, characterised by an invasion of polymorphonuclear leukocytes that release proteases and oxidants that break down cytokines and the extracellular matrix disrupting the local wound environment (Eming et al., 2007). One of the fundamental principles of wound healing is to reduce the bioburden in the wound bed and studies have demonstrated that as wounds heal, bacterial numbers start to fall (Trengove et al., 1999, 2000). Wound cleansing is one way of reducing the bioburden as it helps to remove loosely adherent microorganisms, cellular debris, wound exudate and dressing residue from the surface of the wound.

Temperature

In 1979, Locke demonstrated that optimal mitotic activity occurred in a wound when a stable temper-

ature of 37°C was maintained. This study showed that it could take as long as 40 minutes for wound to return to normal temperature following cleansing with a cold solution. Low temperatures in the wound bed reduce oxygenation and leukocyte activity thereby increasing the risk of infection and delaying healing (Feinstein and Miskiewicz, 2010). Thus, the use of warmed cleansing solutions and selection of dressings that increase wear time and insulate the wound is recommended.

Types of wound cleanser

Wound cleansing solutions must be non-toxic, reduce the number of microorganisms, not cause sensitivity reactions and be cost-effective and widely available (Main, 2008). Normal saline is most commonly used as a wound cleanser as it is an isotonic solution which does not disrupt the physiological process of healing. For many years, clinicians have discussed if tap water is as effective as normal saline for cleansing. A recent Cochrane review concluded that its use as a cleanser in acute wounds does not increase infection rates. However, the reviewers found no strong evidence that wound cleansing was better than not cleansing and concluded that where tap water is of high quality (drinkable), it may be as good as other methods such as sterile water or saline and more cost-effective (Fernandez et al., 2008).

For many years, community nurses have cleaned leg ulcers in buckets filled with warm tap water. However, a study by Johnson et al. (2009) found that 98% of wash basins in a hospital environment were contaminated by multi-resistant bacteria. It would therefore seem sensible to continue to cleanse complex, non-healing wounds that are known to be colonised by pathogenic bacteria with sterile saline unless buckets can be lined with plastic liners to minimise the risk of cross-infection. Consideration should always be given to the quality of tap water used for cleansing so that it does not increase the risk of infection. This will vary depending on the environment as even storage tanks of domestic and health care facilities in developed countries may be stagnant and contaminated with organisms such as Legionella. A sensible precaution is to run a tap or shower for a short time prior to use.

The routine use of antiseptics in wound management is controversial and is now considered inappropriate (Atiyeh et al., 2009). Many authors now advise against the use of antiseptics on open wounds due to concerns about toxicity and recommend that they be used in specific circumstances (Drosou et al., 2003; Wilson et al., 2005; Main, 2008).

Despite cytotoxicity data, most antiseptics have not been shown to delay healing, especially newer formulations like cadexomer iodine, polyhexanide and silver which are an appropriate choice for hard-to-heal wounds to remove biofilms (Khan and Naqvi, 2006), although these days they are likely to be administered as dressings rather than antiseptic solutions. However, the superiority of one antiseptic agent over another has not been shown.

Method of cleansing

A systematic review by Fernandez et al. (2004) to assess the effectiveness of different wound cleansing solutions indicated that there is no difference in infection or healing rates in wounds cleansed with tap water or normal saline and found no evidence to support the efficacy of different cleansing methods such as swabbing or scrubbing. However, this review concluded that an irrigation pressure of 13 pounds per square inch (psi) was effective for cleansing wounds and reducing infection without causing tissue trauma supporting the most frequently cited wound irrigation pressures of 8–15 psi Halvorson, 2007).

Indiscriminate wound cleansing can damage fragile new tissue in the wound bed and should not be performed routinely especially in acute wounds where exudate is known to promote healing. Cleansing in any type of wound is only indicated to remove excess exudate or surface contaminants or if there are clinical signs of infection.

Controlling bacterial burden: wound debridement

It is generally believed that that the presence of necrotic/sloughy tissue disrupts the normal process of wound healing by providing the right conditions for bacterial growth although there is limited data to support this (Bradley et al., 1999). The removal of adherent, devitalised tissue from wounds is thought to be essential to reduce the bacterial burden of the wound and minimise the risk of wound infection (see Chapter 6).

Box 5.1   Factors influencing choice of debridement method

Wound debridement: clinical considerations

- Patient general condition
- Wound aetiology
- Adequate tissue perfusion
- Extent/type of tissue damage
- Wound location
- Wound size
- Exudate production

Wound debridement: practical considerations

- Availability of resources
- Clinician competence
- Cost-effectiveness
- Time available
- Care setting: hospital or community
- Patient preference

There are various ways of debriding wounds and several factors must be considered when deciding on the most appropriate method; these are summarised in Box 5.1.

The most common debridement methods are briefly described below.

Autolytic debridement

Autolytic debridement can be performed at the bedside using semi-occlusive dressings such as film dressings, hydrocolloids and hydrogels. These create a moist wound–dressing interface which enhances the activity of endogenous proteolytic enzymes within the wound, liquefying and separating necrotic tissue from healthy tissue. This technique is particularly useful if, for technical or medical reasons, more invasive procedures are not suitable for the patient.

Enzymatic debridement

Enzymatic agents are popular in some countries and are derived from either proteolytic enzymes extracted from bovine plasma or pancreas, fruit and plants such as papain from papaya or bromelain from pineapple or bacterial collagenase derived from the *Clostridium histolyticum* sp. These exogenous enzyme preparations are applied to the wound bed and are recommended if a hard, dry eschar is present. Enzymatic preparations are usually applied to the eschar edge, encouraging it to separate from the granulation tissue, but penetration of thick, necrotic tissue can be slow and may require cross-hatching with a scalpel which needs to be performed by competent clinicians.

Biosurgical debridement

The use of sterile fly larvae in the treatment of a range of wounds has become popular in the recent years. The sheep blowfly *Lucilia sericata* (Diptera: Calliphoridae) is the only maggot currently used for this purpose. The larvae secrete collagenase and trypsin which liquefies necrotic tissue in wounds which the maggots then ingest along with microorganisms. The *L. sericata* maggot has been found to be effective against *Clostridium welchii*, methicillin-resistant *Staphylococcus aureus* and *Pseudomonas* sp. (Courtenay et al., 2000). Larvae secretions also contain chemicals with inherent antimicrobial properties, which may help to combat infection and increase the pH of the wound, which has an inhibitory effect on bacterial growth (Dumville et al., 2009). Some patients and carers are averse to the use of maggots and larvae as they may drown in deeper, highly exudating wounds. Contraindications include bleeding wounds due to the potential risk of blood vessel erosion by larvae enzymes, and they are not suitable for use in fistulae or wounds that might connect with vital organs.

Mechanical debridement

Types of mechanical debridement include use of wet-to-dry gauze dressings, hydrotherapy or wound irrigation to physically remove tissue from the wound bed. These techniques are painful but are common in some clinical environments. Wet-to-dry gauze uses saline soaked gauze which dries and adheres to the wound surface facilitating mechanical removal of tissue at dressing change. These techniques cause pain and carry the risk of damaging healthy tissue. The introduction of a disposable pad that is moistened and gently rubbed across the wound bed in a rotational movement to mechanically remove devitalised tissue from the wound surface provides an alternative approach to traditional mechanical debridement. Initial results are encouraging as practitioners can control the amount of tissue rubbed away and stop if the patient experiences any discomfort.

Sharp debridement

Sharp debridement is the quickest way to remove necrotic tissue from wounds. This technique requires advanced skills and must always be performed by a competent practitioner.

Conservative sharp debridement

It is the removal of loose necrotic tissue at the bedside and may be performed by a competent health professional, who has undergone appropriate training. This technique should not be performed at home due to the risk of complications, e.g. bleeding complications. Box 5.2 summarises the contraindications to conservative sharp debridement.

Surgical debridement

Surgical debridement usually takes place in an operating theatre environment and should be used when there is an urgent need to remove devitalised tissue, e.g. advancing cellulitis or sepsis. There is increasing evidence that chronic wounds benefit from aggressive debridement as senescent cells, which slow down the tissue repair process, are removed together with necrotic tissue and bacteria converting a chronic wound into an acute one

---

Box 5.2 Contraindications to conservative sharp debridement

- Lack of access to sterile surgical instruments;
- Densely adherent necrotic tissue; interface between viable and non-viable tissue cannot be clearly identified;
- Friable wounds with an increased tendency of haemorrhage, e.g. fungating wounds;
- Impaired clotting mechanism (anticoagulant or antiplatelet medications);
- Increased risk of bleeding, e.g. deep pressure ulcers;
- Risk of anatomical hazards (tendons, nerves, blood vessels), e.g. wounds on hands, feet;
- Risk of ischemia: insufficient tissue oxygenation to support wound healing, e.g. diabetic foot ulcer, patient receiving palliative care.

(Schultz et al., 2003). It should be noted that following surgical or sharp debridement of larger chronic wounds there may be a short-term bacteraemia which may justify administration of antibiotic prophylaxis to prevent sepsis and septic shock.

Despite these advantages, pain caused by sharp debridement and the risk of bleeding and damage to associated structures, e.g. tendons, must be carefully considered. Sharp debridement is contraindicated if tissue perfusion is limited and should be only performed by a suitably trained practitioner.

Hydrosurgical debridement

This method of debridement uses either pressurised water or saline as a precise fluid dissector of devitalised tissue. The pressure is controlled via a handset so that the jet of fluid both cuts and removes tissue whilst irrigating the wound. The technique is quick and can be used in ward, clinic areas or in theatre and should only be used by a trained clinician. A study by Mosti et al. (2005) demonstrated improved healing rates and decreased hospital stay in patients with hard-to-heal leg ulcers when compared to debridement with moist wound dressing controls. Most wounds were adequately debrided with a single application. In trained hands, it is an effective alternative to sharp debridement.

Ultrasound (acoustic pressure wound therapy)

Two low-frequency ultrasound debridement techniques exist for use with hard-to-heal wounds. Both have different modes of application. One uses a low-energy, low-intensity ultrasound to the wound bed through a continuous saline mist which transmits ultrasonic energy to the wound bed to stimulate healing by the removal of slough, exudate and bacteria. The other uses a single-use ultrasound probe, which combines a cleansing system that removes devitalised tissue and bacteria from the wound surface. Results for both systems are reported to be immediate and effective (Cole et al., 2009; Haan and Lucich, 2009), although appraisal of the current evidence base, like so many wound therapies, indicates that the quality of the evidence is insufficient to recommend routine use (NICE, 2011).

In addition to clinical factors previously discussed, there are other practical considerations to be taken into account when debriding a wound.

The availability of resources is determined by the care environment. Access to team members who possess the appropriate technical skills is an important consideration and may be restricted in the community setting where the use of more conservative debridement methods may be more realistic. The advantages and limitations of the different types of wound debridement are listed in Table 5.1.

However, the length of time taken to achieve debridement is an important variable when considering the overall cost-effectiveness of treatment. The patient's wishes should be of primary concern when deciding how best to remove devitalised tissue as co-operation with treatment obviously influences the final outcome.

Regulating moisture balance

Chronic wound fluid is known to have a detrimental effect on healing outcomes and has been described as a 'corrosive biological fluid' (Bishop et al., 2003). Chronic wounds are often associated with copious exudate which causes leakage, skin problems, electrolyte imbalance, infection, odour and psychological problems. On the other hand, minimal exudate delays autolytic debridement, inhibits epithelialisation and causes pain on dressing removal. One of the essential principles of wound management is to maintain moisture balance at the wound–dressing interface whilst avoiding desiccation and maceration of the wound or periwound skin. The surface of the skin does not tolerate excess moisture and barrier function is soon impaired which may result in pressure damage or incontinence-associated dermatitis as the stratum corneum breaks down (see Chapter 2).

Wound dressings have always been the first-line management option for controlling moisture balance in wounds although new technologies offer the clinician a variety of alternatives, e.g. NPWT. The use of indirect fluid handling strategies such as compression therapy, wound drainage and use of barrier products to protect the skin are an important adjunct to wound dressings.

It is important that whichever treatment modality is used to regulate moisture balance, it should maintain a relatively constant level of moisture at the wound–dressing interface and absorb excess exudate so that wound fluid does not have prolonged contact with the skin and the potential to do damage. One of the most important considerations when selecting a dressing is to establish

Table 5.1   Advantages and limitations of different types of wound debridement

	Autolytic	Surgical	Conservative sharp	Mechanical	Enzyme	Larvae	Hydrotherapy	Ultrasound
Selective debridement				×	Depends on product			
Expensive	×		×	×		×		
Time-consuming		×	×			×	×	×
Easy to perform		×	×	×				
Requires advanced skills	×			×		×		
May cause trauma in healthy tissues					×	×		
May cause pain/discomfort	×				×	×	×	×
May cause inflammation/sepsis						×	×	×
May require analgesia/ anaesthetic	×				×	×	×	×
May require secondary dressing								

the type, viscosity and volume of wound fluid being produced as dressing choice is dependent on its absorbent capacity. Once saturated, leakage increases the risk of infection and may cause skin damage and wound deterioration. Dressing materials vary greatly in their fluid-handling capacity, so it is important to understand how different dressing materials function in order to make an appropriate choice.

Wound dressings

This section will provide a summary of generic dressing types and provide broad indications for use. As many of the dressing products reviewed have been established for a long time, there are comparatively few large, well-randomised studies to support their use (Thomas, 2010). A Cochrane review found insufficient evidence 'that any one dressing speeds up healing of surgical wounds healing by secondary intention more than another' as the published data consist of small, poor-quality studies (Vermeulen et al., 2004) and is consistent with other systematic reviews (Chaby et al., 2007; MeReC Bulletin, 2010).

The information provided about dressing use is not intended as a detailed guide. The reader is advised to follow local recommendations together with manufacturer's guidelines for use of specific dressing products. Further guidance on dressing selection for specific wound types such as fungating wounds can be found in the relevant chapter under the heading: *Wound Dressings: special considerations*.

Dressing selection

There are many factors that influence the choice of dressings and wound treatments. Personal experience and the influence of colleagues continue to be a dominant influence when choosing wound dressings. Many practitioners still rely on a small range of treatment approaches with which they have had good results in the past. Traditional knowledge and practice successfully pass down through generations of practitioners and can perpetuate poor practice and myths (Flanagan, 2005). Although aware of a growing evidence base in relation to wound management, some clinicians consider this to be irrelevant to clinical practice.

The choice of dressing product for optimal wound management is not straightforward and should be based on a consideration of the patient and the local wound environment. There are many interrelated factors that influence the selection of wound dressings (Figure 5.2). Use of a framework such as the WBP model (Sibbald et al., 2000; Schultz et al., 2003) can help clinical decisions in relation

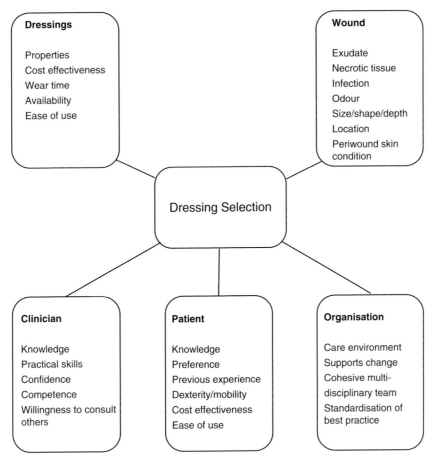

Dressings

Properties
Cost effectiveness
Wear time
Availability
Ease of use

Wound

Exudate
Necrotic tissue
Infection
Odour
Size/shape/depth
Location
Periwound skin
condition

Dressing Selection

Clinician

Knowledge
Practical skills
Confidence
Competence
Willingness to consult
others

Patient

Knowledge
Preference
Previous experience
Dexterity/mobility
Cost effectiveness
Ease of use

Organisation

Care environment
Supports change
Cohesive multi-
disciplinary team
Standardisation of
best practice

Figure 5.2   Factors influencing selection of wound dressings.

to dressing choice as it helps prioritise the aims of treatment and establish the primary function of dressing products.

The selection of wound dressings has become more complicated as different types of products become available. It is important to understand how each dressing product works and its specific indications for use. Some dressing combinations can be detrimental to wound healing. For example, an absorptive secondary foam dressing may remove the moisture from a hydrogel and dehydrate the wound bed.

The characteristics of the ideal dressing were identified many years ago by Scales (1956) and Turner (1985) and more recently by Leaper (2006) which manufacturers have been trying to emulate ever since (Box 5.3). Over the years, there has been a gradual recognition that patient-centred concerns are important to improve adherence with treatment

and reflect the criteria that clinicians consider as the ideal dressing.

The ideal dressing has yet to be developed; so each year as more products are launched into an already crowded market, the choice of dressings becomes more confusing. Despite the development of numerous dressing formularies, protocols and logarithms, dressing selection can be difficult.

Types of wound dressings

Advances in technology mean that today different dressing products have specific indications for use. Choice of the wrong dressing for the particular conditions in the wound may result in ineffective treatment and wound deterioration.

Dressings are often classified in generic groups according to their function, although this is continually evolving and is subject to change. They can

Box 5.3   Characteristics of an ideal dressing (patient and clinician criteria)

Clinician criteria	Patient criteria
Barrier to external contaminants	Prevents infection
High moisture vapour permeability	Minimises risk of skin damage
Create a moist wound–dressing interface	Reduces pain between dressing changes
High absorbing capacity	Controls exudate leakage
Promotes autolytic debridement	Reduces risk of infection
Ability to thermally insulate wound	Comfortable to wear
Non-sensitising and non-toxic	Minimises skin irritation
Eliminates dead space	Speeds up healing
Good adhesion to surrounding skin	Extended wear times
Non-adherence at wound surface	Pain-free dressing change
Cost-effective	Value for money
Conformable to body contours	Discreet and easy to use

Source: Data from Scales (1956), Turner (1985) and Leaper (2006).

be divided into two broad groups (Weller and Sussman, 2006):

- Passive inert products
  - ○ Absorbing
  - ○ Non-absorbing
- Interactive products
  - ○ Absorbing
  - ○ Non-absorbing
  - ○ Moisture donating

Passive inert dressings

For hundreds of years, most dressings were passive wound coverings such as lint and gauze and met few of the requirements of an ideal dressing. These traditional products are not the dressing of choice as a primary wound contact layer but may be useful as secondary dressings. They have limited use in superficial wounds with low exudate as they may adhere to the wound surface and be painful to remove.

Advances in technology have produced modern inert dressings which incorporate relatively inexpensive low-adherent, highly absorbent materials that can be used either as primary or secondary dressings in moderate to highly exudating wounds.

Passive inert absorbent dressings

The properties of products in this group vary significantly and range from simple absorbent dressings which retain fluid until pressure is applied to newer superabsorbent cellulose and polymer dressings with advanced fluid-retention properties allowing for extended wear time. Technological advances in wound contact materials have allowed this group of dressings to improve but they should be considered as low adherent rather than non-adherent and may cause trauma on removal especially in drier wound environments.

Absorbent passive inert dressings:

- are permeable to bacteria;
- have varying absorbent capacity;
- may require a secondary dressing;
- may dry out the wound surface;
- causing trauma on removal;
- are available in various formulations:
  - ○ adhesive/non-adhesive;
  - ○ low profile (thin) – improved flexibility for difficult-to-dress areas.

Indications for use	Contraindication
Moderate to highly exudating wounds	Take care under compression therapy to prevent adherence in drier wounds
Wide range of wound types including those healing by primary intention, e.g. post-operative wounds	May allow exudate to be in prolonged contact with skin under compression

Passive inert non-absorbent dressings

Paraffin gauze (tulle) dressings are non-absorbent passive inert dressings that were developed in 1915 during the First World War (Thomas, 2010). They provide a waterproof layer of paraffin across the wound surface which may lead to maceration as transepidermal water loss (TEWL) is restricted. Today, there are modern alternatives comprising tightly meshed, synthetic materials that allow moisture evaporation and reduce the risk of skin maceration.

Non-absorbent passive inert dressings:

- are permeable to bacteria;
- causing trauma on removal;
- require a secondary dressing;
- require frequent changing;
- may adhere to the wound;
- are available in various formulations:
  - combined with topical antimicrobials, e.g. silver.

Indications for use	Contraindication
Clean wounds	Infected wounds
Superficial wounds	Extensive tissue loss/sinus
Low exudating wounds	Moderate-to-high exudating wounds

Interactive dressings

Interactive dressings modify the local wound environment to promote moisture balance by absorbing and/or retaining wound exudate. The first moist interactive dressings were polyurethane films that were used in Winter's seminal study on moist wound healing (Winter, 1962). Following the development of polyurethane film dressings, a number of more absorbent moist wound dressings were developed and a plethora of products emerged in the 1990s including hydrocolloids, foams, alginates and hydrogels.

Non-absorbent interactive dressings

Polyurethane film dressings

These consist of a thin, polyurethane membrane coated with a layer of acrylic adhesive and were introduced as wound dressings in the early 1970s (Thomas, 2010). Film dressings adhere to the surrounding skin and trap moisture at the wound surface. They can be used as either a primary or secondary wound contact layer and are popular as a secondary dressing to retain amorphous hydrogels at the wound–dressing interface to promote autolytic debridement of eschar or slough. Film dressings provide some pain relief by preventing dehydration and bathing exposed nerve endings in wound fluid. Strong adhesive bonds in film dressings may cause skin damage on removal, unless the adhesive bond is weakened by stretching the dressing laterally and parallel to the wound surface before trying to remove it.

Polyurethane film dressings:

- are impermeable to bacteria;
- are gas/water vapour permeable;
- create a moist wound–dressing interface;
- do not absorb moisture;
- may adhere to the wound, causing trauma on removal;
- are conformable and flexible;
- provide pain relief;
- are transparent;
- are available in various formulations:
  - combined with an absorbent pad with low-adherent wound contact layer;
  - combined with topical antimicrobials, e.g. silver.

Indications for use	Contraindication
Clean wounds	Infected wounds
Superficial wounds	Extensive tissue loss/sinus
Low exudating wounds	Highly exudating wounds
Prevention of friction/shear over high-risk sites, e.g. heels	Fragile/compromised periwound skin
Retention of cannula/drains or protection around catheters and PEG sites	
Useful secondary dressing over alginates or hydrogels	

Silicone/polyurethane wound contact materials

Silicone or polyurethane products gently adhere to the wound and surrounding skin but are designed to minimise trauma on removal. Soft silicone dressings rely on a hydrophobic soft silicone layer that is tacky to touch but prevents the dressing from adhering to the wound surface by maintaining contact without causing friction and shear. This type of primary wound contact layers are not absorbent but allow exudate to pass into a moisture-retentive secondary dressing. They have been proven to reduce wound pain (Dykes et al., 2001; White and Morris, 2009) and are particularly useful for superficial wounds where there is a loss of epidermis, e.g. blistering diseases, burn wounds.

Silicone gel sheets are thicker and do not require a secondary dressing. They are designed to be applied over healed scars and should be worn continuously to help soften and flatten scar tissue. There is growing evidence that silicone gel sheet dressings are effective on both hypertrophic scars and minor keloid scars, although the mode of action is not fully understood (Mustoe et al., 2002). These dressings have similar adhesive properties as silicone primary wound contact layers and are tacky but do not leave an adhesive residue, so they can be lifted from the skin and repositioned without losing their adherent properties.

Silicone/polyurethane wound contact layers are:

- waterproof;
- do not absorb moisture;
- minimise pain at dressing change;
- conform well to body contours without leaving adhesive residues on skin;
- soften and flatten scar tissue;
- available in various formulations:
  - wound contact layer: allows free passage of exudate into secondary dressing;
  - silicone gel sheeting: used on healed wounds.

Indications for use: wound contact layers	Contraindication
Wide range of low to highly exudating wounds	Patients with a known allergy to silicone
Skin graft fixation	Bleeding wounds
Wounds with epidermal loss, e.g. abrasions, blisters, epidermolysis bullosa (EB), skin tears, superficial pressure ulcers, partial thickness burns	
Fragile periwound skin, e.g. skin tears	

Indications for use: silicone gel sheeting	Contraindications
Healed wounds with raised or hypertrophic scars	Patients with a known allergy to silicone
	Open wounds

Absorbent interactive dressings

Alginate dressings

Alginate dressings increased in popularly in the early 1980s due to their superior absorbency compared to other dressings available at the time. They are derived from calcium or sodium/calcium salts of alginic acid, composed of mannuronic and guluronic acids obtained from seaweed (Piacquadio and Nelson, 1992). On contact with wound fluid, sodium salts in the exudate exchange with the calcium in the alginate dressing to form a soft hydrophilic gel which maintains a moist environment at the wound surface. Alginates absorb exudate laterally into their fibres to transform into a soft gel, but if they become supersaturated they may cause maceration of the periwound skin so they should be cut to the shape of the wound. A transient burning sensation may be felt if alginates are applied to dry wounds and sometimes adhere to drier areas of the wound and should be loosened by irrigating with normal saline.

The calcium–sodium ion exchange at the wound surface allows calcium ions to be released into the wound. As calcium is a normal part of the coagulation response, this release of calcium assists in haemostasis (Segal et al., 1998). There is increasing evidence to suggest that alginates are clinically beneficial as a haemostat to stop bleeding in a variety of wounds including donor sites and tooth extraction (O'Donoghue et al., 1997; Kaneda et al., 2008).

Alginate dressings:

- are highly absorbent;
- form a non-adherent gel in exuding wounds;
- create a moist wound–dressing interface;
- promote autolytic debridement in moist wounds;
- may assist control minor bleeding;
- may provide pain relief;
- are easily removed from exuding wounds;
- may adhere to dry wounds;
- are conformable and flexible;

- usually require a secondary dressing;
- are available in various formulations:
  - flat sheets;
  - packing rope for cavities/sinus;
  - combined with silver to increase antimicrobial activity;
  - combined with charcoal to reduce odour.

Indications for use	Contraindication
Infected wounds or wounds with increased risk of infection	Wounds with dry eschar
Flat, cavity wounds and sinus	
Moderate to heavily exudating wounds	Dry wounds
Bleeding wounds, e.g. donor sites	
Suitable for irregular-shaped wounds, e.g. malignant wounds, sinus cavities	Do not tightly pack narrow sinus as alginate will expand when absorbing exudate

Hydrocolloid dressings

Hydrocolloid technology was first used for wounds in the 1980s. Hydrocolloids consist of an adhesive rubber matrix containing a gel-forming colloidal suspension such as sodium carboxymethyl cellulose or gelatine, containing fluid-absorbing particles (Thomas, 2008). By the 1990s, new presentations were introduced and today, approximately 45 different hydrocolloids are available. All look similar and have the same clinical indications, despite minor differences in structure and composition.

Hydrocolloids:

- are impermeable to bacteria;
- are impermeable to gas/water vapour;
- create a moist wound–dressing interface;
- absorb low-to-moderate levels of exudate;
- promote autolytic debridement;
- are conformable and flexible;
- provide pain relief;
- are available in various formulations:
  - paste (increased absorbency for small cavities/sinus);
  - powder (increased absorbency);
  - shaped sacral or heel dressings;

- thin – improved flexibility for difficult-to-dress areas;
- combined with silver – increased antimicrobial activity.

Indications for use	Contraindication
Clean wounds	Infected or excessively sloughy wounds due to increased exudate production
Flat, smaller cavities and sinus	Cavities with extensive tissue loss
Low to moderate exudating wounds	Highly exudating wounds
Removal of hard eschar	Over-granulating wounds
Protection of periwound skin	Fragile/compromised periwound skin
Securing nasal tubes and drains	

Hydrofibre dressings (gelling fibres)

The first hydrofibre dressing was launched in 1997 and they are popular due to their ability to absorb high levels of wound exudate. A new category of dressings was created and the name 'hydrofibre' trademarked. As similar dressings cannot refer to themselves as hydrofibres, this dressing category may become renamed gelling fibres. A hydrofibre is a soft, sterile, non-woven pad or ribbon dressing composed of sodium carboxymethylcellulose which absorbs wound fluid and transforms into a soft gel (Queen, 1992). Hydrofibres and alginate dressings are sometimes confused as they look and perform in a similar way and share the same clinical indications.

Hydrofibre dressings:

- are absorbent;
- form a non-adherent gel in exuding wounds;
- create a moist wound–dressing interface;
- promote autolytic debridement in moist wounds;
- are conformable and flexible;
- are available in various formulations:
  - flat sheets;
  - packing rope for cavities/sinus;
  - combined with silver to increase antimicrobial activity.

Indications for use	Contraindication
Infected wounds or wounds with increased risk of infection	Wounds with dry eschar
Flat, cavity wounds and sinus	
Moderate to heavily exudating wounds	Dry wounds

Hydrogels

Hydrogels are a group of complex insoluble polymers with a high water content between 30% and 90%. They are available as amorphous gels or in a flat sheet form consisting of a cross-linked polymer and water held in a backing sheet. Reformulation of second-generation hydrogels has improved their ability to absorb wound fluid as well as rehydrate dry tissue. Hydrogels are most frequently used to promote autolytic debridement of sloughy wounds or those with a dry necrotic eschar and can be used in a variety of clinical situations without harming granulation tissue.

Hydrogels:

- absorb moderate amounts of wound exudate;
- rehydrates dry tissue;
- promote autolytic debridement;
- create a moist wound–dressing interface;
- have a cooling/soothing effect;
- are easily removed;
- are conformable and flexible;
- are available in various formulations:
  - flat sheets;
  - amorphous hydrogels for cavities/sinus (required secondary dressing);
  - combined with silver to increase antimicrobial activity.

Indications for use	Contraindication
Sloughy wounds or those with dry necrotic tissue	Should not be used with absorbent secondary dressings, e.g. polyurethane foams, hydrofibres, alginates
Wide range of low to moderately exuding lesions including rehydration of excoriated skin, small burns	Effectiveness of amorphous hydrogels limited under compression therapy

Protease modulating dressings

Elevated protease activity in chronic wounds is known to delay healing (Trengove et al., 1999). Dressing products composed of collagen and oxidised regenerated cellulose (ORC) have been designed to control proteolytic activity by absorbing wound fluid and trapping proteases within their structure to render them inactive (Cullen et al., 2004; Smeets et al., 2008). On contract with exudate, the dressing forms a soft biodegradable gel which binds with growth factors protecting them from degradation by MMPs. As protease-modulating dressings correct a specific biochemical imbalance in wounds, they are not suitable for routine use in non-healing wounds.

MMP modulating dressings:

- are absorbent;
- form a non-adherent gel in exuding wounds;
- create a moist wound–dressing interface;
- may assist control minor bleeding;
- are easily removed from exuding wounds;
- may adhere to dry wounds;
- usually require a secondary dressing.

Indications for use	Contraindication
Suitable for all stages of wound healing	Dry wounds require an semi-occlusive secondary dressing
Wounds with increased risk of infection	Contraindicated where anaerobic infection is suspected as hydrogels can support the growth of microorganisms Excess exudate may cause leakage

Indications for use	Contraindication
Suitable for clean, chronic non-healing wounds	Wounds covered with a dry eschar or scab; infected wounds
Can be used in conjunction with compression therapy	Dry wounds require dressing to be moistened with saline prior to application
	Known hypersensitivity to either ORC or collagen

Polyurethane foam dressings

These are soft, open-celled, polyurethane dressings that may be single or multiple layered. They are low adherent, highly absorbent and provide thermal insulation to the wound and became popular in the 1980s due to the introduction of hydrophilic polyurethane materials (Thomas, 2010). Most have an outer semi-permeable membrane that allows fluid to pass into the insulating foam. Foam dressings may adhere to the wound bed if exudate is low under compression therapy (Malone, 1987).

Polyurethane foam dressings:

- are impermeable to bacteria;
- are waterproof;
- are gas/water vapour permeable;
- create a moist wound–dressing interface;
- are highly absorbent;
- reduce risk of maceration;
- are thermally insulating;
- may adhere to dry wounds or fragile skin;
- are available in various formulations:
  - adhesive/non-adhesive;
  - shaped cavity devices for cavity wounds;
  - shaped sacral or heel dressings;
  - thin – improved flexibility for difficult-to-dress areas;
  - combined with silver or PHMB to increase antimicrobial activity;
  - combined with charcoal to reduce odour.

Indications for use	Contraindication
Wide range of wound types/clinical environments	Do not conform well to irregular convex wounds, e.g. tumours
Infected wounds or wounds with increased risk of infection	
Moderate to heavily exudating wounds	Dry wounds or those with minimal exudate
Can be used under compression therapy	Take care under compression therapy to prevent adherence in drier wounds

Antibacterial dressings

The application of a topical antimicrobial dressing is one method of reducing the bioburden in critically colonised or infected wounds. Identifying critical colonisation is not easy but may be indicated by an increase in slough (which is not responsive to standard debridement techniques), malodour and a delay in healing in a wound despite appropriate treatment. Newer slow-release antimicrobial dressings enable control of resistant microbial species such as MRSA and vancomycin-resistant enterococci and have low toxicity and are less likely to induce resistance than antibiotics (Parsons et al., 2005) (see Chapter 6). However, dressings containing antimicrobials should not be routinely applied to wounds just in case.

Cadexomer iodine dressings

Cadexomer iodine was developed in the 1980s and consists of cadexomer polysaccharide polymer and iodine (0.9%). These products are applied directly to the wound surface so that wound exudate combines with the polymer and is absorbed as iodine is slowly released. They form a gel as they absorb fluid and release iodine into the tissues at a low concentration which is non-toxic.

Cadexomer iodine dressings:

- are effective against bacterial, protozoal and fungal infections;
- are highly absorbent;
- create a moist wound–dressing interface;
- promote autolytic debridement;
- are conformable and flexible;
- may require a secondary dressing;
- are available in various formulations:
  - flat sheets;
  - paste for cavities/sinus;
  - ointment paste.

Indications for use	Contraindication
Critically colonised or infected wounds including:	Known sensitivity to iodine Thyroid disease (caution)
Moderate to highly exuding wounds	Pregnancy/lactating women Children under 6 months
Flat, cavity wounds and sinus	Do not exceed 3 months continuous use (risk of systemic absorption)
	Maximum single application: 50 g
	Maximum weekly application: 150 g

Honey dressings

Honey has been used in wounds since ancient times but medical-grade honey dressing was developed in the late 1990s. Honey has a broad spectrum of activity against bacteria, including MRSA and VRE (Cooper and Jenkin, 2012). Antimicrobial activity is thought to be due to a number of factors including the ability of honey to produce low levels of hydrogen peroxide in the wound, the provision of an acidic wound environment (pH 3) and sugar molecules bind to water molecules removing the bacterial food source.

Medical-grade honey dressings:

- are antimicrobial;
- reduce wound odour;
- absorb low-to-moderate exudate;
- promote autolytic debridement;
- are effective debriding agents;
- create a moist wound–dressing interface;
- are conformable and flexible;
- are sometimes associated with localised pain;
- require no secondary dressing;
- are available in various formulations:
  - sheets;
  - paste (increased absorbency for small cavities/sinus);
  - ointment;
  - combined with alginates (increased absorbency for cavities/sinus).

Indications for use	Contraindication
Critically colonised or infected wounds including:	Patients with known allergy to bee stings
Low to moderate exudating wounds	Highly exudating wounds: potential for maceration
Appropriate for use in diabetic patients; no need for increased frequency of blood sugar monitoring	May cause stinging sensation, if so, discontinue

Silver dressings

A variety of antimicrobial dressings containing silver are available for clinical use. However, the silver content and physical and chemical properties of these dressings vary greatly. A study comparing *in vitro* antibacterial activity of seven widely available silver dressings against *S. aureus* and *Pseudomonas aeruginosa* demonstrated that silver content and the rate of silver release did not correlate with antibacterial efficacy (Parsons et al., 2005). This study showed that specific silver dressings have different antibacterial and fluid-handling properties that make them more or less appropriate for different clinical indications highlighting the need to select dressings based on overall performance characteristics rather than silver content and ability to release silver alone.

However, a Cochrane review evaluating efficacy of silver dressings (mostly in burn patients) reported that because most studies were small and of poor quality there was insufficient evidence to support the use of silver dressings as they did not demonstrate improved wound healing or prevent wound infection (Storm-Versloot et al., 2010). These results are consistent with findings from a recent Canadian Health Technology Assessment (Canadian Agency for Drugs Technologies in Health, 2010) and a British Drugs and Therapeutics Review (Iheanacho, 2010).

Silver dressings:

- are effective against bacterial and fungal infections;
- have variable fluid-retention properties;
- create a moist wound–dressing interface;
- are conformable and flexible;
- may require a secondary dressing;
- are available in various formulations:
  - flat sheets;
  - combined with hydrogels, alginates, hydrofibre for increased absorbency.

Indications for use	Contraindication
Critically colonised or infected wounds including:	Use with caution in pregnant or lactating women or children
	Use with caution in patients with hepatic and renal impairment
Flat, cavity wounds and sinus	Discontinue and re-evaluate after 2 weeks if no improvement
Low to moderate exudating wounds	Dry wounds/wounds covered with eschar

Polyhexamethylene biguanide (PHMB)

Although the antimicrobial PHMB has been used in healthcare for many years, it has only recently been introduced into wound management. Relatively few dressing products contain PHMB, but those that do are currently either low–absorbent, perforated, plastic film-faced dressings, foam-based dressings or a biosynthetic cellulose fibre dressing impregnated with PHM (Gray, 2010).

PHMB is recommended for use in critically colonised and locally infected acute and chronic wounds as it has a proven broad antimicrobial action (Wright et al., 2003; Kaehn, 2009; Hubner and Kramer 2010; Dissemond et al., 2011) and is effective against biofilms and fibrin (Gray, 2010).

PHMB dressings:

- are effective against bacterial and fungal infections;
- have a sustained effect;
- have no reports of bacterial resistance to date;
- are conformable and flexible;
- may require a secondary dressing.

Indications for use	Contraindication
Critically colonised or infected wounds including:	During the first 4 months of pregnancy (thereafter, with caution)
	Do not use in joint spaces or if any part of the central nervous system exposed due to potential toxicity
	In patients allergic to PHMB
Flat, cavity wounds and sinus	Discontinue and re-evaluate after 2 weeks if no improvement
Low to moderate exudating wounds	Dry wounds/wounds covered with eschar

Practice point

Has gauze got any place in modern wound management?

Gauze should not be used as a primary wound contact layer as it dehydrates the wound bed and dries out to form a hard mass that causes trauma to newly formed granulation tissue and fresh bleeding when removed (Foster and Moore, 1997). Gauze products are not waterproof and do not provide an effective barrier to invading microorganisms. The pain associated with removal of gauze dressings and packing materials increases patient distress and anxiety and is unnecessary (Moffatt et al., 2005). A Cochrane review concluded that foam dressings are a good alternative to gauze in terms of pain reduction, patient satisfaction and savings in nursing time (Vermeulen et al., 2004). A primary contact dressing with a low-adherent surface should always be used to protect the wound surface. There are many examples of these types of products such as knitted viscose primary dressings, capillary action absorbent dressings and superabsorbent cellulose and polymer dressings. This advice does not relate to gauze used in topical negative pressure therapy systems.

Selection of wound dressings is a complex activity requiring a range of skills that include matching local conditions at the wound bed to the most appropriate dressing and a critical understanding of the principles of dressing management and the evidence supporting manufacturers' claims. The principles of dressing management are summarised in Table 5.2.

Other important considerations are the need to meet dressing formulary and reimbursement requirements whilst addressing patient-centred concerns.

Negative Pressure Wound Therapy

In the past 15 years, NPWT has become established as a popular method of regulating moisture balance and controlling bacterial burden within open wounds such as traumatic wounds, open abdominal wounds and complex diabetic wounds. As clinical experience is growing, NPWT is being used in an increasingly diverse range of wound aetiologies and has in some centres replaced dressings as the modality of choice for the management of some complex wounds such as military wounds (Jeffrey, 2009).

NPWT systems promote healing in open wounds by removing wound exudate, and bacteria by creating a vacuum (negative pressure) at the wound site. NPWT is thought to promote wound healing by stimulating wound contraction and blood flow at the wound edge, improving interstitial fluid flow, wound perfusion, protease profiles, growth factor and cytokine expression leading to improved wound healing (Morykwas et al., 2006).

Table 5.2   Principles of dressings management

Principle	Source
Assess the wound at every dressing change and confirm the appropriateness of the current dressing regimen	Pressure Ulcer Treatment A Quick Reference Guide EPUAP/NAPUAP (2009)
There is no evidence that any one dressing or topical agent speeds up the healing of open wounds healing by secondary intention more than another	Vermeulen et al. (2004)
Evaluate the ability of the dressing to provide a moist but not macerated wound bed at each dressing change and modify dressing regime accordingly	World Union of Wound Healing Societies (2007)
	Pressure Ulcer Treatment: A Quick Reference Guide EPUAP/NAPUAP (2009)
Gauze should be used with caution on wounds healing by secondary intention	NICE (2008) Surgical Site Infection
	EPUAP/NAPUAP l
There is no robust clinical evidence that antimicrobial dressings are more effective than non-medicated dressings for the prevention or treatment of wound infection	Vermeulen et al. (2004)
	MeReC Bulletin (2010)
Reconsider dressing choice if soaking is required for removal or removal causes bleeding/trauma	World Union of Wound Healing Societies (2004)
Select dressings with the ability to stay in place for longer periods to maximise wear time	World Union of Wound Healing Societies (2004)
Follow manufacturer's recommendations	All of the above

NPWT systems consist of a pump that generates a vacuum capable of creating a negative pressure environment within a sealed wound together with dressing materials that fill the wound and create a seal, tubing that drains fluid from the wound and a canister to collect the drainage. There is currently a choice of wound fillers: gauze or a foam dressing, which allows equal distribution of negative pressure across the wound bed and both have been shown to be as effective as each other (Malmsjö and Borgquist, 2010).

NPWT devices have two suction settings: continuous and intermittent. Continuous suction is the most frequently used and is appropriate for highly exudating wounds. The intermittent setting may be used once the amount of wound exudate diminishes (Malmsjö and Borgquist, 2010).

Although rare, complications arising from the use of NPWT have been reported, especially in long-term healthcare facilities and at home (FDA, 2009). Box 5.4 lists the contraindications for NPWT and Box 5.5 lists the factors that should be considered before using NPWT.

The patient's condition, wound status, location and co-morbidities should be evaluated frequently in an appropriate care setting. The use of NPWT should be supervised by a suitable trained clinician, and application particularity in complex wounds requires manual dexterity.

Box 5.4   Contraindications for NPWT

- Necrotic tissue with hard eschar or thick slough;
- Untreated osteomyelitis;
- Malignancy in the wound;
- Exposed vasculature or nerves;
- Non-enteric and unexplored fistulas;
- Exposed anastomotic site;
- Exposed organs.

See http://www.fda.gov/MedicalDevices/Safety/AlertsandNotices/PublicHealthNotifications/ucm190658.htm for the FDA list of contraindications and risk factors.

Practice point

Complications of NPWT include bleeding and infection and may be associated with retained dressing fragments or removal of tissue during dressing change. To help reduce these risks remember the following tips:

- The number of dressing pieces placed in the wound should be carefully monitored.
- Avoid cutting the dressing directly over the wound to prevent dressing fragments falling into the wound.
- Resume NPWT as soon as possible after moving a patient to the home or another care facility so the wound stays moist.
- Do not overfill the wound or compress the foam to reduce the risk of tissue damage on removal or vasoconstriction at the wound–dressing interface.

The development of portable NPWT devices means that some patients may be considered suitable for use of the NPWT system at home. In these circumstances, it is important to teach the patient and caregiver about how to use the system, potential complications and what to do if complications occur and educational resources are available from the system manufacturers to facilitate this.

NPWT should be discontinued once the wound size has diminished, exudate levels fall and granulation tissue has filled the wound bed as at this point an alternative treatment modality should become more suitable.

No one treatment modality is suitable for the management of all types of wound, and very few can cope with conditions in the wound bed throughout all stages of healing. It is therefore appropriate to choose the most cost-effective treatment that meets the requirements of the wound and its stage of healing unless use of a specific treatment can be justified on clinical grounds.

Summary

Strategies that optimise the process of tissue repair have evolved as our knowledge and understanding of wound healing has increased. This chapter has shown that technological advances now offer clinicians a bewildering choice of wound treatments that sometimes lead to ineffective decision-making without a clear rationale to underpin practice. The number of clinical guidelines for chronic wound management is growing and is now accessible via the Internet (EPUAP, 2009; AWMA, 2010) and demonstrates a growing consensus on the principles of wound management that help clinicians disseminate best practice.

The poor quality of evidence and uncertainty about effectiveness of advanced treatment modalities compared to standard care means that for the time being the case for routine adoption of these therapies cannot be supported, although they are likely to offer benefits for patients with complex, non-healing wounds. Good-quality studies and collaborative research are urgently required to demonstrate the clinical effectiveness of the principles of wound management that have been practiced for so long.

Useful resources

Australian Wound Management Association (AWMA). (2010) *Wound Management Standards* (2nd edn). Available at: http://www.awma.com.au/publications/2011_standards_for_wound_management_v2.pdf

European Wound Management Association (EWMA). (2008) Position Document: *Hard-to-Heal Wounds: A Holistic Approach.* London: MEP Ltd. Available at: http://www.woundsinternational.com/pdf/content_45.pdf

World Union of Wound Healing Societies (WUWHS). (2004) *Principles of Best Practise: Minimising Pain at Wound Dressing-related Procedures: a Consensus Document.* London: MEP Ltd. February 1st, 2013.

World Union of Wound Healing Societies (WUWHS). (2007) *Principles of Best Practice: Wound Exudate and the Role of Dressings.* London: MEP Ltd. Available at: http://www.woundsinternational.com

World Union of Wound Healing Societies (WUWHS). (2008) *Principles of Best Practice: Vacuum Assisted Closure: Recommendations for Use. A Consensus Document.* London: MEP Ltd. Available at: http://www.woundsinternational.com/pdf/content_37.pdf

US Food and Drug Administration [FDA]. (2009) Advice for Patients: serious Complications with Negative Pressure Wound Therapy Devices. Issued: November 13, 2009. Available at http://www.fda.gov/MedicalDevices/Safety/AlertsandNotices/PatientAlerts/ucm190476.htm. (accessed 16 June 2012).

References

Atiyeh, B.S., Dibo, S.A., Hayek, S.N. (2009) Wound cleansing, topical antiseptics and wound healing. *International Wound Journal*, 6(6), 420–430.

Atiyeh, B.S., Ioannovich, J., Al-Amm, C.A., El-Musa, K.A. (2002) Management of acute and chronic open wounds: the importance of moist environment in optimal wound healing. *Current Pharmaceutical Biotechnology*, 3(3), 179–195.

Australian Wound Management Association. (2010) *Pan Pacific Clinical Practice Guideline for Pressure Injury Prevention and Management*. Osborne Park, WA: Australian Wound Management Association.

Bishop, S.M., Walker, M., Rogers, A.A., Chen, W.Y. (2003) Importance of moisture balance at the wound–dressing interface. *Journal of Wound Care*, 12(4), 125–128.

Bradley, M., Cullum, N., Sheldon, T. (1999) The debridement of chronic wounds: a systematic review. *Health Technology Assessment*, 3(17), iii-iv, 1–78, 28.

Bowler, P.G. (2002) Wound pathophysiology, infection and therapeutic options. *Annals of Medicine*, 34, 419.

Canadian Agency for Drugs Technologies Health [CADTH] (2010) Silver dressings for the treatment of patients with infected wounds: a review of clinical and cost-effectiveness. Ottawa, Canada: CADTH.

Chaby, G., Senet, P., Vaneau, M., et al. (2007) Dressings for acute and chronic wounds: a systematic review. *Archives of Dermatology*, 143, 1297–1304.

Cole, P.S., Quisberg, J., Melin, M.M. (2009) Adjuvant use of acoustic pressure wound therapy for treatment of chronic wounds. A retrospective analysis. *Journal of Wound, Ostomy and Continence Nursing*, 36(2), 171–177.

Cooper, R., Jenkin, R.E. (2012) Synergy between oxacillin and manuka honey sensitizes methicillin-resistant *Staphylococcus aureus* to oxacillin. *Journal of Antimicrobial Chemotherapy*. dks071 first published online March 1, 2012 doi:10.1093/jac/dks071.

Courtenay, M., Church, J.C., Ryan, T.J.J. (2000) Larva therapy in wound management. *The Royal Society of Medicine*, 93(2), 72–74.

Cullen, B., Kemp, L., Essler, L., et al. (2004) Rebalancing wound biochemistry improves healing: a clinical study examining effect of PROMOGRAN. *Wound Repair and Regeneration*, 12(2), A4.

Dissemond, J., Assadian, O., Gerber, V., et al. (2011) Classification of wounds at risk and their antimicrobial treatment with polihexanide: a practice-oriented expert recommendation. *Skin Pharmacology and Physiology*, 24(5), 245–55.

Drosou, A., Falabella, A., Kirsner, R.S. (2003) Antiseptics on wounds: an area of controversy. *Wounds*, 15, 149–166.

Dumville, J.C., Worthy, G., Bland, J.M., et al. (2009) Larval therapy for leg ulcers (VenUS II): randomised controlled trial. *British Medical Journal*, 19(338), b773.

Dykes, P.J., Heggie, R., Hill, S.A. (2001) Effects of adhesive dressings on the stratum corneum of the skin. *Journal of Wound Care*, 10(1), 7–10.

Eming, S.A., Krieg, T., Davidson, J.M. (2007) Inflammation in wound repair: molecular and cellular mechanisms. *Journal of Investigative Dermatology*, 127, 514–525.

Enoch, S., Harding, K. (2003) Wound bed preparation: the science behind the removal of barriers to healing. *WOUNDS*, 15(7), 213–229.

European Pressure Ulcer Advisory Panel; National Pressure Ulcer Advisory Panel (2009) *Prevention and Treatment of Pressure Ulcers: Quick Reference Guide*. Washington, DC: National Pressure Ulcer Advisory Panel. Available at: www.npuap.org and www.epuap.org, retrieved on 23 February 2012.

Falanga, V. (2000) Classifications for wound bed preparation and stimulation of chronic wounds. *Wound Repair and Regeneration*, 8, 347–352.

Feinstein, L., Miskiewicz, M. (2010) Perioperative hypothermia: review for the anesthesia provider. *The Internet Journal of Anesthesiology*, 27(2) (last accessed 1 May.2012).

Fernandez, R., Griffiths, R., Ussia, C. (2004) Effectiveness of solutions, techniques and pressure in wound cleansing. *JBI Reports*, 2, 231–270.

Fernandez, R., Griffiths, R., Ussia, C. (2008) Water for wound cleansing. *Cochrane Database of Systematic Reviews*, Issue 1. Art. No.: CD003861. DOI: 10.1002/14651858.CD003861.pub2.

Flanagan, M. (2005) Barriers to the implementation of best practice in wound care. *Wounds UK Journal*, 1(3), 74–82.

Foster, L., Moore, P. (1997) The application of cellulose fibre dressings in surgical wounds. *Journal of Wound Care*, 6(100), 169–173.

Gray, D. (2010) PHMB and its potential contribution to wound management. *Wounds, U.K.*, 6(2), 40–46.

Haan, J., Lucich, S. (2009) A retrospective analysis of acoustic pressure wound therapy: effects on the healing progression of chronic wounds. *Journal of the American College of Certified Wound Specialists*, 1, 28–34.

Halvorson, E.G. (2007) Wound irrigation in the emergency room: a simple, effective method. *Plastic and Reconstructive Surgery*, 119, 2345–2346.

Hubner, N.O., Kramer, A. (2010) Review on the efficacy, safety and clinical applications of polihexanide, a modern wound antiseptic. *Skin Pharmacology and Physiology*, 23(Suppl), 17–27.

Iheanacho, I. Drug and Therapeutics Bulletin (2010) Silver dressings: do they work? *Drug and Therapeutics Bulletin*, 48(4), 38–42.

Jeffrey, S. (2009) Advanced wound therapies in the management of severe military lower limb trauma: a new perspective. *Eplasty*, 9, e28.

Johnson, D., Lineweaver, L., Maze, L.M. (2009) Patients' bath basins as potential sources of infection: a multicenter sampling study. *American Journal of Critical Care*, 18, 31–40.

Kaehn, K. (2009) An *in-vitro* model for comparing the efficiency of wound rinsing solutions. *Journal of Wound Care*, 18(6), 229–236.

Kaneda, K., Kuroda, S., Goto, N., Sato, D., Ohya, K., Kasugai, S. (2008) Is sodium alginate an alternative haemostatic material in the tooth extraction socket? *Journal of Oral Tissue Engineering*, 5(3), 127–133.

Khan, M.N., Naqvi, A.H. (2006) Antiseptics, iodine, povidone iodine and traumatic wound cleansing. *Journal of Tissue Viability*, 16, 6–10.

Leaper, D.J. (2006) Silver dressings: their role in wound management. *International Wound Journal*, 3, 282–294.

Locke, P.M. (1979) *The Effects of Temperature on Mitotic Activity at the Edges of Experimental Wounds*. Chatham, UK: Lock Laboratories Research.

Main, R.C. (2008) Should chlorhexidine gluconate be used in wound cleansing? *Journal of Wound Care*, 17, 112–114.

Malmsjö, M., Borgquist, O. (2010) NPWT settings and dressing choices made easy. *Wounds International*, 1(3), Available at: http://www.woundsinternational.com. (last accessed 7 November 2012).

Malone, W.D. (1987) Wound dressing adherence: a clinical comparative study. *Archives of Emergency Medicine*, 4(2), 101–105.

MeReC Bulletin (2010) Evidence-based prescribing of advanced wound dressings for chronic wounds in primary care. Vol. 21, No. 1; June 2010. Available at: http://www.npc.nhs.uk/merec/therap/wound/merec_bulletin_vol21_no1.php.

Moffatt, C.J., Franks, P., Hollinworth, H. (2005) Understanding wound pain and trauma: an international perspective. In: *Pain at Wound Dressing Changes*, EWMA, London: MEP Ltd.

Morykwas, M.J., Simpson, J., Punger, K., et al. (2006) Vacuum-assisted closure: state of basic research and physiologic foundation. *Plastic and Reconstructive Surgery*, 117(7 Suppl), 121S–126S.

Mosti, G., Iabichella, M. L., Picerni, P., Magliaro, A., Mattaliano, V. (2005) The debridement of hard to heal leg ulcers by means of a new device based on Fluidjet technology. *International Wound Journal*, 2, 307–314.

Mustoe, T.A., Cooter, R.D., Gold, M.H., et al. (2002) International clinical recommendations on scar management. *Plastic and Reconstructive Surgery*, 110, 560–571.

NICE (2008) Prevention and treatment of surgical site infection. Clinical guideline (CG74)–surgical site infection. Available at: www.nice.org.uk, retrieved on February 1st, 2013.

NICE (2011) MTG5 MIST Therapy system for the promotion of wound healing in chronic and acute wounds: guidance. Available at: http://guidance.nice.org.uk/MTG5/Guidance/pdf/English, retrieved on July 27, 2011.

O'Donoghue, J.M., O'Sullivan, S.T., Beausang, E.S., et al. (1997) Calcium alginate dressings promote healing of split skin graft donor sites. *Acta Chirurgiae Plasticae*, 39(2), 53–55.

Parsons, D., Bowler, P.G., Myles, V., Jones, S. (2005) Silver antimicrobial dressings in wound management: a comparison of antibacterial, physical, and chemical characteristics. *Wounds*, 17(8), 222–232.

Piacquadio, D., Nelson, D.B. (1992) Alginates. A "new" dressing alternative. *Journal of Dermatologic Surgery and Oncology*, 18(11), 992–995.

Queen, D. Understanding hydrofiber technology. *Wounds International*, 1(5). Available at: http://www.woundsinternational.com/journal.php?issueid=328, retrieved on 1 May 2012.

Scales, J.T. (1956) Development and evaluation of a porous surgical dressing. *British Medical Journal*, 2, 962–981.

Schultz, G., Sibbald, R., Falanga, V., et al. (2003) Wound bed preparation: a systematic approach to wound management. *Wound Repair and Regeneration (Supplement)*, 11 (2S), S1–S28.

Segal, H.C., Hunt, B.J., Gilding, K. (1998) The effects of alginate and non-alginate wound dressings on blood coagulation and platelet activation. *Journal of Biomaterials Applications*, 12, 249–257.

Sibbald, R.G., Williamson, D., Orsted, H.L., et al. (2000) Preparing the wound bed – debridement, bacterial balance and moisture balance. *Ostomy/Wound Management*, 46(11), 14–35.

Smeets, R., Ulrich, D., Unglaub, F., et al. (2008) Effect of oxidized regenerated cellulose/collagen matrix on proteases in wound exudate of patients with chronic venous ulceration. *International Wound Journal*, 5(2), 195–203.

Storm-Versloot, M.N., Vos, C.G., Ubbink, D.T., Vermeulen, H. (2010) Topical silver for preventing wound infection. *Cochrane Database of Systematic Reviews*, Issue 3. Art. No.: CD006478. DOI: 10.1002/14651858.CD006478.pub2.

Trengove, N.J., Stacey, M.C., Macauley, S., et al. (1999) Analysis of the acute and chronic wound environments: the role of proteases and their inhibitors. *Wound Repair and Regeneration*, 7, 442.

Trengove, N.J., Bielefeldt-Ohmann, H., Stacey, M.C. (2000) Mitogenic activity and cytokine levels in non-healing and healing chronic leg ulcers. *Wound Repair and Regeneration*, 8, 13.

Thomas, S. (2008) Hydrocolloid dressings in the management of acute wounds: a review of the literature. *International Wound Journal*, 5(5), 2–13.

Thomas S. (2010) *Surgical Dressings and Wound Management*. United Kingdom: Medetec Publications.

Turner, T. (1985) Which dressing and why? In: *Wound Care* (ed S. Westerby). London: Heinemann Medical Books.

Vermeulen, H., Ubbink, D.T., Goossens, A., de Vos, R., Legemate, D.A., Westerbos, S.J. (2004) Dressings and topical agents for surgical wounds healing by secondary intention. *Cochrane Database of Systematic Reviews*, Issue 2. Art. No.: CD003554. DOI: 10.1002/14651858.CD003554.pub2.

Weller, C., Sussman, G. (2006) Wound dressing update. *Journal of Pharmacy Practice and Research*, 36(4), 318–324.

White, R., Morris, C. (2009) Mepital:a non adherent wound dressing with Safetac technology. *British Journal of Nursing*, 18(1), 58–64.

Wilson, J.R., Mills, J.G., Prather, I.D., Dimitrijevich, S.D. (2005) A toxicity index of skin and wound cleansers used on in vitro fibroblasts and keratinocytes. *Advances in Skin & Wound Care*, 18, 373–378.

Winter, G. (1962) Formation of the scab and the rate of epithelialisation of superficial wounds in the skin of the young domestic pig. *Nature*, 193, 293–294.

Wright, J.B., Lam, K., Olson, M.E., Burrell, R.E. (2003) Is antimicrobial efficacy sufficient? A question concerning the benefits of new dressings. *Wounds*, 15(3). Available at: www.woundsresearch.com/article/1583, retrieved April 2010.

6 Wound Infection

Valerie Edwards-Jones[1] and Madeleine Flanagan[2]
[1]School of Research, Enterprise and Innovation, Faculty of Science and Engineering,
Manchester Metropolitan University, Manchester, UK
[2]School of Life and Medical Sciences, University of Hertfordshire, Hertfordshire, UK

Overview

- In clinical practice, wound infection can be difficult to identify and may be mismanaged causing treatment delays and avoidable serious complications.
- Different wound types exhibit different signs and symptoms of infection, so clinicians need to familiarise themselves with the characteristics of infection in the wound aetiologies that they manage most frequently.
- The principles of managing wound infection aim to optimise the patient's ability to fight infection and reduce the number of microbes in the wound.
- Infected or heavily colonised wounds typically produce large amounts of exudate and an offensive odour and are painful. Treatment aimed at reducing the bacterial burden of the wound should alleviate these unpleasant symptoms.
- Antimicrobial therapy should be considered when wound healing is delayed or clinical signs of infection are observed, but indiscriminate use of antimicrobial agents must be avoided.

Introduction

Wound infection is associated with delayed wound healing and increased morbidity. These infections are often difficult to treat and can complicate illnesses, cause distress to patients and their family and may even be fatal. Early recognition and prompt management of infected wounds is therefore important to reduce the associated health and financial consequences.

Patients with wound infections cost more to treat than uninfected patients, and escalating antibiotic resistance is making some infections difficult to treat. Coello et al. (2005) estimated that the cost to treating a surgical site infection is on average £3200 per case. In one study of patients with complicated malignant head and neck wounds, the additional cost of wound infection was three times higher for patients with methicillin-resistant *Staphylococcus aureus* (MRSA) than without MRSA (Watters et al., 2004).

Diagnosing infection in acute wounds is often straightforward because the patient will display clinical signs of inflammation, the first immune

---

Wound Healing and Skin Integrity: Principles and Practice, First Edition. Edited by Madeleine Flanagan.
© 2013 John Wiley & Sons, Ltd. Published 2013 by John Wiley & Sons, Ltd.

response to an attack by microorganisms. These are increased pain, exudate, temperature, redness and swelling. Many of these symptoms are activated by components of the microorganism. There are strict definitions for reporting surgical site infections which help with diagnosis and are categorised as those affecting superficial tissues (skin and subcutaneous layer) and those affecting deeper tissues (deep incision and organ space) based on the Centres for Disease Control and Prevention (CDC) definitions (Horan et al., 1992). However, diagnosis of infection in chronic wounds is made more difficult because the wound is often heavily colonised by mixed microorganisms and the patient does not always elicit a host response. The characteristics for identifying wound infection are summarised in Figure 6.1. The laboratory will report the presence (and approximate numbers) of potential pathogens with associated antibiotic sensitivities but they cannot determine whether the presence of the microorganism actually indicates active infection.

Bacterial invasion of the skin

Skin provides a variety of microenvironments for a diverse range of microorganisms existing in a balanced relationship and form the normal (commensal) flora. The types and abundance of normal skin flora varies in different areas of the body and this is dependent upon the microenvironment. For example, the perineum, axilla and toe webs have increased levels of moisture and surface lipids. This leads to increased diversity and a higher number of microorganisms than the rest of the body. Typical microorganisms found on the skin are members of the Micrococcaceae, coryneforms, *S. aureus, Staphylococcus epidermidis, Staphylococcus lugdunensis, Staphylococcus hominis,* alpha haemolytic streptococci and *Propionobacterium* spp. (Evans et al., 1950).

Commensal floras do not break the natural skin barrier unless the host is injured or becomes immunosuppressed. Transient microorganisms may affect the dynamic interrelationship with resident normal flora, upsetting the ecological balance and may predispose to infection, especially if they are invasive pathogens. Once the epithelial barrier is breached, the normal host response is initiated with local inflammation, which protects the host (patient) and initiates healing. If the injury is extensive, infection may develop as microorgan-

isms that previously colonised the skin invade the tissues. The exact relationship between microorganisms in the wound and delayed healing is still poorly understood and requires further research (Percival et al., 2012).

Chronic wounds are known to have an elevated bioburden (Siddiqui and Bernstein, 2010). As bacterial load increases, wound healing is significantly delayed as the normal inflammatory response excessively releases cytotoxic enzymes, free oxygen radicals and inflammatory mediators that cause extensive collateral damage to the host tissue (Bowler, 2003; Han et al., 2011). Pathogenic microorganisms responsible for wound infection prolong healing by producing endotoxins that cause broad damage to the host by destroying cells and disrupting normal cellular metabolism producing further tissue necrosis (Han et al., 2011). This results in a prolonged inflammatory response which increases matrix metalloproteinases (MMPs) production and breaks down the extracellular matrix (ECM), interrupting wound contraction, reduces tensile strength and delays epithelialisation." Invading microorganisms or their toxins may overwhelm this local protective response causing local tissue damage (necrosis) progressing to systemic sepsis and death. Synergistic mixed aerobic and anaerobic bacteria can have a greater net pathogenic effect and are often present in chronic wounds (Bowler, 2003).

Wound pathogens

Different wound types do not provide identical conditions and so support different communities of microorganisms. Common wound pathogens can be broadly divided into Gram-positive and Gram-negative aerobic and anaerobic bacteria, occasional fungi and very occasionally specific viral pathogens.

Depending upon the specific pathogen, the clinical symptoms of wound infection may differ due to the virulence of the microorganism and the immune response of the host. For example, *S. aureus* produces an array of virulence factors such as coagulase which breaks down fibrinogen to fibrin causing abscesses; protein A which attracts macrophages; type A haemolysin which kills leucocytes, lyses platelets and red blood cells. *Pseudomonas aeruginosa* typically produces a green pigment (pyocyanin) which is cytotoxic and also produces exotoxin A

Acute Wounds
e.g. surgical or traumatic wounds or burns

Localised infection	Spreading infection

• Classical signs and symptoms
     – New or increasing pain
     – Erythema
     – Local warmth
     – Swelling
     – Purulent discharge
 • Pyrexia – in surgical wounds, typically five to seven days post-surgery
 • Delayed (or stalled) healing
 • Abscess
 • Malodour
	As for localised infection PLUS:
	 • Further extension or erythema
	 • Lymphangitis
	 • Crepitus in soft tissues
	 • Wound breakdown/dehiscence

Notes
- Burns – also skin graft rejection; pain is not always a feature of infection in full thickness burns
- Deep wounds – induration, extension of the wound unexplained increased white cell count or signs of sepsis may be signs of deep wound infection
- Immunocompromised patients – signs and symptoms may be modified and less obvious

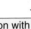

Systemic infection

Sepsis – documented infection with pyrexia or hypothermia, tachycardia, tachypnoea, raised or depressed white blood cell count
↓
Severe sepsis – sepsis and multiple organ dysfunction
↓
Septic shock – sepsis and hypotension despite adequate volume resuscitation
↓
Death

N.B. Other sites of infection should be excluded before assuming that systemic infection is related to wound infection

Chronic Wounds
e.g. diabetic foot ulcers, venous leg ulcers, arterial leg/foot ulcers or pressure ulcers

Localised infection	Spreading infection
• New increased or altered pain* • Delayed (or stalled) healing • Peri wound oedema • Bleeding or friable (easily damaged) granulation tissue • Distinctive malodour or change in odour • Wound bed discolouration • Increase or altered/purulent exudate • Induration • Pocketing • Bridging	As for localised infection PLUS: • Wound breakdown • Erythema extending from wound edge • Crepitus, warmth, induration or discolouration spreading into peri wound area • Lymphangitis • Malaise or other non-specific deterioration in patient's general condition

Notes
- In patients who are immunocompromised and/or who have motor or sensory neuropathies, symptoms may be modified and less obvious. For example, in a diabetic patient with an infected foot ulcer and peripheral neuropathy, pain may not be a prominent feature
- Arterial ulcers – previously dry ulcers may become wet when infected
- Clinicians should also be aware that in the diabetic foot, inflammation is not necessarily indicative of infection. For example inflammation may be associated with Charcot's arthropathy

*Individually highly indicative of infection. Infection is also highly likely in the presence of two or more of the other signs listed

Figure 6.1   Criteria for identifying wound infection (WUWHS, 2008). Reproduced with permission from Wounds International.

which inhibits protein synthesis. *S. aureus* delays wound closure by secreting anti-angiogenic factors and anti-inflammatory properties and inhibits leukocyte function (Athanasopoulos et al., 2006). *Streptococcus pyogenes* (group A strep) is a dangerous wound pathogen because the invasive properties of many of the virulence factors produced cause cellulitis and occasionally necrotising fasciitis. This devastating infection can spread rapidly and destroy skin, fat, muscle tissue and fascia (Green et al., 1996). Management should consist of immediate resuscitation, radical surgical excision and administration of broad-spectrum intravenous antibiotics.

There are a large number of rarer bacterial pathogens that can cause skin infections, and the clinician should always be mindful of these, especially if the patient is associated with animals, has recently travelled to the tropics or has unusual hobbies or occupations. For example, *V. vulnificus* can cause radical fasciitis and if not treated promptly can be fatal. Infection is seen in traumatic wounds acquired in or associated with coastal waters and seafood (Horseman and Surani, 2011). Fish Fanciers Finger is caused by a minor abrasion becoming infected with *Mycobacterium marinum* which is found frequently in fish tanks. The incubation time is variable (2–89 weeks) and small papules form which enlarge and ulcerate forming granulomatous lesions (Bhatty et al., 2000). *M. ulcerans* is found less frequently but can cause Buruli's ulcers which often start as painless nodular swellings that progress to extensive destruction of skin and soft tissue with the formation of large ulcers on the legs or arms. Delayed treatment may cause irreversible deformity or long-term functional disability (Nakanaga et al., 2011).

Factors increasing the risk of wound infection

Some individuals are actually more susceptible to chronic wound infections because they have other complications that weaken the immune system such as diabetes, renal impairment or even surgery (James et al., 2008). Extremes of age are also considered an important factor, with neonates and the elderly at particular risk of cutaneous infection. Nutritional status and lifestyle choices such as alcohol and drug abuse, smoking and lack of exercise or sleep can create stress, which can have an adverse affect on the immune system, predisposing certain individuals to an increased risk of infection.

Endogenous host factors and exogenous bacterial factors cause an imbalance of the production and degradation of the ECM of the wound bed and becomes static. The loss of skin integrity and exposure of underlying tissue provides a nutritious, moist, warm microenvironment that encourages bacterial multiplication and proliferation. The type and abundance of microorganisms depends on the location of the wound, depth, oxygen supply, host factors and level of tissue perfusion (Dowd et al., 2008). Devitalised tissue facilitates microbial proliferation especially if there is an accumulation of associated foreign material and increases the bioburden to inhibit wound healing. The wound becomes static and continues in a state of chronicity until something breaks the cycle (Bjarnsholt et al., 2008; James et al., 2008).

Specific wound characteristics also increase the likelihood of infection making particular types of wounds susceptible to infection such as chronic wounds and contaminated traumatic wounds.

The significance of bacteria within wounds

The complete removal of bacteria from a wound is not possible or necessary as despite being colonised by bacteria most wounds heal uneventfully. The microorganisms capable of causing cutaneous infection can be derived from endogenous or exogenous sources and superficial infection will normally occur in the outer layers of the skin. However, some microorganisms may invade the deeper, subcutaneous layers depending upon their ability to causing disease by breaking down the protective mechanisms of the host. This is called the virulence or pathogenicity of the microorganism (Bowler et al., 2001). Virulence factors can be divided into surface-associated virulence and excreted virulence factors. Surface-associated virulence is a general term used to describe the way in which bacteria adhere to the cell surface during the first stage of the infectious process. Examples of these include hydrophobicity of cell surface, capsules, glycocalyx, slime layers, fimbriae, lipopolysaccharide (LPS) outer membrane proteins (OMPs) and other adhesins. Excreted virulence factors include toxins

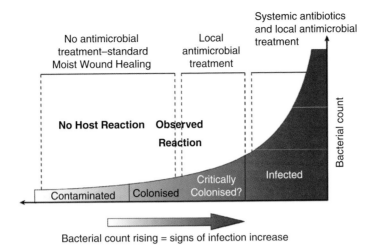

Figure 6.2   Clinical significance of bacteria in wounds.

or enzymes excreted into the surrounding environment to allow the microorganism to invade into deeper tissues. This array of toxins and enzymes varies depending upon the microorganism but can kill phagocyte cells, destroy cell membranes, inhibit complement and cause metabolic imbalance of the cell (Edwards-Jones, 2010).

Factors determining the effects of bacterial multiplication on the tissue surrounding a wound are unclear, but critical factors include the number, type and virulence of the invading microorganisms as well as the ability of the individual's immune system (host resistance) to fight the organisms. The clinical significance of bacteria in wounds is shown in Figure 6.2.

Microorganisms are likely to enter the wound from three main sources: the surrounding skin, mucous membranes of the host and the external environment.

Bacteria within a wound lead to three outcomes:

● contamination;
● colonisation;
● infection.

Contamination

Contamination of a wound begins shortly after the skin barrier is breached usually by exogenous or endogenous organisms. The organisms do not increase in number as the wound environment or nutrients are not available to support multiplication so there is no host response (no signs of inflammation or other signs of overt infection) and the organisms are transient. The wound is not affected by the presence of these organisms and exhibits no signs of infection.

Colonisation

Bacterial colonisation is where the organisms become established in the wound environment but still does not elicit a host response. The microorganisms begin to multiply but slow down due to the host response or a lack of nutrients resulting in an equilibrium between growth and death of the microorganism. Wound healing is not impaired and no tissue damage occurs. At this point, the microorganisms can either slow replication or produce virulence factors (if capable) to release other nutrients. This is sometimes called critical colonisation and refers to wounds in which the bacterial burden is increased above superficial contamination levels but below overt infection, and wound healing is delayed (Jørgensen et al., 2005; Leaper, 2006). Further research is required to demonstrate if critical colonisation represents the transition from colonisation to infection, or the transition between acute and chronic inflammation.

Practice point

Critical colonisation is usually associated with a static, painful wound but without a noticeable host reaction which makes it difficult to identify in clinical practice. Signs to look for are subtle but may include an increase in adherent slough that is difficult to remove from the wound bed, the presence of friable and discoloured granulation tissue and increasing odour and serous exudate. Wound debridement and application of topical antimicrobial treatments could help tip the balance in favour of colonisation by reducing the number of bacteria present in the wound.

Infection

Only pathogens capable of producing toxins and enzymes can invade the tissues and cause true infection. If the wound environment provides the right conditions (nutrients, warmth), the microorganisms will multiply and the bioburden increases as they begin to invade and damage the surrounding tissues and initiate a host response. At this point, the wound begins to show signs of infection which may be difficult to detect (Edwards-Jones, 2010). If left untreated, the bacteria will cause spreading infection and septicaemia which can be fatal.

Significance of biofilms

Bacteria in wounds attach and colonise surfaces through a variety of different mechanisms and can form microcolonies and complex communities referred to as biofilms, which are more common in chronic wounds (James et al., 2008). Biofilms are thought to be the 'natural habitat' of bacteria often consisting of several different species of bacteria (but can be a single species) embedded in a polysaccharide matrix which is excreted by the microbe and creates a physical barrier that prevents phagocytosis by inflammatory cells (James et al., 2008). Bacteria in biofilms are dynamic and can alter their structure and develop a slower metabolic rate and growth pattern. This, alongside the protective effect of the ECM, makes bacteria growing in a biofilm more resistant to host defences and conventional antimicrobial therapy is less effective (Mitchell et al., 2011). *Pseudomonas* species are particularly effective at forming biofilms and treatment is complicated further by their ability to rapidly acquire antibacterial resistance (Wu et al., 2011). Figure 6.3 shows a venous leg ulcer with

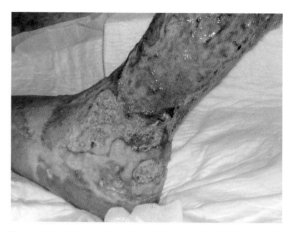

Figure 6.3   Venous leg ulcer with extensive biofilm on the wound surface caused by *Pseudomonas*. Photo courtesy of Shiu-Ling Briggs.

extensive biofilm on the wound surface caused by *Pseudomonas*.

Once the mature biofilm forms, individual free-floating bacterial cells (planktonic cells) can separate from the biofilm through a process called dispersion and colonise other susceptible sites, e.g. a biofilm in the mouth (plaque) can release streptococci which get into the bloodstream and colonise the heart valves to cause endocarditis. Although biofilms have been implicated in wound infections, there is little *in vivo* data showing their role in the pathogenesis of wound infection and this is an area where further research needs to be undertaken (Thomson, 2011). Biofilms allow the bacteria to live in a state of equilibrium and unless there is some form of disruption such as wound debridement (physical disruption) or antiseptic cleansing (chemical disruption), they will continue *ad infinitum*.

Identifying wound infection

When the skin barrier is breached an acute inflammatory response is initiated that leads to the familiar signs of redness, elevated temperature, localised swelling and pain. Apart from the physical barrier there are a number of cells such as keratinocytes, dendritic cells, mast cells, macrophages and Langerhans cells which release chemical signals that lead to the production of antibodies. The diagnosis of wound infection is primarily a clinical skill based on evaluation of the external characteristics of the wound, the surrounding skin and the patient.

Microbiological data should be used to supplement the clinical diagnosis (Cooper, 2005). However, wound infection is often over- or underdiagnosed, even when positive wound cultures have been obtained. Accurate diagnosis of wound infection relies on an accurate history and examination of the patient and consideration of the factors likely to increase the risk of infection. The criteria for identifying wound infection can be seen in Figure 6.1 (WUWHS, 2008).

Clinical signs and symptoms

The clinical signs of wound infection may differ from individual to individual so require close examination of the wound and surrounding skin over a period of time so that subtle changes can be identified and documented. To ensure early detection and prompt treatment of wound infection, clinicians need to correlate the clinical features of infection with patient outcomes and microbiological data (EWMA, 2005; WUWHS, 2008). Wound infection in patients with a healthy immune response is typically easy to identify; however, in immune-compromised individuals with chronic wounds, diagnosis may be more difficult as local signs of infection may be subtle or absent.

The classic signs of infection include localised erythema, pain, heat, oedema and can be seen in Figure 6.4 which shows an infected venous leg ulcer with extending cellulitis.

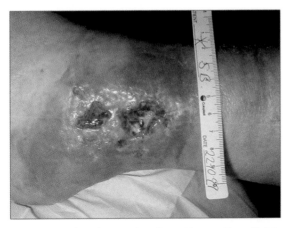

Figure 6.4   Infected venous leg ulcer with spreading cellulitis. Photo courtesy of Ray Norris.

Additional criteria are evolving as evidence accumulates that infection produces specific signs and symptoms in different types of wounds (Cutting and Harding, 1994; EWMA, 2005; WUWHS, 2008).

Reliable signs of infection, even in immune-compromised patients, are wounds that bleed easily or are very painful (Gardner et al., 2001; Reddy et al., 2012).

Microbiological assessment of wounds

The clinical diagnosis of wound infection can be difficult. Any evidence of cellulitis or wound breakdown needs immediate response and appropriate antimicrobial therapy. Laboratory confirmation of acute infection is helpful, when deciding on the appropriate antibiotic therapy. This is especially the case when there is evidence of infection at a surgical site.

In general, it has been shown that acute wounds tend to be colonised by a single pathogen, if infected. However, diagnosis of infection in a chronic wound is more difficult as there are often multiple microorganisms present growing in a biofilm and their pathogenicity is not easy to determine due to an interaction of a number of different microorganisms (Dowd et al., 2008; James et al., 2008). Isolation of a single pathogen from a heavily contaminated wound does not necessarily mean that it is causing an infection as it may have become part of the resident contaminating flora.

Obtaining accurate wound cultures

Laboratory testing by the microbiology department is undertaken to identify known pathogens responsible for wound infection and to determine likely susceptibility to specific antimicrobial agents. The process is called microscopy, culture and sensitivity (C&S). The pathology request form should be completed with as much relevant information as possible to improve the result. Table 6.1 shows the minimum data required for pathology wound culture request.

The most commonly used technique for obtaining a wound swab samples the wound by zigzagging across the surface of the wound (Z swab technique). Another sampling method is the Levine technique, which involves rotating a sterile swab

Table 6.1   Minimum data required for pathology wound culture request

Patient details	Name, age, gender, record
Wound type	Acute, chronic, e.g. venous leg ulcer, surgical incision (hip replacement)
Wound/surgical site details	Anatomical location (indicate left or right side of the body), wound size, chronicity (duration)
Risk factors	Comorbidities, e.g. diabetes, malnutrition, haematoma, foreign bodies
Clinical concerns	Delayed healing, wound dehiscence, increased pain, bleeding granulation tissue, pus formation
Treatment details	Specify any oral/intravenous antibiotics, antimicrobial dressings used in past 48 hours; immunosuppressive agents, recent surgical debridement
Specific tests required	*Pseudomonas*, MRSA

over a 1 cm^2 area of the wound whilst applying local pressure to extract exudate from wound bed (Levine et al., 1976). Studies comparing sampling techniques have shown that a more accurate assessment of bacterial numbers and diversity of species in the wound was obtained using the Levine method over the Z swab technique. Furthermore, specimens obtained using the Levine technique were found to be accurate when compared with tissue cultures obtained by punch biopsy, which is an invasive, painful procedure (Gardner et al., 2006; Angel et al., 2011).

Practice point

What is the most accurate method of taking a wound culture to determine susceptibility to specific antimicrobial agents?

Current consensus indicates that wounds should be cleaned before taking a sample for microbiological analysis and any superficial necrotic tissue removed, as the bacteria deeper within the wound bed will cause the infection rather than bacteria on the surface of the wound. However, there is limited evidence to recommend which is the best method of collecting microbiological samples, although the Levine method is currently considered to be the most accurate. Cleansing is also important as residues from topical antiseptic agents or dressings may contami-

nate the swab and inhibit the growth of microorganisms if the wound is not thoroughly cleaned before the sample is taken. If possible, fresh pus or wound exudate should be expressed (facilitated using the Levine approach) and the swab tip moistened with normal saline or the clear medium in the swab container to increase effectiveness. The swab should be taken by pressing the centre of the wound bed for 15 seconds over an area of clear, exposed granulation tissue.

The swab container should be carefully labelled and the pathology request form completed. Many laboratories will not accept an unlabelled or partially labelled swab and will discard them. The wound swab should be transported at room temperature and not in a fridge. They should be sent to the microbiology laboratory as soon as possible – preferably within 24 hours, but no later than 48 hours – as there is often microbial overgrowth of those with a rapid growth rate compared to those with a slower rate. The swabs contain culture medium that will maintain the viability of the organism and absorb toxic products that could kill them *in situ*. However, microbiologists need to receive swabs as soon as possible because some organisms overgrow and overwhelm others, e.g. coliforms grow more quickly than staphylococci.

The role of the wound biopsy as a sampling technique is controversial and the original work and validation was undertaken in acute burn wounds. Quantitative assessment and histological investigation were included and it was showed that bacterial counts were consistently over 10^5 cfu/g and depth of invasion could be detailed. However, acute burn wounds are typically infected with a single bacterial species (or occasionally two species) and although tissue biopsy gives extremely important information to aid diagnosis in burn wounds, it is not advisable to try to reproduce this diagnostic technique in chronic wounds due to problems with interpretation of results. Most clinical microbiology laboratories will not process wound biopsies because this technique is outside normal standard operating procedures.

The accuracy of culturing the bacteria from a wound swab is determined by the method used, the skill of the operator and the time taken between collection and analysis of results. The whole exercise is futile if the results are not followed up and acted upon.

Practice point

What happens to a wound swab once it is sent to the microbiology laboratory?

Processing of the swab in the laboratory is relatively standard unless the person assessing the wound indicates the need for a certain microorganism to be screened, e.g. MRSA or *Mycobacterium* sp or for further tests. In the laboratory the swab is streaked onto a variety of solidified culture media and streaked out to allow for growth of single colonies of bacteria or fungi. This helps with isolation of certain pathogens.

Many of the primary culture media contain selective agents to allow certain pathogens to grow, for example MRSA. The plates are incubated for up to 48 hours at 37°C to allow growth of bacteria and also are placed in different environments to allow growth of anaerobic organisms should they be present. Special cultures for slow-growing organisms, such as fungi or mycobacteria, may require several weeks.

Interpretation of results

The limitations of bacterial isolation are numerous and interpretation of results from the laboratory has to be done in conjunction with the clinical appearance of the wound and the condition of the patient. It is very important to follow up the results from the wound swab to identify which organisms have been isolated and the appropriate sensitivities even if the wound appears to be improving.

In chronic wounds such as pressure ulcers and leg ulcers, there may be mixed populations of the same species in the wound which can affect virulence and the potential to cause infection (Hansson et al., 1995). The interaction of the microorganisms and their potential synergistic virulence in chronic wounds is never investigated because this is not the remit of most clinical laboratories.

Practice point

How should I interpret the results reported on the pathology form?

Following 48 hours of incubation, the culture plates are inspected for growth. In the case of an acute wound, there is often only a single organism which will be identified and reported with an antibiotic sensitivity. However, in the case of a chronic wound, there is often a heavy, mixed growth of a variety of different microbes. In this case, the biomedical scientist will look for known potential wound pathogens, e.g. *S. aureus*, *Pseudomonas* sp, *E. coli*, and report with an appropriate antibiotic sensitivity. The other microbes in the mixture will be reported as mixed skin flora (e.g. micrococci, diphtheroids and coagulase-negative staphylococci) or mixed faecal organisms (indicating they are probably contaminating the wound bed and have been derived from the gut). Some laboratories restrict the reporting of the antibiotic sensitivity

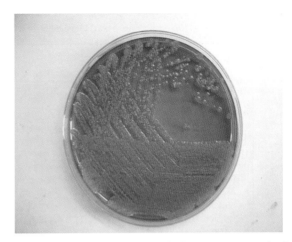

Figure 6.5   A cultured wound swab showing +++ growth of mixed bacteria. Photo courtesy of Valerie Edwards Jones.

because of inappropriate use and overuse of antibiotics, and those laboratories which do report antibiotic sensitivities expect the clinician will only prescribe if the patient requires them. Qualitative data are provided to indicate the numbers of bacteria present with + indicating a light growth, ++ a moderate growth and +++ a heavy growth. Figure 6.5 shows a cultured wound swab showing +++ growth of mixed bacteria.

Principles of managing infected wounds

Many superficial bacterial infections will resolve on their own without treatment, however others may require treatment with a topical antimicrobial. Deep infection which is spreading will require antibiotic therapy. Close monitoring of any wound suspected to be critically colonised or infected is important so that appropriate treatment can be implemented and specialist referral instigated (if required). The principles of managing wound infection are summarised in Figure 6.6.

The principles of managing infected wounds aim to restore the balance between the patient's immune status and the infecting microorganism(s) by:

- improving the patient's general health by optimising management of comorbidities and minimising factors increasing the risk of infection;
- reducing the bioburden of the wound by preventing further contamination, debriding

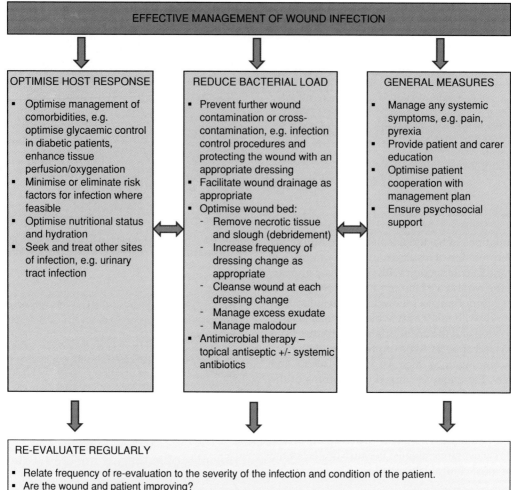

EFFECTIVE MANAGEMENT OF WOUND INFECTION

OPTIMISE HOST RESPONSE

- Optimise management of comorbidities, e.g. optimise glycaemic control in diabetic patients, enhance tissue perfusion/oxygenation
- Minimise or eliminate risk factors for infection where feasible
- Optimise nutritional status and hydration
- Seek and treat other sites of infection, e.g. urinary tract infection

REDUCE BACTERIAL LOAD

- Prevent further wound contamination or cross-contamination, e.g. infection control procedures and protecting the wound with an appropriate dressing
- Facilitate wound drainage as appropriate
- Optimise wound bed:
  - Remove necrotic tissue and slough (debridement)
  - Increase frequency of dressing change as appropriate
  - Cleanse wound at each dressing change
  - Manage excess exudate
  - Manage malodour
- Antimicrobial therapy – topical antiseptic +/- systemic antibiotics

GENERAL MEASURES

- Manage any systemic symptoms, e.g. pain, pyrexia
- Provide patient and carer education
- Optimise patient cooperation with management plan
- Ensure psychosocial support

RE-EVALUATE REGULARLY

- Relate frequency of re-evaluation to the severity of the infection and condition of the patient.
- Are the wound and patient improving?
- Is the wound starting to heal?
- Systemic monitoring and recording of symptoms is helpful in detecting improvement or deterioration. Consider use of an appropriate assessment tool. Serial clinical photographs or tracking changes in markers of inflammation (e.g. erythrocyte sedimentation rate (ESR), C-reactive protein (CRP), white blood cell count) may be useful in registering subtle deterioration or improvement, especially in chronic wounds.

Figure 6.6   Management of wound infection. Reproduced with permission from Wounds International.

necrotic tissue, removing excess exudate and by the commencement of antimicrobial treatment;
- effectively managing symptoms associated with cutaneous infection, e.g. pyrexia, pain, cellulitis.

Improving immune status

Consideration of an individual's host resistance is an important aspect of patient assessment. Patients receiving immunosuppressive agents and steroids as well as those with protein-calorie malnutrition have increased susceptibility to bacterial infection usually controlled by the inflammatory response. In reality, most seriously ill patients will have an altered immune response and decreased host resistance making wound infection more likely. Effective management of patients with infected wounds requires a multidisciplinary team approach that should actively involve microbiologists, infection control specialists and senior management.

Referral to specialist medical colleagues particularity in relation to management of comorbidities is essential to improve the patient's resistance to microorganisms.

Reducing wound bioburden

Meticulous attention to infection-control policies will minimise contamination or cross-contamination of the wound and should be routinely adopted by healthcare professional regardless of whether patients are known to have an infection. Effective handwashing is the single most important infection-control measure and should be carried out after every patient contact.

The surface of any wound thought to be infected needs to be cleaned or debrided to ensure that organic matter such as slough, extracellular products, biofilm and exudate are removed as they are the ideal growth media for microorganisms. The most effective wound cleanser has not yet been identified (Moore and Cowman, 2005; Fernandez and Griffiths, 2008). There are a number of methods available for debridement and choice needs to consider assessment of the patient and the wound. Studies have shown that there is a brief period immediately after wound debridement when organism numbers are reduced and the biofilm is disrupted. At this point the application of a topical antimicrobial dressing may help stimulate wound healing (Wolcott et al., 2010).

The accumulation of pus, slough and wound fluid within a wound will encourage multiplication of microorganisms. Drainage methods are dependent on resource availability and will include absorbent dressings, insertion of wound drains, topical negative pressure therapy and surgical intervention. These local measures may be sufficient to reduce the bioburden to allow healing to resume without the need for systemic antibiotic therapy.

Antimicrobial treatment

If it is suspected that the wound infection is spreading or becoming systemic then antimicrobial therapy may be required. Antimicrobial is a general

term to describe substances used to treat infection and includes antiseptics and antibiotics. Antibiotics act selectively on a specific target site, whereas topical antiseptics have multiple targets with a broad spectrum of activity and associated toxicity. Therefore, the choice of antiseptic used in wound care should be one that provides sustained antimicrobial activity, does not impede healing and has the least potential for local or systemic toxicity. In addition, there should be limited accumulation of the antimicrobial agent in the surrounding tissues that may cause harm systemically to the patient. Antibiotics are able to selectively target bacteria, so can be used in low concentrations.

Antimicrobial agents should not be used indiscriminately and must be used for limited periods of time and effectiveness should be frequently reviewed. Factors influencing choice of topical antimicrobials for treatment of infected wounds should be based on (EWMA, 2006; WUWHS, 2008):

- clinical efficacy;
- cost and reimbursement issues;
- availability;
- ease of use.

The clinical indications for use of topical antimicrobials and systemic antibiotics for wound management are described in Table 6.2.

Worries about the toxic effects of topical antiseptics in animal studies have restricted their use despite an inconclusive evidence base (EWMA, 2006; Leaper, 2011). Meta-analyses and systematic reviews on the use of topical antimicrobials in chronic wounds have revealed a lack of evidence to support their use which is likely to be due to the challenges of conducting outcomes research in patients with chronic wounds and recruitment difficulties rather than clinical ineffectiveness (Leaper, 2011).

If chronic wounds become critically colonised or infected, newer formulations of topical antimicrobials such as silver, iodine, honey and polyhexamethylene biguanide (PHMB) impregnated into dressings can help reduce the bioburden and prevent infection without inhibiting wound healing (WUWHS, 2008; Leaper, 2011) (see Chapter 5).

Antimicrobial treatments must show activity against microorganisms that are typically isolated

Table 6.2   Indications for use of antimicrobial therapy in wounds

	Topical antimicrobials	Systemic antibiotics
Prevention of wound infection or recurrence in high-risk patients[a]	✓	✕
Superficial wound infection	✓	✕
Deep wound infection	✕	✓
Localised infection	✓	✕
Spreading infection, e.g. cellulitis, lymphangitis	In combination with systemic antibiotics	✓
Wound infection + systemic symptoms, e.g. bacteraemia, sepsis	In combination with systemic antibiotics	✓
Beta-haemolytic streptococci[b]	✕	✓
Bone involvement[c]	✕	✓
Presence of antibiotic resistant bacteria	✕	✓

[a]Contaminated surgical wounds, dirty traumatic wounds, e.g. degloving injuries.
[b]Even in the absence of clinical signs of infection.
[c]These conditions may require extended oral treatment and/or treatment with intravenous antibiotics.

from wounds such as *S. aureus* (including MRSA), *P. aeruginosa*, *Streptococcus pyogenes* and other haemolytic streptococci. Topical antimicrobials incorporated into wound dressings should release the antimicrobial agent slowly or affect a targeted release. If there is no alteration in the wound condition after 10–14 days, then a change in antimicrobial treatment should be considered together with further debridement and a wound culture should be sent for C&S. If the wound is progressing well and signs of infection have resolved, wound management should follow the principles of best practice and antimicrobial therapy be discontinued.

When appropriately used, systemic antibiotics effectively treat infection and prevent serious complications. In addition to the criteria listed above, selection of antibiotic for treatment of a wound infection will depend on antibiotic susceptibility of the known or suspected pathogen(s), severity and degree of spread of infection, patient factors, e.g. allergies, comorbidities and local treatment policies.

Unless the patient has systemic signs and symptoms or a limb is at risk, microbiology results should be waited for before deciding to use antibiotics. If it is necessary to commence treatment before identifying antibiotic susceptibility, a broad-spectrum antibiotic should be selected and the results of C&S reviewed as soon as possible.

Practice point

Are topical antibiotics effective at preventing wound infection?

Topical antibiotics have been used as prophylaxis for post-operative wound care for many years, despite a lack of evidence to support their use. There is growing evidence, although studies are small, that topical antibiotics do not improve wound healing for the treatment of clean surgical wounds and are an unnecessary expense, can produce contact dermatitis, increase drug resistance and can, rarely, cause anaphylaxis (Draelos et al., 2011; Trookman et al., 2011).

There is also no convincing evidence demonstrating the superiority of topical antibiotics over the use of topical antimicrobials for management of chronic wounds. Topical antibiotics are not able to penetrate deep wound infections and may be systemically absorbed when applied to larger wounds. Topical antibiotics may cause hypersensitivities. The common causes of sensitivity reactions include neomycin, framycetin, gentamicin and sodium fusidate (Draelos et al., 2011). The risks of toxicity, sensitization and bacterial resistance outweigh any benefits that topical antibiotics might have in the treatment of wound infection.

Patients with chronic wounds receive significantly more antibiotic prescriptions (both systemic and topical) than age- and sex-matched patients (Howell-Jones et al., 2005). Current guidelines for antibiotic prescribing for wounds are often based on expert opinion rather than scientific evidence. The relationships between antibiotic resistance, chronic wound microbiology and the rationale for antibiotic therapy have yet to be determined. As a result, published guidelines do not recommend the use of topical antibiotics for chronic wounds (IWGDF, 2007; EPUAP, NPUAP, 2009).

Symptom management

Infected or heavily colonised wounds carrying a high microbial load tend to generate a large amount of exudate and an unpleasant odour. Choice of appropriate dressings should be based on their ability to absorb exudate, contain odour and control microbial contamination which will increase wear time and necessitate fewer dressing changes (see Chapter 5).

Pain is one of the earliest symptoms of wound infection and occurs before any clinical signs of infection are evident in the wound. This makes it a reliable indicator of wound infection which should not be ignored (Gardner et al., 2001). The inflammatory response initiated by invading microorganisms is the underlying cause of the wound pain which is often described as a tender or intense, throbbing pain. The release of inflammatory mediators in the infected wound and surrounding tissues results in oedema and tissue damage which stimulates the peripheral pain receptors to produce pain of increasing intensity. Patients will often notice that infection-related pain feels different to previously felt wound pain (Cutting et al., 2005). Any change in type of wound pain or sudden onset of pain is therefore a significant indicator for infection. Treatment aimed at reducing the bacterial burden of the wound should help to alleviate infection-related wound pain. The use of broad-spectrum antimicrobial dressings and anti-inflammatory analgesia can be particularly effective.

Summary

Management of patients with infected wounds requires an understanding of the significance of microorganisms in wounds, a knowledge of the criteria to identify localised and systemic infection and the ability to select appropriate treatment options. Adoption of the infection control and management measures described in this chapter will result in lower rates of wound infection, decreased morbidity, shorter duration of treatment and a more rapid return to health for patients. For healthcare organisations this will help to prevent the spread of infection, reduce treatment costs and avoid litigation.

Future research into rapid diagnostic methods of wound infection may well include self-diagnostic dressings where biosensors detect metabolic products from the host or bacteria that are indicative of a non-healing wound due to infection or wound stasis induced by high bacterial bioburden. This is an area of huge research potential as the increasing number of elderly patients with chronic wounds creates a financial burden for the healthcare environment.

Useful resources

Wound infection and pain management made easy. (2010) *Wounds International*. Available at: http://www.woundsinternational.com/made-easys/wound-infection-and-pain-management-made-easy

Biofilms made easy. (2010) *Wounds International*. Available at: http://www.woundsinternational.com/made-easys/biofilms-made-easy

Wound infection in clinical practice: an international consensus. (2008) *World Union of Wound Healing Societies*. Available at: http://www.woundsinternational.com/clinical-guidelines/wound-infection-in-clinical-practice-an-international-consensus

Clinical Knowledge Summaries: nail and skin: boils, carbuncles, whitlows. Available at: http://www.cks.nhs.uk/home

References

Angel, D.E., Lloyd, P., Carville, K., Santamaria, N. (2011) The clinical efficacy of two semi-quantitative wound-swabbing techniques in identifying the causative organism(s) in infected cutaneous wounds. *International Wound Journal*, 8, 176–185.

Athanasopoulos, A.N., Economopoulou, M., Orlova, V.V., et al. (2006) The extracellular adherence protein (Eap) of *Staphylococcus aureus* inhibits wound healing by interfering with host defense and repair mechanisms. *Blood*, 107, 2720–2727.

Bhatty, M.A., Turner, D.P., Chamberlain, S.T. (2000) *Mycobacterium marinum* hand infection: case reports and review of literature. *British Journal of Plastic Surgery*, 53, 161–165.

Bjarnsholt, T., Kirketerp-Møller, K., Jensen, P.Ø., et al. (2008) Why chronic wounds will not heal: a novel hypothesis. *Wound Repair and Regeneration*, 16, 2–10.

Bowler, P.G. (2003) The 10(5) bacterial growth guideline: reassessing its clinical relevance in wound healing. *Ostomy Wound Management*, 49, 44–53.

Bowler, P.G., Duerden, B.I., Armstrong, D.G. (2001) Wound microbiology and associated approaches to wound management *Clinical Microbiology Reviews*, 14, 244–269.

Coello, R., Charlett, A., Wilson, J., Ward, V., Pearson, A., Borriello, P. (2005) Adverse impact of surgical site infections in English hospitals. *Journal of Hospital Infection*, 60, 93–103.

Cooper, R.A. (2005) Understanding wound infection European Wound Management Association (EWMA). Position Document. In: *Identifying Criteria for Wound Infection*. London: MEP Ltd.

Cutting, K., White, R.J., Mahoney, P., Harding, K.G. (2005) Clinical identification of wound infection: a Delphi approach. European Wound Management Association (EWMA). Position Document. In: *Identifying Criteria for Wound Infection*. pp. 6–9. London: MEP Ltd.

Cutting, K.F., Harding, K.G. (1994) Criteria for identifying wound infection. *Journal of Wound Care*, 3, 198–201.

Dowd, S.E., Sun, Y., Secor, P.R., et al. (2008) Survey of bacterial diversity in chronic wounds using pyrosequencing, DGGE, and full ribosome shotgun sequencing. *BMC Microbiology*, 8, 43.

Draelos, Z.D., Rizer, R.L., Trookman, N.S. (2011) A comparison of postprocedural wound care treatments: Do antibiotic-based ointments improve outcomes? *Journal of the American Academy of Dermatology*, 64, S23.

Edwards-Jones, V. (2010) The science of infection. *Wounds UK*, 6(2), 86–93.

European Pressure Ulcer Advisory Panel and National Pressure Ulcer Advisory Panel (2009) *Treatment of Pressure Ulcers: Quick Reference Guide*. Washington, DC: National Pressure Ulcer Advisory Panel.

European Wound Management Association (EWMA) (2005) *Position Document: Identifying Criteria for Wound Infection*. London: MEP Ltd.

European Wound Management Association (EWMA) (2006) *Position Document: Management of Wound Infection*. London: MEP Ltd.

Evans, C.A., Smith, W.M., Johnston, E.A., Giblett, E.R. (1950) Bacterial flora of the normal human skin. *The Journal of Investigative Dermatology*, 15, 305–324.

Fernandez, R., Griffiths, R. (2008) Water for wound cleansing. *Cochrane Database of Systematic Reviews*, (1). Art. No.: CD003861. DOI: 10.1002/14651858. CD003861.pub2.

Gardner, S.E., Frantz, R.A., Doebbeling, B. (2001) The validity of the clinical signs and symptoms used to identify localized chronic wound infection. *Wound Repair and Regeneration*, 9, 178–186.

Gardner, S.E., Frantz, R.A., Saltzman, C.L., Hillis, S.L., Park, H., Scherubel, M. (2006) Diagnostic validity of three swab techniques for identifying chronic wound infection. *Wound Repair and Regeneration*, 14, 548–557.

Green, R.J., Dafoe, D.C., Raffin, T.A. (1996) Necrotizing fasciitis. *Chest*, 110, 219–229.

Han, A., Zenilman, J.M., Melendez, J.H., et al. (2011) The importance of a multifaceted approach to characterizing the microbial flora of chronic wounds. *Wound Repair and Regeneration*, 19, 532–541.

Hansson, C., Hoborn, J., Moller, A., Swanbeck, G. (1995) The microbial flora in venous leg ulcers without clinical signs of infection. *Acta Dermato-Venereologica*, 75(1), 24–30.

Horan, T.C., Gaynes, R.P., Martone, W.J., Jarvis, W.R., Emori, T.G. (1992) CDC definitions of nosocomial surgical site infections, 1992: a modification of CDC definitions of surgical wound infections. *Infection Control and Hospital Epidemiology*, 13(10), 606–608.

Horseman, M.A., Surani, S. (2011) A comprehensive review of *Vibrio vulnificus*: an important cause of severe sepsis and skin and soft-tissue infection. *International Journal of Infectious Diseases*, 15, 157–166.

Howell-Jones, R.S., Wilson, M.J, Hill, K.E., Howard, A.J., Price, P.E., Thomas, D.W. (2005) A review of the microbiology, antibiotic usage and resistance in chronic skin wounds. *Journal of Antimicrobial Chemotherapy*, 55, 143–149.

International Working Group on the Diabetic Foot (2007) International Consensus on the Diabetic Foot and Practical Guidelines on the Management and the Prevention of the Diabetic Foot. Amsterdam, the Netherlands, on CD-ROM (www.idf.org/bookshop).

James, G.A., Swogger, E., Wolcott, R., et al. (2008) Biofilms in chronic wounds. *Wound Repair and Regeneration*, 16, 37–44.

Jørgensen, B., Price, P., Anderson, K.E., et al. (2005) The silver-releasing foam dressing, Contreet foam, promotes faster healing of critically colonised venous leg ulcers: a randomised, controlled trial. *International Wound Journal*, 2, 64–73.

Leaper, D. (2011) Topical antiseptics in wound care: time for reflection. *International Wound Journal*, 8, 547–549.

Leaper, D.J. (2006) Silver dressings: their role in wound management. *International Wound Journal*, 3, 282–294.

Levine, N.S., Lindberg, R.B., Mason, A.D., Pruitt, B.A. (1976) The quantitative swab culture and smear: a quick simple method for determining the number of viable aerobic bacteria on open wounds. *Journal of Trauma*, 16(2), 89–94.

Mitchell, R.J., Lee, S.K., Kim, T., Ghim, C.M. (2011) Microbial linguistics: perspectives and applications of microbial cell-to-cell communication. *BMB Reports*, 44, 1–10.

Moore, Z.E.H., Cowman, S. (2005) Wound cleansing for pressure ulcers. *Cochrane Database of Systematic Reviews*, (4). Art. No.: CD004983. DOI: 10.1002/14651858. CD004983.pub2.

Nakanaga, K., Hoshino, Y., Yotsu, R.R., Makino, M., Ishii, N. (2011) Nineteen cases of Buruli ulcer diagnosed in Japan, 1980–2010. *Journal of Clinical Microbiology*, 49, 3829–3836.

Percival, S.L., Emanuel, C., Cutting, K.F., Williams, D.W. (2012), Microbiology of the skin and the role of biofilms in infection. *International Wound Journal*, 9, 14–32.

Reddy, M., Gill, S.S., Wu, W., Kalkar, S.R., Rochon, P.A. (2012) Does this patient have an infection of a chronic wound? *JAMA*, 307(6), 605–611.

Siddiqui, A.R., Bernstein, J.M. (2010) Chronic wound infection: facts and controversies. *Clinics in Dermatology*, 28, 519–526.

Thomson, C.H. (2011) Biofilms: do they affect wound healing? *International Wound Journal*, 8, 63–67.

Trookman, N.S., Rizer, R.L., Weber, T. (2011) Treatment of minor wounds from dermatologic procedures: a comparison of three topical wound care ointments using a laser wound model. *Journal of the American Academy of Dermatology*, 64, S8.

Watters, K., O'Dwyer, T.P., Rowley, H. (2004) Cost and morbidity of MRSA in head and neck cancer patients: what are the consequences? *Journal of Laryngology and Otology*, 118, 694–699.

Wolcott, R.D., Rumbaugh, K.P., James, G., et al. (2010) Biofilm maturity studies indicate sharp debridement opens a time-dependent therapeutic window. *Journal of Wound Care*, 19, 320–328.

World Union of Wound Healing Societies (WUWHS) (2008) *Principles of Best Practice: Wound Infection in Clinical Practice. An International Consensus.* London: MEP Ltd. Available at: www.mepltd.co.uk

Wu, D.C., Chan, W.W., Metelitsa, A.I., Fiorillo, L., Lin, A.N. (2011) Pseudomonas skin infection: clinical features, epidemiology, and management. *American Journal of Clinical Dermatology*, 12, 157–169.

7 Psychological Impact of Skin Breakdown

Patricia Price
School of Healthcare Studies, Cardiff University, Cardiff, UK

Overview

- Patients with skin breakdown and open wounds can experience a wide range of symptoms that affect their ability to live their lives as they wish.
- Many patients adapt to a progressive illness which may require lifelong behaviour change.
- Some patients will experience psychological problems (e.g. anxiety or depression) which will require health professionals to develop strong therapeutic relationships with patients and their carers to help patients cope with their skin problems.
- The relationship between stress and healing is not fully understood: initial findings suggest that experiencing stress may delay wound healing.
- There are few studies that have fully evaluated psychological interventions in patients with skin breakdown, although initial work is promising.
- Health professionals must recognise that dealing with psychological or emotional problems may require additional or specialist training, and should be aware of their own stress levels – particularly when working in healthcare systems with few options for referral to specialist centres.

Introduction

Health psychology is a very substantial area of study; important concepts can only be discussed briefly in this chapter, which will focus on those topics that are most directly related to individuals with skin breakdown.

Many areas of health psychology overlap and have been artificially divided in order to structure this chapter. However, it is important to remember that none of these issues can be considered in isolation; for example it is difficult to discuss issues of adherence to treatment without knowing about the personal and demographic factors of a patient, their belief systems about health and pain, the stress experienced, the amount of social support and the coping strategies available. Many healthcare services/facilities have very limited access to health or clinical psychologists – often due to funding or resource issues, so other professional groups have to incorporate psychological aspects of care into their routine practice even though they may find this stressful, as they feel underprepared to take on these additional roles (Wilkes et al., 2003; Kornhaber and Wilson, 2011).

Psychological impact on the individual and society

The relationship between loss of skin integrity and psychological status, in terms of causing skin breakdown or preventing it from healing, has always been controversial. However, it is quite clear that people with skin disorders and open wounds often experience a range of psychological problems associated with alterations in physical appearance and daily symptom management.

Problems often focus on three key areas:

(1) The visibility of the skin condition means that social situations, in particular, become very difficult.
(2) Changes in body image resulting from the skin problem can lead to psychological distress, and high levels of psychological morbidity.
(3) Living with symptom management on a daily basis can lead to the skin condition/wound dominating daily living experiences, so individuals can become isolated and depressed as they manage their pain, lack of mobility, wound leakage and associated malodour.

However, these experiences are part of a broader phase of adapting to a state of illness, including the associated stress and the coping with change that come with accepting lifelong changes in behaviour which may be needed, and for some, recognising that a life of dependency on others may lie ahead.

Adaptation to chronic illness

Chronic illness is a generic term that covers a wide range of illnesses, diseases and conditions. Many of those working with patients with dermatological conditions and wounds are aware that patients are at different points in the process of adapting to their condition and that a range of factors will affect how this process occurs.

Practice point

What type of questions could I ask to help understand what someone is feeling when living with a chronic, non- healing wound or skin conditio?

You could consider asking:

- How does your wound/skin condition make you feel?
- Do you want to know more about the symptoms you might experience?
- Are there friends or family that you would like to be present when we review treatment options? What do you think they will be concerned about?
- How do you fit treatment into your everyday life?
- What do think may lie ahead?

These questions may start a discussion where the patient can lead the conversation to areas of concern, but it is really important to build such questions into developing (and maintaining) a positive therapeutic relationship with the patient. You will need to ensure that you are fully engaged in the conversation – with no distractions (such as your mobile phone ringing, or taking notes) – so that you are *actively* listening to what the patient has to say. Often the patient will ask 'Why me?' questions and it is important to realise that they may not expect a direct answer, but they do want someone to hear their voice.

Stress and skin disease

The link between emotional state and illness has been the focus of debate for many years, and raises a number of interesting questions, e.g. why does the same stressful situation result in such a range of responses from individuals? One clear reason is that the perception of the same situation varies between individuals, as does the predisposition towards disease/health condition. Having a predisposition towards a disease/condition does not mean that it is inevitable that an individual will develop it, as the stress part of the relationship can account for how the predisposition translates into the presentation of the disorder; for example, atopic eczema has a genetic component, but that is not the whole story – a deeply held fear of developing such a condition may evoke a chronic stress response, which impacts on your immune system and makes you more susceptible to the environmental factors that also play a role. As yet, we do not have a detailed understanding of the links between psychological health and skin disorders, or the mechanisms that activate a predisposition into actual disease progression.

Recent work has highlighted the multidimensional nature of 'stress' as it comprises physiological, psychological and sociological factors (Soon and Action, 2006). From a physiological perspective, stress can result in raised levels of the hormone cortisol, which if raised for prolonged periods of time can affect both immunity and inflammatory responses (Segerstrom and Miller, 2004). Recent reviews have focused on the potential stress related to managing the symptoms associated with skin breakdown, particularly for those living with chronic wounds (Solowiej et al., 2009), whilst Walburn et al. (2009) concluded from their meta-analysis of human wound healing that the negative impact of stress ($r = -0.42$, medium effect) is broadly consistent across a wide range of wound types. Their work shows that increased stress is associated with both impaired healing and dysregulation of biomarkers across acute and chronic wounds. However, this work only includes one study on patients with a chronic wound as very little work has been completed in this area to date, with data on other skin conditions yet to be collected.

The poor clinical outcomes associated with patients with diabetic foot ulcers (DFU) has prompted a detailed investigation of the role of stress in this patient group, with the work of Vileikyte and colleagues (2007, 2010) and Vedhera et al. (2010) demonstrating the complexity of the relationship between stress and tissue repair, as researchers search for the mechanism of action. Further work is needed to confirm whether the relationship between stress and healing is consistent; this is particularly important given the known relationship between stress and behaviours such as poor sleep patterns, poor nutrition, less exercise and abuse of alcohol, cigarettes and drugs (Baum and Posluszny, 1999).

Depression

Anecdotally, clinicians report that patients with chronic wounds present with depression but the data are inconclusive. Jones and colleagues (2006) explored the prevalence of anxiety and depression in 190 patients with chronic venous ulceration in England, using the Hospital Anxiety and Depression Scale (HADS). They reported that 52 (27%) people were reported as depressed, while 50 (26%)

scored as anxious, with the symptoms of pain and odour most closely related to both anxiety and depression. This research was followed by qualitative interviews (Jones et al., 2008, p. 56) which demonstrated that, particularly for those with a first leg ulcer, leakage and odour had an 'all-consuming impact on people's ability to get on with everyday living'.

For patients with diabetes who have already developed peripheral neuropathy, a study by Gonzalez et al. (2010) that followed 333 patients for 18 months (63 developed a foot ulcer) concluded that self-reported depression is associated with an increased risk of developing a first foot ulcer. Also in 2010 Williams et al. published an American population-based prospective cohort study of 3474 adults with type 2 diabetes and no prior DFU or amputations, who were followed up for a mean of 4.1 years. In this study, major and minor depression was assessed by the Patient Health Questionnaire-9 at baseline and followed up by a review of medical records: these results suggest that whilst 80% of patients reported no depression, there was a twofold risk of developing a foot ulcer in those with major depression.

However, a study by Vedhera et al. (2010) concludes that neither depression nor anxiety predicted healing at 24 weeks in a study of 93 patients with *active* DFU. Winkley et al. (2007) observed that depression predicts mortality over 18 months, but was not associated with DFU recurrence or amputation, in contrast to the findings of Monamy et al. (2008) who concluded that DFU healing at 6 months and recurrence over 12 months were associated with greater depression in patients with diabetes. These contradictory results support the idea that depression may play a different role in the *prevention* of ulceration rather than actual *healing*, and support a call for psychological interventions that address depressive symptoms before skin breakdown occurs (Vedhera et al., 2010).

We must also be aware that those individuals with mental health problems may also experience wound problems; many fall outside those routinely included in wound healing literature (e.g. factitious or self-harming wounds) (see Chapter 17). Kilroy-Finlay (2010) concludes that many of the tissue viability issues experienced by patients with mental health issues may be exactly the same as those who present routinely in the primary care setting; however, the management of such patients requires practitioners to be much more innovative in working with patients to find ways to help them adhere to treatment.

Adjustment to physical change/disfigurement

Whether a patient has lived with their skin condition from childhood or acquired the condition as an adult, all individuals will undergo a period of adjustment. Many of those who experience such changes to their physical self can experience shock, denial, anger and sadness before coming to terms with their 'new' face or body.

However, it is important to remember that not everyone reacts in exactly the same way – sometimes this is due to the severity of the condition, although research has shown that those with less 'severe' changes often experience more psychological distress than those with more severe changes (Robinson, 1997). There are also other factors that can relate to adjustment – the situation is so complex, that many of the following factors interact with each other, as shown in Figure 7.1.

Some individuals will cope quite successfully due to their own personality and the support of their family and friends, whilst others may need some additional professional support to help them face the problems of living with a skin condition. Neither group is any 'better' in terms of adjustment than the other – they simply have different ways of coping.

Coping strategies

Coping is seen as a process by which individuals try to manage the perceived difference between the demands they experience and the resources they have to deal with these demands. For example, patients can be overwhelmed by the time demands of treatment, having to continually ask for time off work to go for appointments, juggling the needs of their family and may go through phases when they feel they do not have the energy or skills to keep managing everything. The strategies that people use to cope with demanding situations include a range of thought processes (e.g. thinking positively) and actions (e.g. seeking information). These strategies are often grouped into 'approach' (e.g. trying to deal with the problem head on, confronting the problem) or 'avoidance' (e.g. distracting attention) strategies (Moos and Schaefer, 1984). For example, some patients want to find out everything they can about their illness, start making lists of what needs to be done and who can help (these would be seen as 'approach' strategies), whilst others can deny that there is a problem and refuse to change their behaviour, or increase their drinking behaviour to avoid thinking about their new situation (these would be classified as 'avoidance strategies'). Vedhera et al. (2010) suggest that patients who used an 'approach' style of coping may be associated with non-healing in patients with diabetic foot wounds; this is a very surprising result as approach strategies have traditionally been thought to result in positive outcomes, and demonstrates

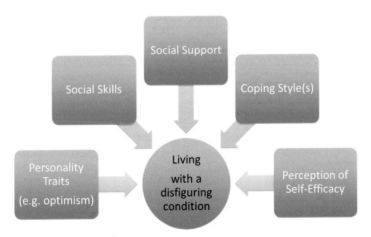

Figure 7.1   Interrelated factors that affect a patient's ability to live successfully with a disfiguring condition.

that we need to know more about coping strategies in patients with skin breakdown.

Many patients report that it is not only 'society' that is unaware of the complexities of their situation, but that often healthcare professionals (HCPs) are unhelpful or dismissive – skin conditions are usually not life-threatening, and the problems are often thought of as purely cosmetic and therefore not that important. Many patients report that the longer they live with their condition, the easier it is to cope with it (Patterson et al., 1993), and that the quality of the social support they receive is also important, with the positive involvement of family and friends making a real difference to patients (Papadopoulos and Bor, 1999).

Social support

Social support is a widely used term that refers to the amount and type of support received by social contacts: 'Social support is the perceived comfort, caring, esteem or help a person receives from other people or groups' (Wills, 1984, p. 34). Although some work has looked at the amount of support an individual receives, many researchers (e.g. Cohen and Wills, 1985) feel that the quality and function of the support experienced is more important than the number of people in an individual's personal network.

Social support can be divided into:

- *emotional support* including the expression of empathy, caring and concern, providing companionship, a shoulder to cry on, etc.; and
- *practical support* including financial assistance, providing information, advice, suggestions, etc.

Positive social support is beneficial to the patient as this can help in the adjustment and coping process. However, individuals do not always receive such support. Some people are unlikely to receive support if they are unsociable, do not help others or do not let others know that they need help – this could be because they are not assertive enough, do not know whom to ask, do not want to lose their independence nor become a burden to others. Some segments of society are at risk of not getting support: men tend to have larger social networks than women, but women use their networks more efficiently, whilst many elderly individuals live alone (Sarafino, 1994).

Body image

We live in a society that is dominated by two key issues related to body image: the 'body beautiful' and 'beauty equals goodness'. You do not have to think for long to realise the extent to which society is dominated by these concepts. An example is the amount of money spent on cosmetics and the pressure in the media to 'look good'. It is important to remember that these values are 'socially constructed'; that is they are defined by the society that we live in and the values are not 'absolute'.

One of the main problems in the literature, particularly outside the area of eating disorders, is that the term 'body image' has been used in an ill-defined way. However, many clinicians are familiar with the definition by Price (1990), who proposed that body image is the totality of how we feel and think about our bodies and its appearance; many of the assumptions behind the model have not been tested empirically, and as a result, writers such as Gournay et al. (1997) state that the model is purely speculative.

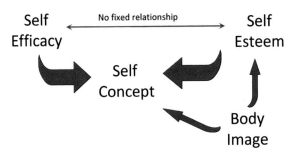

Figure 7.2   'Self' and body image.

Many clinicians report that those with body image difficulties also experience low self-esteem. Self-esteem is a personal resource that may moderate the effects of disfigurement, incapacitating illness and injury or threatening life events. We know that an altered body image can lead to negative self-esteem in patients who experience acute wounds following trauma, those with dermatological conditions and those that live with long-term disfigurement.

However, very often these findings are reported incidentally to the quality-of-life data (e.g. Phillips, 1994; Walshe, 1995). In such studies, the lack of self-esteem that is reported following leg ulceration may be due to any number of symptoms, or related to the overall impact of the experience. The complex ways in which self-esteem, self-efficacy and body image are interrelated are summarised in Figure 7.2.

For those with a skin condition or an open wound it can often be difficult to disguise the fact that their skin is different, especially if exposed areas are affected. Be careful not to assume, however, that those whose condition cannot be seen will have no problems – this is clearly not the case. For example, a female whose skin is affected in those parts of her body that define her sexuality may have extreme problems in developing intimate relationships. Patients with pressure ulcers report the physical changes affected both their self-concept and their body image (Gorecki et al., 2009). Many skin conditions occur intermittently or are progressive, and this element of uncertainty can add to feelings of insecurity about how others will react (Jowett and Ryan, 1985).

For those living with disfigurement or visual scarring, the reaction of society to them because they 'look different' can have serious consequences for their psychological health. Most people are uncertain of how to react when they meet someone who

'looks different', and one of the biggest challenges for individuals with a skin condition is coping with the reactions of others. Although some individuals experience rude comments and intrusive questions, many of the messages from others are non-verbal, such as staring, avoiding eye contact or avoiding the person altogether. Over time such avoidance behaviour can lead to feelings of lack of self-worth, wanting to avoid social situations, difficulties in making new friends or forming new intimate relationships (Porter et al., 1990). Indeed, many individuals who experience such behaviour can become either depressed (and withdraw from society) or angry (and distance people even further).

> **Practice point**
>
> **Stop and think about your own practice – do you stereotype patients or label the patients you care for? If so, ask yourself why? If not, can you think of anyone you work with who has either intentionally or unintentionally stereotyped patients? What impact does this have on the way you and your colleagues work together?**
>
> One of the key factors to address this is that the response from others is not always negative: many people stare initially because they are curious or feel sympathy for the individual. Many avoid making eye contact because they are embarrassed that they will do or say the wrong thing, and are aware that they do not really know how to behave. However, over time this reaction of society can lead to a 'self-fulfilling prophecy', whereby the individual with a skin condition expects to be treated differently and becomes sensitised to such behaviour, and focuses on it when it occurs (Partridge, 1994).

Living with skin breakdown and chronic wounds: symptom management

This chapter has given a clear indication that living with a skin condition can result in a heavy burden in terms of everyday social situations. However, it must also be remembered that the physical symptoms of the condition can also have a major impact; the pain associated with very dry and cracked skin, the itching that can drive individuals to distraction, interrupted sleep and, in some cases, the lack of human contact through touch.

It is also important to remember that the use of medications, treatments and topical preparations can be expensive, and they are difficult and time-consuming to apply, so that the time needed to treat the condition can be considerable. The intermittent and progressive nature of skin conditions can mean that individuals feel they have no control over their condition or their lives. Individuals will go to great lengths to avoid exposing their skin, and restrict their social activities so that they need not expose their skin to others. Such experiences, together with the reactions of others outlined above, indicate a profound effect on everyday living. Qualitative research in this area has highlighted specific issues associated with living with a chronic wound, such as fear about odour and leakage (Hopkins, 2004; Spilsbury et al., 2007), pain and its management (Flanagan et al., 2006; Price et al., 2008), mobility, anxiety, depression and frustration with the healing process (Mudge, 2007), lack of sleep and increased frequency of dressing and bandage changes (Flanagan et al., 2006), which highlight the difficulties associated with symptoms that may dominate a person's everyday life (Price, 2007). Work in this area has shown that an improvement in daily life quality is an important health outcome that may, in the short term, affect a person's motivation to continue with treatment in the long term (Speight et al., 2009).

Although pain is not the only symptom that patients experience, there is little doubt that pain has a major impact on everyday living, as patients with wounds experience high levels of constant, persistent pain, as well the pain from the interventions necessary to care for their wounds (e.g. dressing changes) (Price et al., 2008; Gorecki et al., 2009). Despite the clinical assumption that DFU are not painful, recent work has suggested that this is a genuine problem for many patients which has been underestimated (Benstsson et al., 2008; Yunus and Rajbhandari, 2011; Bradbury and Price, 2011a, 2011b).

In 2002, the European Wound Management Association (EWMA) produced a position document on pain, followed in 2004 by the World Union of Wound Healing Societies consensus statement on key issues related to minimising pain at dressing change. Both these documents represent an important step forward in our understanding of pain as applied to this patient group. Unfortunately, the psychological aspects of pain, its perception and treatment in this special group have yet to be fully investigated. However, a trial of a community intervention programme showed pain-level improvements and improved ulcer healing for those with extra focus on information sharing and preventive care for the patient (Edwards et al., 2005). This approach could be a model to help with the considerable emotional aspects of wound pain.

A synthesis of qualitative studies on patients with leg ulcers (Briggs and Flemming, 2007) clearly demonstrates that living with the physical symptoms associated with an open, chronic wound dominated the data from all 12 studies included in the review. In addition to pain, patients reported odour, itch, leakage and infection as problems. The relationship with the professional was described in both positive and negative ways: positive themes focused on therapeutic value, provision of continuity of care, providing strategies to cope with a chronic condition and whenever possible, aiding the patient to regain control of their lives. The negative comments from the data included disputes between patients and their HCPs, being given conflicting advice, and across a number of studies ($n = 8$) patients perceived there to be a lack of time, trust, empathy and understanding – patients felt they were not listened to, and dissatisfaction with treatment was highlighted. Although not all papers focused on psychological problems, many papers reported feelings of embarrassment associated with the leg ulcer, the negative impact on body image, fear of amputation, negative self-esteem, anger, depression (in some cases linked to suicidal thoughts) and a general sense of loss of identity (as the wound dominated their lives).

The authors conclude that many professionals work to a code of practice whereby the emphasis is on the route to healing, with the assumption that a healed wound will improve quality of life. However, they also note that aiming for healing may not be the most appropriate route for those with large, hard-to-heal wounds or for those whose wound duration is extensive as this may 'initiate a spiral of hopelessness' (Briggs and Flemming, 2007, p. 326).

Measuring impact of skin breakdown

Many of the concepts discussed in this chapter make intuitive sense to clinicians, but for psychological and person-focused concepts to fit into evidence-based clinical practice, they need to be measureable so that we can assess whether treatments/interventions are available to improve the patient experience as well as relevant clinical outcomes. The assessment of health-related quality of life (HRQOL) or health status comes under the general heading of Patient Reported Outcome Measures (PROMs), and has increased in importance since regulatory bodies and governments have emphasised the need to include data on the impact of treatment on the individual patient.

The term health-related quality of life (HRQOL) is a specific term used to measure the effect of chronic health conditions on patients in order to gain a better understanding of how an illness interferes with a person's day-to-day life, and research in this area has been helpful in improving services in some diseases (e.g. cancer; Velikova et al., 2004). However, it is a difficult concept to define because it is such a complex phenomenon. It is therefore considered as being composed of separate domains, such as physical functioning, social life and well-being. HRQOL has been used in the field of wound healing to measure the effect of living with chronic wounds in different patient populations (Persoon et al., 2004; Palfreyman, 2008; Gorecki et al., 2009; Green and Jester, 2010; González-Consuegra and Verdú, 2011); many reviews consistently report that patients with chronic non-healing wounds tend to display lower mean HRQOL domain scores than healthy adults or than patients with healed wounds (Price and Harding, 2000; Armstrong et al., 2008).

In recent years, a number of generic and condition specific instruments have been developed to calculate a person's HRQOL. Generic tools have been designed to compare the impact of a range of health states and so include general questions about health status, whilst condition-specific tools have been designed to measure the impact of a particular condition or illness on those patients. However, no single assessment tool can suit every purpose or application, and therefore it is important to choose an appropriate assessment tool that is both valid and reliable for the patient group under investigation as misinterpretation of results can be detrimental. Recent reviews have attempted to summarise condition-specific tools for certain wound types; for example, Hogg et al. (2012) have provided an overview of current condition-specific tools available for patients with diabetic foot wounds and concluded that there was no one patient-reported outcome identified as a 'gold standard' at this time.

Factors affecting treatment

It is important to stress the importance of the patient–practitioner relationship in helping patients to come to terms with their skin condition or wound. Many patients look to HCPs to provide them with help in dealing with the psychological problems associated with their condition, as well as help with clinical treatment. The importance of good communication patterns cannot be overemphasised as patients, whether adults or children, need someone who will see beyond the skin condition/wound to the person. Through supportive communication, HCPs can help patients to understand their condition, support them through lifelong behaviour change and assist in negotiating agreed care plans. Most problems associated with skin problems are not life-threatening and dermatology/wound issues are often dealt within an outpatient or community setting. Indeed, many patients often try initially to deal with the skin breakdown themselves, under the guidance of family and friends, before approaching a professional caregiver (Briggs and Flemming, 2007), which suggests that we may not be aware of the hidden burden of skin care problems. The increasing recognition of the psychological distress that can be experienced by some patients has lead to the development of multidisciplinary teams, ideally working together to ensure patients are able to manage their treatment as well as the underlying condition.

Compression therapy is the treatment that is advocated with a strong evidence base for the management of patients with chronic venous ulceration, but the major inconvenience accompanying the use of compression bandages creates the need for rigorous adherence over a long period of time (Moffatt, 2004). The proportion of those healing appears to be directly related to adherence, yet for some patients, adherence to compression systems has been reported as poor (Edwards et al., 2002). Patients are also undergoing a wide range of more complex treatments in response to their complex skin conditions; for example, patients with open wounds reported on their experiences using *negative pressure* (Moffatt et al., 2011) and described the negative impact of not understanding why their wounds failed to heal, matched with the positive experiences associated with a treatment that dealt with copious exudate levels. This study highlights the positive change in patient's experience that can follow from a relationship with HCPs who were able to effectively communicate information about the potential positive benefits of interventions, and manage patient expectations appropriately.

A patient's relationship with their HCP has frequently been highlighted in the literature as having an influence on adherence to treatment (Vermeire et al., 2001). A collaborative relationship with the HCP has been shown to encourage more patient control, better self-esteem and improved coping strategies (Douglas, 2001; Hareendran et al., 2005). Nevertheless, HCPs are often accused of not listening to patients or not adequately explaining treatments to patients (Charles, 1995), and there is little research which questions the influence of HCPs' beliefs about patients on their professional decision-making.

Patients' frustration with the healthcare system has been shown to encompass the whole management of their condition ranging from transport difficulties, inconsistency of treatment, lack of confidence in the HCP and a sense of being forced/coerced into treatment strategies, sometimes against their will (Rich and McLachlan, 2003). Two discerning factors that influence patient adherence are a belief that the treatment is worthwhile and a belief that the treatment is uncomfortable (Jull et al., 2004). The main drawback of compression therapy has been described as discomfort and intolerance, which can be exacerbated by incorrect application (Tonge, 1995). Demographic details such as age, sex, marital status, number of people in the household and social class have consistently been observed as poor indicators of treatment adherence (Vermeire et al., 2001). Patients may feel that too many demands are being expected of them and as time passes without 'cure', enthusiasm may wane.

Many patients with wound-healing difficulties are also coping with the management of a chronic disease or chronic condition that requires them to make lifestyle behaviour changes, e.g. managing glucose levels through diet and exercise. Many find it difficult to make such changes, and often experience feelings of powerlessness when faced with such challenges. Motivation is fundamental to adherence and the key to developing individual motivation is personal self-awareness and knowledge (Wilkinson, 1997); hence clinicians often focus on the concept of empowerment when working with patients over extended time periods in order to fully engage them in the process of behaviour change, although there is very little research work underpinning its use in patients with wounds.

'Empowerment' as a concept has been the focus of discussion for the past 20 years, and was defined in 2010 by Anderson and Funnell (p. 277) as 'a process designed to facilitate self directed behaviour change'. However, the definition is not accepted by all. Indeed, some have gone so far as to argue that the whole concept is not well-understood (Asimakopoulou et al., 2011), that there is confusion between 'empowerment' and a 'patient-centred' approach (Holstrom and Roing, 2010) and that some researchers use the term as an alternative to 'compliance', where patients are responsible for their choices and the consequences of those choices (Aujoulat et al., 2008).

> ### Practice point
>
> It can be very difficult to maintain motivation to adhere to treatment or keep to lifelong changes in behaviour. Think about ways in which you could help patients with this ongoing problem.
>
> You might want to think about the following tips:
>
> - Patients are all different and need advice that suits the way they live their lives: a more personal approach often makes it easier for patients to accept advice.
> - Work with patients and listen to the reasons they use to explain their difficulties; this can help to agree on a treatment plan that fits into their everyday lives.
> - Explain that lifelong changes take time; using positive feedback is important to keep patients motivated.
> - Be reasonable – changing everything in one go is impossible; break down the changes into smaller steps with realistic goals, so that patients can see their own success.
> - Avoid giving mixed messages or contradictory advice, as this leads to confusion and patients feel there is little point in changing behaviour, as the 'experts' cannot agree on what is best. This means staff must work as a team, and ensure good communication across the professions involved in patient care.
> - Make sure patients really understand what you have advised them to do: it can help to ask patients to report back to you what they understand has been agreed.

Norris et al. (2001) reviewed the effectiveness of management training in type 2 diabetes and found evidence to support an improvement in patients' knowledge and self-care skills, but this did not necessarily lead to an improvement in glycaemia control or cardiovascular risk factors. In 2010, Dorresteijn et al. published their updated systematic review on patient education for preventing diabetic foot ulceration, and concluded that there is insufficient robust evidence that simple patient education alone can lead to a clinically relevant reduction in ulcer and amputation incidence. This conclusion may reflect the complex and multidimensional nature of patient empowerment that may be needed for sustained behaviour change.

Healthcare systems also need to consider the ways in which self-management can be built into a framework of care, particularly knowing the projected increase in the elderly population (Bloom et al., 2011), many of whom will present with wound problems, and the anticipated worldwide increase in diabetes (and associated complications) (Mainour et al., 2007; Lauterbach et al., 2010). These increases will happen at a time when there is likely to be a reduction in the percentage of skilled HCPs (as a proportion of the population) due to the forecasted balance of numbers in the workplace compared with the proportion of the population of retirement age (Bloom et al., 2011). It is almost inevitable that we will need to develop professional–patient partnerships, increase collaborative care and self-management education and 'empower' people to think critically and make informed decisions in partnership with HCPs.

Interventions

The form of psychological intervention with the most evidence of success is cognitive behavioural therapy (CBT). This is a term used to describe a programme of therapy to work on how people think and behave in relation to problem areas (e.g. pain) and to help the patient manage and cope with the situation. The first principle of cognitive behavioural assessment is that an individual's behaviour is determined by their immediate situation and their interpretation of that situation (e.g. many patients see pain as ruling their lives and cannot see how this can change without pharmacological intervention).

The programme is always time-limited, with clearly agreed-upon goals. A programme should include positive reinforcement of 'well' behaviour, increasing general fitness and developing insight into the nature of self-defeating thought patterns and the 'evidence' that individuals use to justify

them. There have been several systematic reviews of CBT for adults with chronic pain (Malone and Strube, 1988; Flor et al., 1992; Turner et al., 1996; Morley et al., 1999), each of which concluded that there is good evidence of effectiveness, especially when compared with no-treatment controls or education alone. However, there is also evidence that the success of CBT is dependent on the experience and quality of the therapist. Recent work in Canada has shown that a programme of group CBT session led to short-term improvements in anxiety, depression, stress and quality of life for 60 patients with diabetes, with a range of complications (Evans et al., 2010). The evidence for the effectiveness of CBT in patients with psoriasis is now sufficiently strong that researchers are evaluating ways in which the process can be further refined by the inclusion of an understanding of patient schemas (i.e. ingrained cognitive and emotional patterns); initial work is promising, although further work is needed at this stage (Mizara et al., 2011).

HCPs should encourage patients to become involved in coping skills training, behavioural contracts, biofeedback, relaxation and distraction techniques, or social support/self-help groups. Help in organising their day to include exercise, socialisation, TV, music and relaxation can encourage patients to take more control and improve their coping ability. Although there has been little specific research on psychological interventions for pain in wound care, there are lessons that can be learnt from the chronic pain world that show that a few changes to clinical practice can have a beneficial impact on patients. HCPs must be aware that the wound pain experience will not only relate to the acute pain experienced during treatment interventions (e.g. dressing changes, debridement) but may also exist as chronic, persistent pain which dominates the lives of their patients. Awareness of the benefits of psychological interventions, especially as part of a package of pain-related care, may lead to major improvements in the everyday lives of those living with chronic wounds. In 2007, Price et al. (2007) published a Wound Pain Management Model, which highlighted the range of options available to assist in dealing with this difficult symptom (Figure 7.3); such strategies, in addition to good local skin care/wound management and the appropriate use of pharmacological assistance, can help support patients to take control of this aspect of their lives.

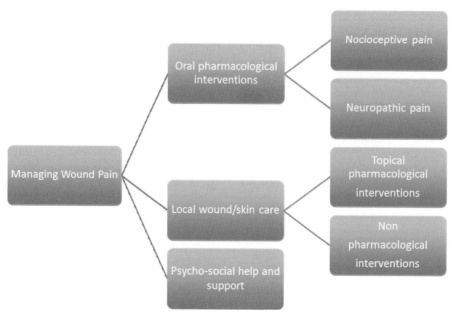

Figure 7.3   Wound pain management.

In recent years, there has been a move to explore whether relaxation and anger management relate to wound healing, with Gouin et al. (2008) reporting in a study ($n = 100$) on the physiological mechanism by which relaxation can facilitate acute wound healing in healthy volunteers. The hypothesis that relaxation would lead to faster healing was not supported, but secondary analysis indicated that those able to control their anger were associated with faster healing (possibly through lower cortisol levels), even when controlled for hostility, negative affectivity, social support and health behaviours. It is unclear at this stage how relevant these findings are for those with chronic wounds, although successful therapeutic strategies are available to help individuals improve control over the expression of their anger (Del Vecchio and O'Leary, 2004) should this become an area of future development. A pilot study to evaluate a 12-week intervention that includes cognitive education on skin and general health issues, together with stress-reducing techniques ($n = 43$), has shown significant improvements in self-reported HRQOL measures after participation in the programme for patients with a range of skin conditions, including those with psoriasis and atopic dermatitis (Lambert et al., 2011).

Although assessment of psychological and patient-focused measures is progressively being recognised as an integral element of holistic chronic wound management, there is still much to learn about these complex processes. In a world of increasing demands and expectations from patients, in terms of the quality of their care and the clinical outcomes associated with interventions, the impact of care provision on health and social gain is becoming an ever more prominent concern for healthcare providers. Further research is required if we are to design strategies to maintain and improve quality of life, everyday living and treatment satisfaction.

Clinical reflection

- Everyday living will be affected for many patients.
- Perceived severity is linked to psychological distress.
- Individuals may vary in how they cope with the associated distress, but the problems are often similar regardless of skin condition/type of wound.
- If you are really concerned about the psychological status of your patient, make sure you discuss the situation in a professional manner with senior colleagues who will have more

experience of working with patients with skin conditions.

- If a patient is self-harming or clearly interfering with the wound, then an immediate referral for specialist help should be made – be careful not to jump to conclusions and blame the patient if a wound/skin condition is not improving, but be aware that for a very small group of patients the underlying condition may be psychiatric.

Summary

Compared with other areas of our understanding of skin breakdown and its management, the issues related to the psychological problems that patients experience are in their infancy. We have strong data that show the quality of life of patients with skin breakdown can be very poor; such patients' lives are often dominated by the physical symptoms they experience, the time-consuming ways of treating their skin breakdown and the fear of future recurrence. Positive relationships with HCPs can help patients make the best of the management of their skin; good communication, consistent information, supportive and active listening and involving patients in making decisions about their care are all ways in which we can routinely ensure that the patient's well-being is at the centre of our thinking. Many, but not all, patients may experience increased stress, anxiety and/or depression; knowing about these conditions and ways in which patients try to cope – often on their own – can aid professional staff in assessing and monitoring patient progress, noting that these emotional experiences may interfere with the patient's ability to adhere to treatment and directly impact their ability to heal. Sometimes relatively straightforward, low costs changes to how we interact with patients can have a positive, enhancing effect on their ability to understand their treatment and get involved in skin management in a way that leads to improved outcomes – and ultimately enables patients to live their lives in the most positive way possible.

Useful resources

Many self-reported questionnaires can be found online using resources such as:

The PROM Group, Oxford. Patient-reported outcome measures (PROMs).

Available at: http://phi.uhce.ox.ac.uk/home.php

Medical Outcomes Trust

Available at: http://http://www.outcomes-trust.org

The Patient-reported Outcome and Quality of Life Instrument Database (PROQOLID).

Available at: http://www.proqolid.org.

Although these are not restricted to PROMs related to skin breakdown, they provide links to generic and condition-specific tools, as well as related publications.

International consensus. (2012) *Optimising Wellbeing in People Living with a Wound. An Expert Working Group Review.* London: Wounds International.

Available at: http://www.woundsinternational.com

References

Anderson, R.M., Funnell, M.M. (2010) Patient empowerment: myths and misconceptions. *Patient Education and Counselling,* 79, 277–282.

Armstrong, D.A., Lavery, L.A., Wrobel, J.S., Vileikyte, L. (2008) Quality of life in healing diabetic wounds: does the end justify the means? *The Journal of Foot & Ankle Surgery,* 47(4), 278–282.

Asimakopoulou, K., Gilbert, D., Newton, P., Scambler, S. (2011) Back to basics: re-examining the role of patient empowerment in diabetes. *Patient Education and Counselling,* doi: 10.1016/j.pec.2011.03.017.

Aujoulat, I., Marcologo, R., Bonadiman, L., Deccache, A. (2008) Reconsidering patient empowerment in chronic illness: a critique of models of self-efficacy and bodily control. *Social Science and Medicine,* 66, 1228–1239.

Baum, A., Posluszny, D.M. (1999) Health psychology: mapping biobehavioral contributions to health and illness. *Annual Review Psychology,* 50, 137–163.

Benstsson, L., Jonsson, M., Apelqvist, J. (2008) Wound related pain is underestimated in patients with diabetic foot ulcers. *Journal Wound Care,* 17(10), 433–435.

Bloom, D., Boersch-Supan, A., McGee, P., Seike, A. (2011) Population aging: fact, challenges and responses. PGDA Working Paper No. 71: The Harvard Initiative for Global Health. Available at: http://www.hsph.harvard.edu/pgda/WorkingPapers/2011/PGDA_WP_71.pdf, last accessed on 17 November 2013.

Bradbury, S., Price, P.E. (2011a) Diabetic foot ulcer pain (part 1): the hidden burden. *EWMA Journal,* 11(1), 11–22.

Bradbury, S., Price, P.E. (2011b) Diabetic foot ulcer pain (part 2): the hidden burden. *EWMA Journal,* 11(2), 25–37.

Briggs, M., Flemming, K. (2007) Living with leg ulceration: a synthesis of qualitative research. *Journal of Advanced Nursing,* 59(4), 319–328.

Brown, T.A., Cash, T.F., Milulka, P.J. (1990) Attitudinal body-image assessment: factor-analysis of the body-self relations questionnaire. *Journal of Personality Assessment*, 55, 135–144.

Charles, H. (1995) The impact of leg ulcers on patients' quality of life. *Professional Nurse*, 10(9), 571–574.

Cohen, S., Wills, T.A. (1985) Stress, social support, and the buffering hypothesis. *Psychological Bulletin*, 98(2), 310–357.

Del Vecchio, T., O'Leary, D.K. (2004) Effectiveness of anger treatments for specific anger problems: a meta-analytic review. *Clinical Psychology Review*, 24, 15–34.

Dorresteijn, J.A., Kriegsman, D.M., Assendelft, W.J., Valk, G.D. (2010) Patient education for preventing diabetic foot ulceration. *Cochrane Database Systematic Reviews*, May 12(5), CD001488.

Douglas, V. (2001) Living with a chronic leg ulcer: an insight into patients' experiences and feelings. *Journal of Wound Care*, 10(9), 355–360.

Edwards, H., Courtney, M., Findlayson, K., et al. (2005) Chronic venous leg ulcers: effect of a community nursing intervention on pain and healing. *Nursing Standard*, 19, 47–54.

Edwards, L.M., Moffatt, C.J., Franks, P.J. (2002) An exploration of patients' understanding of leg ulceration. *Journal of Wound Care*, 11(1), 35–39.

European Wound Management Association (2002) *Pain at Dressing Changes*. EWMA Position Document. London: MEP Ltd.

Evans, G., Lewin, T.J., Bowen, K., Lowe, J. (2010) Dealing with anxiety: a pilot cognitive behavioural therapy program for diabetic clinic outpatient attendees. *International Journal of Diabetes Mellitus*, 2, 51–55.

Flanagan, M., Vogensen, H., Haase, L. (2006) Investigating patients' pain experience with venous leg ulcers. *World Wide Wounds*, http://www.worldwide wounds.com/2006/april/Flanagan/Ibuprofen-Foam-Dressing.html, last accessed on 17 November 2012.

Flor, H., Fydrich, T., Turk, D.C. (1992) Efficacy of multidisciplinary pain treatment centers: a meta-analytic review. *Pain*, 49, 221–230.

Gonzalez, J.S., Vileikyte, L., Ulbrecht, J.S., et al. (2010) Depression predicts first but not recurrent diabetic foot ulcers. *Diabetologica*, 53(10), 2241–2248.

Gorecki, C., Brown, J.M., Nelson, A., et al. (2009) Impact of pressure ulcers on quality of life in older patients: a systematic review. *Journal of American Geriatric Society*, 57, 1175–1183.

Gouin, J.P., Kiecolt-Glaser, J.K., Malarkey, W.B., Glaser R. (2008) The influence of anger expression on wound healing. *Brain, Behaviour, and Immunity*, 22, 699–708.

Gourney, K., Veale, D., Walburn J. (1997) Body dysmorphic disorder: pilot randomised controlled trial of treatment; implications for nurse therapy and practice. *Clinical Effectiveness in Nursing*, 1(1), 38–43.

González-Consuegra, R.V., Verdú, J. (2011) Quality of life in people with venous leg ulcers: an integrative review. *Journal of Advanced Nursing*, 67(5), 926–944.

Green, J., Jester, R. (2010) Health-related quality of life and chronic venous ulceration: part 2. *British Journal of Community Nursing*, 15(3), S4–S14.

Hareendran, A., Bradbury, J., Budd, G., et al. (2005) Measuring the impact of venous leg ulcers on quality of life. *Journal of Wound Care*, 14(2), 53–55.

Hogg, F.R.A., Peach, G., Price, P., Thompson, M.M., Hinchliffe, R.J. (2012) Measures of health-related quality of life in diabetes-related foot disease: a systematic review. *Diabetologica*, 55(3), 552–565.

Holstrom, I., Roing, M. (2010) The relation between patient-centeredness and patient empowerment: a discussion on concepts. *Patient Education and Counselling*, 79, 167–172.

Hopkins, A. (2004) Disrupted lives: investigating coping strategies for non-healing leg ulcers. *British Journal of Nursing*, 13(9), 556–563.

Jones, J.E., Barr, W., Robinson, J., Carlisle, C. (2006) Depression in patients with chronic venous ulceration. *British Journal of Nursing*, 15(11): *Tissue Viability* Supplement: S17–S23.

Jones, J.E., Barr, W., Robinson, J., Carlisle, C. (2008) Impact of exudate and odour from chronic venous leg ulceration. *Nursing Standard*, 22(45), 53–61.

Jowett, S., Ryan, T. (1985) Skin disease and handicap: an analysis of the impact of skin conditions. *Social Science and Medicine*, 20(4), 425–429.

Jull, A.B., Mitchell, N., Aroll, J., et al. (2004) Factors influencing concordance with compression stockings after venous leg ulcer healing. *Journal of Wound Care*, 13(3), 90–92.

Kilroy-Findley, A. (2010) Tissue viability in mental health. *Nursing Standard*, 24(45), 60–67.

Kornhaber, R.A., Wilson A. (2011) Building resilience in burns nurses: a descriptive phenomenological inquiry. *Journal of Burn Care & Research*, 32(4), 481–488.

Lambert, J., Bostoen, J., Geusens, B., et al. (2011) A novel multidisciplinary educational programme for patients with chronic skin diseases: Ghent pilot project and first results. *Archives of Dermatological Research*, 303(1), 57–63.

Lauterbach, S., Kostev, K., Kohlmann, T. (2010) Prevalence of diabetic foot syndrome and its risk factors in the UK. *Journal Wound Care*, 19(8), 333–337.

Mainour, A.G., 3rd, Baker, R., Koopman, R.J., et al. (2007) Impact of the population at risk of diabetes on projections of diabetes burden in the United States: an epidemic on the way. *Diabetologia*, 50(5), 934–940.

Malone, M.D., Strube, M.J. (1988) Meta-analysis of non-medical treatments for chronic pain. *Pain*, 34, 231–244.

Mizara, A., Papadopoulos, L., McBride, S.R. (2011) Core beliefs and psychological distress in patients with psoriasis and atopic eczema attending secondary care: the role of schemas in chronic skin disease. *British Journal of Dermatology*, 166(5), 986–993.

Moffatt, C.J. (2004) Factors that affect concordance with compression therapy. *Journal of Wound Care*, 13(7), 291–294.

Moffatt, C.J., Mapplebeck, L., Murray, S., Morgan, P.A. (2011) The experience of patients with complex wounds and the use of NPWT in a home-care setting. *Journal of Wound Care*, 20(11), 512–527.

Monami, M., Longo, R., Desideri, C.M., Masotti, G., Marchionni, N., Mannucci, E. (2008) The diabetic person beyond a foot ulcer – healing, recurrence and depressive symptoms. *Journal of American Podiatric Medical Association*, 98, 130–136.

Moos, R., Schaefer, J.A. (1984) The crisis of physical illness: an overview and conceptual approach. In: *Coping with Physical Illness: New Perspectives*, Vol. 2 (ed. R.H. Moos), pp. 3–25. New York: Plenum Press.

Moos, R.H. (1990) The coping response inventory. In: *Assessment: A Mental Health Portfolio* (ed. D. Milne). Windsor: NFER.

Morley, S., Eccleston, C., Williams, A. (1999) Systematic review and metaanalysis of randomised controlled trials of cognitive behaviour therapy and behaviour therapy for chronic pain in adults, excluding headache. *Pain*, 80, 1–13.

Mudge, E. (2007) Meeting report. Tell me if it hurts: the patients' perspective of wound pain. *Wounds UK*, 3 (1), 6–7.

Newell, R.J. (1999) Altered body-image: a fear-avoidance model of psycho-social difficulties following disfigurement. *Journal of Advanced Nursing*, 30(5), 1230–1238.

Norris, S.L., Engelgau, M.M., Venkat Narayan, K.M. (2001) Effectiveness of management training in type 2 diabetes: a systematic review of randomised controlled trials. *Diabetes Care*, 24, 561–87.

Palfreyman, S. (2008) Assessing the impact of venous ulceration on quality of life. *Nursing Times*, 104(41), 34–37.

Papadopoulos, L., Bor, R. (1999) *Psychological Approaches to Dermatology*. Leceister: The British Psychological Society.

Partridge, J. (1994) *Changing Faces*. Harmondsworth; Penguin Books.

Patterson, D., Everrett, J., Bombardier, C. (1993) Psychological effects of severe burn injuries. *Psychological Bulletin*, 113, 362–378.

Persoon, A., Heinen, M.M., van der Vleuten, C.J., de Rooij, M.J., van de Kerkhof, P.C., van Achterberg, T. (2004) Leg ulcers: a review of their impact on daily life. *Journal of Clinical Nursing*, 13(3), 341–354.

Phillips, T., Stanton, B., Provan, A., Lew, R. (1994) A study of the impact of leg ulcers on quality of life:

financial, social and psychologic implications. *Journal of American Academy of Dermatology*, 31, 49–55.

Porter, J.R., Beuf, A.H., Lerner, A., Norlund, J. (1990) The effect of vitiligo on sexual relationships. *Journal of the American Academy of Dermatology*, 22, 221–222.

Price, B. (1990) *Body-Image: Nursing Concepts and Care*. New York: Prentice Hall.

Price, P. (2007) Leg ulceration: impact on everyday living and health-related quality of life. *Journal of Wound Care*, 16(4 Suppl), 4–5.

Price, P., Fogh, K., Glynn, C., Krasner, D.L., Osterbrink, J., Sibbald, R.G. (2007) Managing painful chronic wounds: the wound pain management model. *International Wound Journal*, 4(1 Suppl), 14–15.

Price, P.E., Fagervik-Morton, H., Mudge, E.J., et al. (2008) Dressing-related pain in patients with chronic wounds: an international perspective. *International Wound Journal*, 5(2), 159–171.

Price, P.E., Harding, K.G. (2000) Acute and chronic wounds: differences in self-reported health-related quality of life. *Journal of Wound Care*, 9(2), 93–95.

Rich, A., McLachlan, L. (2003) How living with a leg ulcer affects people's daily life: a nurse-led study. *Journal of Wound Care*, 12(2), 51–54.

Robinson, E. (1997) Psychological research on visible difference in adults. In: *Visibly Different: Coping with Disfigurement* (eds R. Lansdown, N. Rumsey, E. Bradbury, T. Carr, J. Partridge). Oxford: Butterworth-Heinemann.

Sarafino, E.P. (1994) *Health Psychology: Biopsychosocial Interactions*, 2nd edn. New York: Wiley.

Segerstrom, S.C., Miller, G.E. (2004) Psychological stress and the human immune system: a meta-analytic study of 30 years of inquiry. *Psychological Bulletin*, 130, 601–630.

Solowiej, K., Mason, V., Upton, D. (2009) Review of the relationship between stress and wound healing: part 1. *Journal of Wound Care*, 18(9), 357–366.

Soon, K., Acton, C. (2006) Pain-induced stress: a barrier to wound healing. *Wounds UK*, 2, (4), 92–101.

Speight, J., Reaney, M.D., Barnard, K.D. (2009) Not all roads lead to Rome – a review of quality of life measurement in adults with diabetes. *Diabetic Medicine*, 26, 315–327.

Spilsbury, K., Nelson, A., Cullum, N., Iglesias, G., Nixon, J., Mason, S. (2007) Pressure ulcers and their treatment and effects on quality of life: hospital inpatient perspectives. *Journal of Advanced Nursing*, 57(5), 494–504.

Tonge, H. (1995) A review of factors affecting compliance in patients with leg ulcers. *Journal of Wound Care*, 4(2), 84–85.

Turner, J.A., Schroth, W.S., Fordyce, W.E. (1996) Educational and behavioural interventions for back pain in primary care. *Spine*, 21, 2851–2859.

Vedhara, K., Miles, J., Wetherell, M., et al. (2010) Coping and depression influence the healing of diabetic foot ulcers: observational and mechanistic evidence. *Diabetologica*, 53(8), 1590–1598.

Velikova, G., Booth, I., Smith, A. (2004) Measuring quality of life in routine oncology practice improves communication and patient well-being: a randomised controlled trial. *Journal of Clinical Oncology*, 22, 714–724.

Vermeire, E., Hearnshaw, H., Van Royen, P., Denekens, J. (2001) Patient adherence to treatment: three decades of research. A comprehensive review. *Journal of Clinical Pharmacy and Therapeutics*, 26, 331–342.

Vileikyte, L. (2007) Stress and wound healing. *Clinical Dermatology*, 25, 49–55.

Vileikyte, L., Shen, B.J., Hardman, M.J., Kirsner, R.S., Boulton, A.J.M., Schneiderman, N. (2010) Emotional distress may impede diabetic foot ulcer healing through elevated levels of interleukin-6: preliminary findings. *Diabelolgica*, (Suppl 1), 1153–1158.

Walburn, J., Vedhera, K., Hankins, M., Rixon, L., Weinman, J. (2009) Psychological stress and wound healing in humans: a systematic review and meta-analysis. *Journal of Psychosomatic Research*, 67, 253–271.

Walshe, C. (1995) Living with a venous leg ulcer: a descriptive study of patients' experiences. *J Advanced Nursing*, 22, 1092–1100.

Wilkes, L., Boxer, E., White, K. (2003) The hidden side of nursing: why caring for patients with malignant malodorous wounds is so difficult. *Journal of Wound Care*, 12(2), 76.

Wilkinson, J. (1997) Understanding motivation to enhance patient compliance. *British Journal of Nursing*, 6(15), 879–884.

Williams, L.H., Rutter, C.M., Katon, W.J., et al. (2010) Depression and incident diabetic foot ulcers: a prospective cohort study. *The American Journal of Medicine*, 123, 748–754.

Wills, T.A. (1984) Supportive functions of interpersonal relationships. In: *Social Support and Health* (eds S. Cohen, L. Smye). New York: Academic Press.

Winkley, K., Stahl, D., Chalder, T., Edmonds, M.E., Ismall, K. (2007) Risk factors associated with adverse outcomes in a population-based prospective cohort study of people with their first diabetic foot ulcer. *Journal Diabetes and Complications*, 21, 341–349.

World Union of Wound Healing Societies (2004) *Principles of Best Practise: Minimising Pain at Wound Dressing-Related Procedures: A Consensus Document*. London: MEP Ltd.

Yunus, Y.M., Rajbhandari, S.M. (2011) Insensate foot of diabetic foot ulcer can have underlying silent neuropathic pain. *International Wound Journal*, 8(3), 301–305.

Section 2

Challenging Wounds

8 Pressure, Shear and Friction

Keryln Carville

Assoc Professor Domiciliary Nursing Silver Chain Nursing Association & Curtin University of Technology

Overview

- Pressure ulcers are a serious health issue: they cause considerable pain and suffering to patients and place a significant financial burden on healthcare systems.
- Inconsistencies in pressure injury prevalence and incidence data mean that comparison is difficult across different clinical settings and geographical areas.
- Non-blanchable erythema, lymphopenia, immobility, dry skin, decreased body weight and a previous history of pressure injury are significant risk factors for pressure ulceration in patients whose activity is limited to the bed or chair.
- The principles of management can be broadly directed towards preventing further pressure damage, optimising the health and potential healing of the individual and optimising the local wound healing environment.
- There is a high level of agreement among international guidelines on the prevention and management of pressure ulcers.
- There is currently no evidence to support the increased effectiveness of one higher-specification foam mattress over another, but they appear to be more effective in preventing pressure ulcers than standard hospital foam mattresses.
- Education of clinicians, carers and individuals is fundamental for preventing pressure ulceration and optimising healing. High-risk individuals living independently should receive regular instruction on how to conduct self skin inspections on a regular basis.

Introduction

Florence Nightingale was a visionary and one of the earliest authors to appreciate the importance of preventative skin care and the concept of risk of skin breakdown (Baly, 1991). It was to be another 100 years before nurses were using risk assessment tools for predicting pressure injury. It proved to be equally as long, before clinicians and researchers engaged in rigorous endeavours to ascertain the pathophysiology of pressure injuries and determine the best evidence for their prevention and management.

In Nightingale's era, time spent in bed was deemed to be the cause of the problem and thus, the resultant issue was termed a 'bed sore'. Over succeeding generations, other terms such as decubitus ulcer (from the Latin *decumbere*, which means 'to lie down'), pressure area, pressure sore, pressure ulcer, pressure necrosis and, more recently, pressure

Wound Healing and Skin Integrity: Principles and Practice, First Edition. Edited by Madeleine Flanagan.
© 2013 John Wiley & Sons, Ltd. Published 2013 by John Wiley & Sons, Ltd.

injury have been employed as synonymous terms. Whilst pressure ulcer is perhaps the most commonly embraced term, many consider it as failing to adequately describe a stage I lesion. Technically, an ulcer is a wound that breaches the epidermis and extends into the dermis or presents as erosion of the mucosa, and stage I 'ulcers' present as intact non-blanching skin. It is because of this confusion that the term 'pressure injury' is gaining in popularity in some countries (AWMA, 2011), as the term is more definitive, and indicates that injuries are largely preventable.

Regardless, a pressure ulcer (and its various synonymous terms) has been defined as a 'localised injury to the skin and/or underlying tissue usually over a bony prominence, as a result of pressure, or pressure in combination with shear and/or friction'.

Pressure injuries are considered by most to be largely preventable wounds (Orsted et al., 2010). However, they continue to pose significant health issues for susceptible individuals and health providers. Pressure ulcers have been reportedly found on ancient Egyptian mummies (Thompson, 1961) and Nightingale's nurses during the Crimean War reported the presence of extensive bed sores amongst wounded soldiers who had been left for days on frozen battlefields or bare boat boards during transport to Scutari (Richardson, 1977). When one considers the quantum leap in contemporary knowledge and state-of-the-art pressure offloading equipment developed since the late 1880s, it is astonishing that pressure ulcers continue to be such common and problematic wounds. Pressure ulcers significantly impact on the global healthcare burden. However, the impact on individuals has far-reaching consequences due to increases in morbidity and mortality and lessening of quality of life.

Prevalence and incidence

Prevalence measures the number of people with an existing pressure ulcer at a given point in time, whilst incidence measures the number of individuals with a new pressure ulcer within a specified population and over a specified period. Pressure ulcer prevalence and incidence rates, when reported, vary across clinical settings both nationally and internationally. However, benchmarking is made difficult by inconsistencies in data collection and analysis methods. For instance, some health facilities report stage I pressure damage whilst others do not. Some facilities conduct skin inspections to ascertain the existence of pressure ulcers, whilst others conduct data audits of case notes. Of considerable concern is the fact that some surveys exclude psychiatric, maternity and paediatric populations. Some report point prevalence whilst others period prevalence, and challenges for determining incidence abound. Although an increasing number of national and international health providers collect prevalence and incidence data, the opportunity for effective benchmarking is sadly lost because of this dearth of agreement in regards to methodology employed.

However, limited insight into the scope of the international problem can be glimpsed in published reports. A Welsh study conducted across orthopaedic units in National Health Service Trusts in 2007 and amongst orthopaedic patients in community hospitals in 2008 reported a pressure ulcer prevalence of 13.9% and 26.7%, respectively (James et al., 2010). Whilst a clinical audit, conducted across 44 acute NHS trusts in England and Wales over 3 years (2005–2007) revealed an overall prevalence of 10.3%, and 50% of the ulcers were hospital acquired (Phillips and Buttery, 2009). A Swedish survey conducted amongst adult medical and surgical patients in an university hospital and a general hospital found a pressure ulcer prevalence of 17.6% and 9.5%, respectively, and when comparisons were made with the Collaborative Alliance for Nursing Outcomes, a benchmarking registry in the United States, the latter group reported 6.3–6.7% prevalence (Gunningberg et al., 2011). In Australia, pressure ulcer prevalence in 10 national acute care facilities ranged from 4.5% to 27%[11]. However, these *ad hoc* findings serve little collective good unless clinicians and administrators can undertake benchmarking activities. Thus, what is urgently required is a standardised approach to the collection of prevalence and incidence data, and a willingness to share that data for benchmarking purposes.

Pathophysiology

A network of vascular and lymphatic vessels carries the nutrients and oxygen necessary for cell metabolism and epidermal mitosis to the skin and its underlying tissues. This network is also active in temperature regulation and the removal of waste products (Bridel, 1993). Damage to tissues results from excessive or sustained compression of the vascular and lymphatic network. When compression exceeds the perfusion pressure and structural resistance of the capillaries, oxygenation and nutrient supply to the skin and underlying tissue is compromised. This results in localised tissue ischaemia, hypoxia, acidosis, oedema and necrosis.

Capillary-closing pressure, or the pressure required to collapse capillaries and prevent blood flow, was cited in 1930 by Landis as 32 mmHg. However, capillary-closing pressure will vary between individuals, depending on vessel structure, adipose tissue deposition overlying bony prominences, blood pressure and general health status (Landis, 1930). Capillaries are compressed when external pressure is applied and all individuals are constantly affected by pressure being applied to a body surface when it comes in contact with an object or a hard surface. Healthy, cognitively aware individuals spontaneously react to the discomfort related to sustained pressure and resultant capillary compression and tissue hypoxia by moving or repositioning the body in order to relieve the discomfort. The immediate reperfusion response in the tissues when pressure is relieved is termed reactive hyperaemia. The affected tissues become bright red until reperfusion is optimised and skin tone returns to normal.

Failure to adequately relieve tissue pressure results in the following sequelae: vessel occlusion, tissue hypoxia, pallor, ischaemia, increased capillary permeability and resultant accumulation of metabolic wastes and proteins in the interstitial space and oedema (Pieper, 2007). The resultant oedema further impairs tissue and skin perfusion and a pressure ulcer results.

Pressure

Pressure is the major cause of pressure ulcers, and pressure is defined as perpendicular force (or force applied at right angles) applied to an anatomical surface per unit area of application (Taalajasjo et al., 2010). However, damage to the skin can also result from shearing and friction forces, and often in conjunction with pressure. Shear or sheer stress is defined as parallel or tangential force. Shear produces distortion of the tissues, causing two adjacent internal tissues to deform in the transverse plane (Reger et al., 2010). Shear can occur when the individual is lying flat (Reger et al., 2010), but is

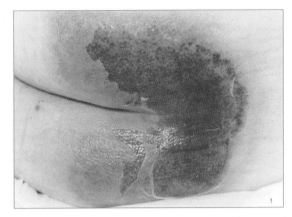

Figure 8.1 Sacral pressure ulcer caused by a combination of friction and shear. Photo courtesy of Madeleine Flanagan.

more commonly associated with sliding or pulling activities. There is an increased risk of shear injury amongst elderly or dehydrated individuals when skin turgor and elasticity is reduced and tissues are more flaccid. Shear stress more readily deforms flaccid skin and subdermal tissues with resultant capillary compression and occlusion, when gravitational force causes the individual laying or sitting in a semi-recumbent position, to slide down the bed or chair (Reger et al., 2010). Although capillaries are more commonly affected by shear, deeper and larger blood vessels can also be affected which in turn extends the tissue damage into adjacent tissues such as muscle. Figure 8.1 shows a pressure ulcer caused by a combination of friction and shear.

Friction

Friction is generally referred to as rubbing of one surface against another (NPUAP, 2007) or the 'force that resists the relative motion of two objects that are touching' (Reger et al., 2010). The force applied to the 'patient–support surface interface is dependent on the perpendicular force and the coefficient of friction of the skin and the contact surface' (Reger et al., 2010). The coefficient of friction is described as 'a measurement of the amount of friction existing between two surfaces' (Reger et al., 2010), and is dependent upon the contact surface material, the skin or surface moisture and the ambient humidity (Carville, 2007). The coefficient of friction is higher in the presence of macerated skin or wet support surfaces and when the skin is in contact with rough or wrinkled textiles or bedding. The resultant injury presents as a blister or abrasion. Blisters all too commonly occur on the heels of individuals with a fractured femur, because they tend to find it too painful to lift their heels when repositioning, and associated pressure, shear and friction injuries occur as they fail to relieve pressure under their heels and drag their heels against the support surface.

The development of a pressure ulcer is dependent upon the intensity of pressure applied to the tissues, the duration of applied pressure and the tissue tolerance or capacity of the skin and underlying tissues to endure the pressure without harmful effects (Burman, 1994; Carville, 2007; AWMA, 2011).

Risk factors

Risk factors associated with pressure ulceration are those factors that influence the intensity and duration of pressure applied, or the skin and tissue's capacity to tolerate the pressure (AWMA, 2011). Clinical practice guidelines report risk factors as being either intrinsic or extrinsic in nature. Numerous intrinsic and extrinsic factors have been associated with pressure ulceration (Ayello and Lyder, 2008, 2009; AWMA, 2011). Intrinsic risk factors are predominately those that reduce the skin and its supporting structure's tolerance to pressure because of vascular, lymphatic, nutritional, perfusion, temperature regulation, excess moisture, sensory, mobility and activity compromise.

Commonly reported intrinsic and extrinsic factors are summarised below:

Intrinsic factors

- advancing age over 65 years and more especially over 75 years is a common demographic;
- chronic illnesses such as diabetes, carcinoma, peripheral arterial disease, cardiopulmonary disease, lymphoedema, renal impairment or failure, hypotension and anaemia;
- smoking;
- immobility and inactivity deficits that impair repositioning and movement;
- sensory deficits due to cognitive or neurological impairment, sedative medications or anaesthetics;
- malnutrition and dehydration and associated extremes in weight;
- dry skin;
- non-blanchable erythema;

- elevated skin temperature due to raised core body temperature, elevated ambient temperature or skin contact with materials that reduce air flow such as plastic and vinyl surfaces.
  (Ayello and Lyder, 2008, 2009; AWMA, 2011)

Extrinsic factors

- shear;
- friction;
- moisture from increased ambient humidity, urinary or faecal incontinence, diaphoresis, spilled fluids and uncontrolled wound exudate.
  (Ayello and Lyder, 2008, 2009; AWMA, 2011)

Pressure, shear and friction are closely linked to soft tissue breakdown, especially when over a bony prominence. The relationship between these forces is complex and depends on local conditions (microclimate) at the skin–support surface interface such as humidity, moisture control and skin temperature (Clarke et al., 2010).

Psychological impact

In recent years, researchers have started to demonstrate the full extent of the psychological impact that pressure ulcers have on individuals with pressure damage. A systematic review by Gorecki et al. (2009) focusing on the impact of pressure ulcers on HRQL evaluated the responses of 2463 adults with pressure ulcers in hospital, community and long-term care settings across Europe, the United States, Asia and Australia.

The conclusion highlighted that pressure ulcers and treatment cause substantial distress to patients and their families and have a significant impact on patients HRQL. This review highlights the social isolation that results from having a large pressure ulcer, as patients are fearful of others' reaction to exudate leakage and smell.

Clinicians are aware that pressure ulcers cause patients pain and discomfort which affects their everyday lives. However, a recent systematic review by Gorecki et al. (2011) demonstrates that even relatively minor skin damage can cause patients excruciating pain that interferes with sleep, appetite and causes significant anxiety and distress. Patients described unrelenting background pain originating from their pressure ulcers that is not well controlled by analgesia and not effectively managed by health professionals. This finding supports the earlier work by Hopkins et al. (2006) that found that elderly people with severe pressure ulcers reported that pain was constant and unremitting and relieved by keeping still. Studies in this area are consistent and demonstrate that pressure damage has a major and lasting psychological impact on those unfortunate to suffer skin breakdown and that clinicians struggle to acknowledge these issues and manage them effectively (Spilsbury et al., 2007; Gorecki et al., 2009, 2011).

Current best practice

The management of an individual with a pressure ulcer requires an interprofessional and collaborative approach. The principles of management can be broadly directed towards preventing pressure damage, optimising the health and potential healing of the individual and optimising the wound healing environment.

Assessment outcomes will determine short-term goals of care and deficits in nutrition, hydration, mobility, activity and skin condition will need to be remedied. Optimisation of the wound healing environment is dependent upon evidence-based wound management interventions which should be directed towards:

- redistribution of pressure and elimination of shear and friction;
- maintenance of a stable wound temperature and pH;
- debridement of nonviable tissue;
- preservation of moisture balance;
- prevention or management of infection.

The effective management of patients at risk of, or suffering from pressure ulceration is dependent upon organisational support, adequate resources and implementation of best clinical practice that addresses redistribution of pressure, nutritional assessment continence management and pain control.

Prevention strategies

There is no better implementation of the old adage 'prevention is better than cure' than when guiding strategies for pressure ulcer prevention. Although prevention costs are difficult to ascertain, the implicit and explicit costs associated with the treatment of pressure ulcers are considerable and far outweigh costs associated with prevention (Lapsey and Vogels, 1996; Lyder et al., 2002).

The costs associated with treating pressure ulcers in the United Kingdom in 2004 were determined to be £1.4 to £2.1 billion (Bennett et al., 2004). In the United States, the annual cost of treating hospital-acquired pressure ulcers was estimated to be $11 billion between 2007 and 2009[23, 24, 25], and in that country, there was found to be a 79% increase in hospital-acquired pressure ulcers between 1993 and 2006 (Ayello and Lyder, 2009).

In Australia, in common with other countries, it has been determined that pressure ulcers increase the average length of hospital stay by 4 days (Graves et al., 2005), which places a significant and unnecessary burden on health providers and individuals. Therefore, identification of individuals at risk of pressure ulcers and the implementation of strategies to eliminate or reduce the risks underpins principles for best practice.

Pressure ulceration: assessment considerations

As is the case with all types of wounds, individuals with pressure ulcers require a comprehensive and systematic assessment of the person, their skin, wound and healing environment. Assessment of the person should provide documented evidence of:

- health history;
- age and age-related changes;
- medication history;
- psychosocial implications of wounding;
- skin status;
- nutritional status;
- sensitivities and allergies;
- pain;
- relevant diagnostics and investigations;
- vital signs;
- the individual's perceptions and wound healing goals and their ability to participate in self-care.

Biochemical, microbiological or histopathological diagnostic investigations may be required to support a clinical diagnosis.

Assessment of the pressure injury includes the staging of the damage as outlined in Figure 8.2.

Category/Stage I: Non-Blanchable Erythema

Intact skin with non-blanchable redness of a localised area usually over a bony prominence. Darkly pigmented skin may not have visible blanching; its colour may differ from the surrounding area.

The area may be painful, firm, soft, warmer or cooler as compared to adjacent tissue. Category/Stage I may be difficult to detect in individuals with dark skin tones. May indicate 'at risk' persons (a heralding sign of risk).

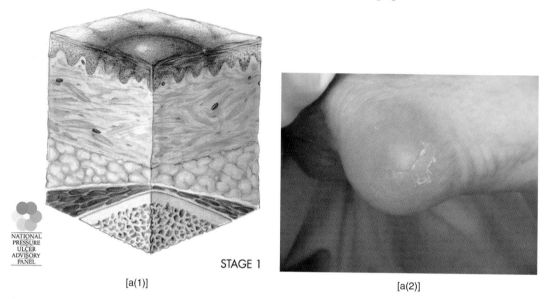

[a(1)]   STAGE 1   [a(2)]

Category/Stage II: Partial Thickness Skin Loss

Partial thickness loss of dermis presenting as a shallow open ulcer with a red pink wound bed, without slough. May also present as an intact or open/ruptured serum-filled blister.

Presents as a shiny or dry shallow ulcer without slough or bruising*. This Category/Stage should not be used to describe skin tears, tape burns, perineal dermatitis, maceration or excoriation.

*Bruising indicates suspected deep tissue injury.

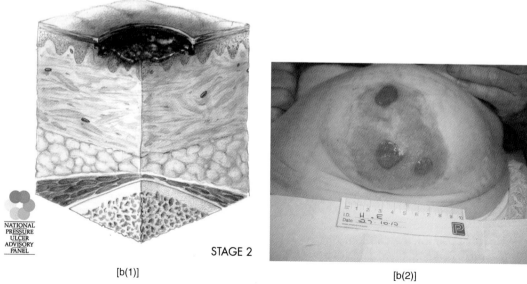

[b(1)]   STAGE 2   [b(2)]

Figure 8.2 International NPUAP–EPUAP Pressure Ulcer Classification System (http://www.npuap.org/resources.htm). Used with permission of the National Pressure Ulcer Advisory Panel, August 2012. © NPUAP. Photos courtesy of Caryn Carr (a2 and b2), Madeleine Flanagan (c2 and f2) and Lorraine Grothier (d2 and e2). (*Continued*)

Category/Stage III: Full Thickness Skin Loss

Full thickness tissue loss. Subcutaneous fat may be visible but bone, tendon or muscle are not exposed. Slough may be present but does not obscure the depth of tissue loss. May include undermining and tunnelling.

The depth of a Category/Stage III pressure ulcer varies by anatomical location. The bridge of the nose, ear, occiput and malleolus do not have subcutaneous tissue and Category/Stage III ulcers can be shallow. In contrast, areas of significant adiposity can develop extremely deep stage III pressure ulcers. Bone/tendon is not visible or directly palpable.

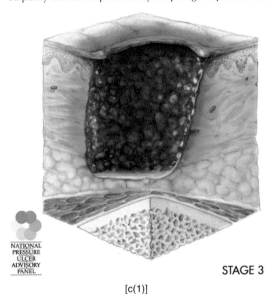

STAGE 3

[c(1)]

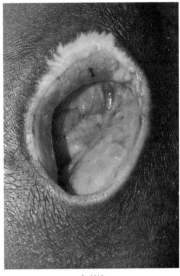

[c(2)]

Category/Stage IV: Full Thickness Tissue Loss

Full thickness tissue loss with exposed bone, tendon or muscle. Slough or eschar may be present on some parts of the wound bed. Often includes undermining and tunnelling.

The depth of a Category/Stage IV pressure ulcer varies by anatomical location. The bridge of the nose, ear, occiput and malleolus do not have subcutaneous tissue and these ulcers can be shallow. Category/Stage IV ulcers can extend into muscle and/or supporting structures (e.g. fascia, tendon or joint capsule) making osteomyelitis possible. Exposed bone/tendon is visible or directly palpable.

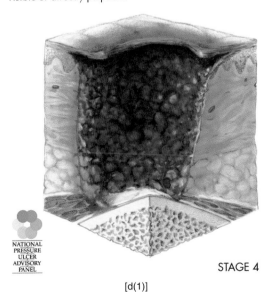

STAGE 4

[d(1)]

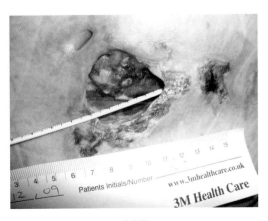

[d(2)]

Figure 8.2   (Continued)

Unstageable: Depth Unknown

Full thickness tissue loss in which the base of the ulcer is covered by slough (yellow, tan, grey, green or brown) and/or eschar (tan, brown or black) in the wound bed.

Until enough slough and/or eschar is removed to expose the base of the wound, the true depth, and therefore Category/Stage, cannot be determined. Stable (dry, adherent, intact without erythema or fluctuance) eschar on the heels serves as 'the body's natural (biological) cover' and should not be removed.

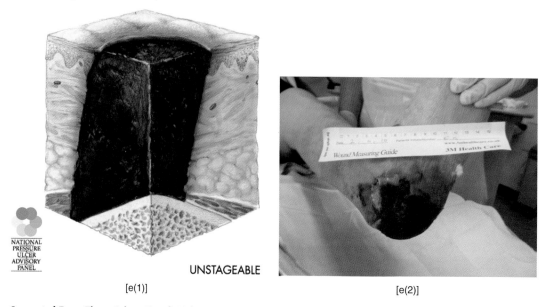

UNSTAGEABLE

[e(1)]   [e(2)]

Suspected Deep Tissue Injury: Depth Unknown

Purple or maroon localised area of discoloured intact skin or blood-filled blister due to damage of underlying soft tissue from pressure and/or shear. The area may be preceded by tissue that is painful, firm, mushy, boggy, warmer or cooler as compared to adjacent tissue.

Deep tissue injury may be difficult to detect in individuals with dark skin tones. Evolution may include a thin blister over a dark wound bed. The wound may further evolve and become covered by thin eschar. Evolution may be rapid, exposing additional layers of tissue even with optimal treatment.

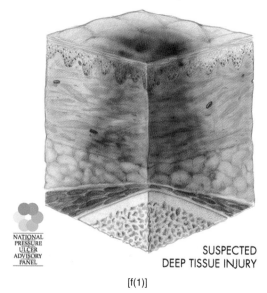

SUSPECTED
DEEP TISSUE INJURY

[f(1)]

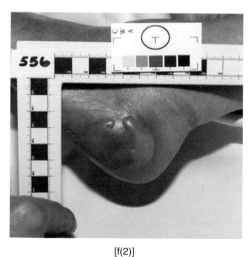

[f(2)]

Figure 8.2   (Continued)

Assessment and documentation of the parameters of wound assessment includes

- pressure ulcer aetiology (eliminate other aetiologies such as incontinent dermatitis, ecchymosis, senile purpura, malignancy, etc.);
- duration of ulcer;
- location;
- dimensions (length, width, depth and undermining);
- clinical characteristics of the wound bed (agranular, granular, necrosis, slough, exposed bone or tendon, epithelium);
- wound edges (raised, rolled, undermined, coloured);
- wound exudate (amount, colour, consistency, odour);
- peri-ulcer skin appearance (induration, erythema, oedema, maceration);
- signs of overt or covert infection.

(NPUAP, 2007)

Assessment of the individual's healing environment should identify factors and behaviours that could impact healing or potentially lead to new episodes of pressure ulceration. Transfer and support equipment should be examined to ensure appropriate use and condition. Self-care abilities for activities of daily living need to be ascertained and support services instigated, if required. Optimal infection control practices need to be implemented and breaches identified and corrected.

Classification of pressure ulcers

The earliest classification system for pressure ulcers was devised by Guttman in 1955 (Black et al., 2007). However, a four-stage classification system was developed by Shea in 1975 (Shea, 1975), which classified according to the degree of soft tissue damage and established a precedent for other classification systems that followed. In 1988, the International Association of Enterostomal Therapists (IAET), now known as the Wound, Ostomy, Continence Nurses Society (WOCN, 2010), devised a four-stage pressure ulcer classification, and another classification was developed by the National Pressure Ulcer Advisory Panel (NPUAP) in 1989 (Black et al., 2007). The latter group refined their system on several occasions during the intervening

years and the most recent modification was undertaken in partnership with the European Pressure Ulcer Advisory Panel (EPUAP) and National Pressure Ulcer Advisory Panel (NPUAP) in 2009. This partnership did much to advance a consensus for defining the four main categories of pressure injury across North America and Europe; however, they failed to reach a consensus on two additional categories and a standard descriptor for categorising degrees of tissue damage.

The NPUAP included two additional categories termed 'unstageable' and 'suspected deep tissue injury' but the EPUAP did not. The NPUAP embraced the term 'stage' and the EPUAP the 'category' of ulcer. More recently, a Pan Pacific Alliance between Australia, New Zealand, Hong Kong and Singapore has led to the development of *Clinical Practice Guidelines for the Prevention and Treatment of Pressure Injuries* (AWMA, 2011) and this group has adopted the NPUAP six-stage classification system and the term 'stage' in an effort to expand an international consensus.

Risk assessment

A comprehensive risk assessment should be conducted on admission and discharge as clinically indicated by change in an individual's condition or as indicated by the specific healthcare agency protocol. A risk assessment should include a comprehensive clinical history for intrinsic and extrinsic risk factors, mobility and activity screening, nutritional screening, continence assessment and a systematic skin inspection and assessment. A validated pressure ulcer risk assessment tool should be employed in conjunction with the skin inspection and appropriate education of clinicians and carers should inform the appropriate use of these tools.

Risk assessment tools have gradually increased in number and use since the early 1960s. The most commonly employed risk assessment tools for adult populations include the Norton Scale (Norton et al., 1962), the Waterlow Score (Waterlow, 1985), the Braden Scale (Braden and Bergstrom, 1988), and for paediatric populations, the Braden Q (AWMA, 2011). A variety of other tools exist for specific populations such as the Glasgow Scale and Cubbin and Jackson Scale which are designed for intensive care populations, and the Neonatal Skin Risk Assessment Scale, Burn Pressure Ulcer Skin Risk Assessment Scale, Starkid Skin Scale and Glamorgan Scale for paediatric populations (AWMA, 2011). However, amongst these risk assessment tools there is no agreed consensus on subscales assessed, nor their ranking. Furthermore, methodological testing for reliability, sensitivity, specificity or predictive value rating differs to such an extent amongst these tools that comparisons have become difficult. Some clinical practice guidelines recommend that a validated risk assessment tool should be used in conjunction with informed clinical judgement (AWMA, 2011). The outcome of skin inspections and risk assessments need to be appropriately documented.

> **Practice point**
>
> An assessment of a patient's at-risk status is only beneficial if it is documented and a pressure ulcer prevention strategy is implemented, monitored and evaluated. In an acute care setting, initial pressure ulcer risk assessment should be carried out on admission then reassessed every 48 hours or whenever the patient's condition changes (i.e. improves or deteriorates). Long-term care reassessment of risk status should be done weekly for the 4 weeks then monthly to quarterly after that, and whenever the resident's condition changes.

Skin inspection

A comprehensive skin inspection should be conducted to ascertain the presence of pressure ulcers or observable pressure-related changes of intact skin such as blanching or non-blanching erythema, changes in skin temperature (warmth and coolness), tissue consistency (induration or boggy feel), alterations in sensation (pain, itching) and oedema. Skin colour changes due to erythema or hypoxia may not be so obvious on darkly pigmented skin and the assessor will need to palpate the skin to identify changes in temperature and tissue consistency as compared to adjacent anatomical tissues.

Skin inspection should also take into account the presence of medical devices such as compression stockings, tubes, cervical collars, callipers, contact casts, external prostheses and restraints. Although pressure ulcers most commonly occur over bony prominences such as the sacrum, ischial tuberosities, heels, trochanters and occiputs, they can also occur in soft tissues, such as ears and male genitalia when these tissues are compressed between contracted limbs or hard contact surfaces. Skin inspections should be conducted and documented

by educated clinicians and carers. High-risk individuals living independently, especially those with spinal cord or other neurological deficits, should receive regular instruction as to how to conduct self-inspections on a daily or more frequent basis and be advised of processes to be followed for off-loading and reporting identified skin damage.

> **Practice point**
>
> The use of vigorous skin rubbing or massage is contraindicated as a method of pressure ulcer prevention as this may be painful and stimulates an acute inflammatory response and increases the likelihood of damage to the microcirculation and fragile skin (AWMA, 2011).

Nutritional screening and assessment

Malnutrition-related extremes of body mass index such as morbid obesity or cachexia will increase the individual's predisposition to pressure ulcers. Individuals with morbid obesity have large amounts of poorly vascularised adipose tissue, and the capillaries in adipose tissue are particularly vulnerable to shear stress[17]. Furthermore, morbid obesity compromises movement and activity, and thus increases the risk of prolonged interface pressure. Cachexic individuals, on the other hand, have little adipose tissue deposition over bony prominences, which reduces the skin's tolerance to pressure. In addition, individuals with malnutrition and pressure ulcers can be expected to have impaired healing.

Although there are several validated nutritional screening tools for assessing malnutrition, none have been specifically validated for populations with pressure ulcers. However, those in existence provide a framework for assessment and can guide interventions to address identified deficits in body mass index, nutritional intake, swallowing, drug food interactions and access issues.

Treatment strategies: pressure ulcers

Skin care

Optimal healthy skin care is fundamental for skin protection. The goal is to maintain the normal slightly acidic pH of the skin (averages 5.5) and optimise the skin microclimate. The latter term relates to the temperature of skin or tissues and the humidity or skin-surface moisture (Clark et al., 2010). The acid mantle of the skin discourages bacterial colonisation and reduces the risk of opportunistic infection. Skin pH can best be maintained by avoidance of alkaline soaps and cleaners in favour of those that are perfume-free and pH neutral. Gentle skin cleansing practices and the use of tepid water will assist in preventing skin trauma and the use of skin barrier creams, emollients and protective barrier films can provide additional skin protection against urinary or faecal incontinence or excessive wound exudate.

Increases or decreases in skin temperature are closely aligned to changes in core body temperature; however, local increases in skin temperature can occur due to contact with plastic- or vinyl-covered support surfaces or the use of excessive amounts of bed linen, clothing or plastic-covered incontinence pads. Elevated body temperatures have been demonstrated to increase the risk of pressure ulcers and an increased body temperature of 1°C raises the metabolic demands of tissues by approximately 10% (Fisher et al., 1978). Therefore, it has been proposed that individuals with pyrexia and associated increased tissue metabolic demands may be even more susceptible to pressure ulcers when lesser amounts of pressure are applied for shorter duration (Fisher et al., 1978; Knox et al., 1994; Sae-Sia et al., 2005). Increased susceptibility to pressure ulcers has also been proposed by some researchers when localised skin temperatures are elevated, although more research is in this area is warranted (Fisher et al., 1978; Knox et al., 1994; Sae-Sia et al., 2005).

Excessive skin moisture or excessive skin dryness can alter the skin's tensile strength and resilience to pressure and shear forces. Interventions for optimising skin hydration and reducing dryness involve regular applications of moisturisers and adequate fluid intake. Interventions for reducing excessive skin moisture involve continence management if incontinence is an identified problem, containment of wound fluids and the use of skin barrier creams, emollients and protective barrier films. Environmental regulation of ambient room temperatures and good skin hygiene practices will assist in reducing the effects of excessive perspiration on the skin microclimate.

> **Practice point**
>
> If left in contact with vulnerable skin, exudate from pressure ulcers can lead to the development of irritant dermatitis (see Chapter 2) and new areas of skin breakdown. Erythematous maceration can be extremely painful, so treatment should be prompt and can benefit from application of a moderately potent, topical corticosteroid for a limited time to reduce local inflammation prior to the use of a barrier preparation.

Repositioning

Various methods of pressure redistribution are used to minimise the combined effects of pressure, friction and shear on the subcutaneous tissues as shown in Figure 8.3. The cognitively and neurologically aware individual will spontaneously

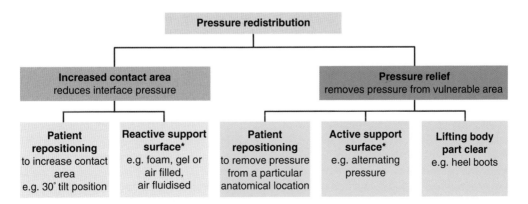

*A **reactive** support surface has the capability to change its load distribution properties only in response to applied load; an **active** support surface is able to change its load distribution properties with or without applied load.

Figure 8.3   Uses of pressure-redistributing support surfaces. Reprinted with permission from Wounds International, 2010.

reposition themselves when confronted by discomfort associated with prolonged interface pressure. Individuals with cognitive or neurological deficits, on the other hand, will need regular prompting or manual or mechanical device assistance with repositioning. The use of repositioning devices such as slide sheets and hoists can reduce the impact of shear and friction whilst repositioning. The frequency of repositioning is entirely dependent upon the individual's tissue tolerance to pressure and not times that suit care routines. Routine skin inspection on repositioning for signs of pressure compromise, such as erythema or warmth, will indicate if the individual is being repositioned as frequently as needed or the need for dynamic support surfaces, although continued repositioning is required even when pressure-redistribution surfaces are used.

It is important to avoid positioning an individual directly onto a bony prominence such as the iliac crests, trochanters or heels; and pillows, cushions or foam wedges may assist in maintaining correct positioning. Even minor changes in positioning can increase comfort and reduce the impact of pressure. To prevent shear stress, the head of the bed should be lowered to 30° or less an hour after feeding, unless medically contraindicated[15]. Heels require special attention and additional heel off-loading support, as the tissue density over the calcaneus is thin and support surfaces vary in their ability to off-load heel pressures adequately. Medical grade natural sheepskin can reduce friction and shear under heels and stabilise the microclimate (Jolley et al., 2004).

Pressure-redistribution support surfaces

Pressure-redistribution support surfaces are used in the prevention of pressure ulcers and the management of individuals with pressure ulcers. Numerous and increasingly more sophisticated support surfaces are available. A support surface has been defined as 'a specialised device for pressure redistribution designed for management of tissue loads, microclimate, and/or other therapeutic functions'[19]. Support surfaces include mattress or trolley overlays, mattress replacements, mattress and integrated bed systems, cushion overlays and replacement cushions. Support surfaces can be static (non-powered) and dynamic (powered) and are comprised of a variety of media, such as high-specification viscoelastic foam, elastic foam, gel, air or combinations of these media. Pressure-redistribution support surfaces can be broadly classified as either powered or non-powered constant low-pressure support surfaces (also referred to as reactive devices) and powered alternating support surfaces (also referred to as active devices) (Carville, 2007; AWMA, 2011).

Constant low-pressure support surfaces maintain a constant interface pressure while the individual remains in the same position, and the interface pressure is considered lower than a 'standard' mattress (AWMA, 2011). Although specifications or assumptions as to what constitutes a standard mattress vary considerably across different health settings and countries, generally any mattress that falls short of standards or recommendations for a high-specification foam mattress is considered a standard mattress. There is strong evidence for the efficacy of high-specification foam mattresses (contoured foam support surfaces) for pressure ulcer prevention (McInnes et al., 2008). So the reader is advised to check local recommendations for high-specification foam mattresses, and these recommendations should cover: design features such as type and multilayering of foam, foam density/hardness, support properties, mattress depth and cover features such as waterproof factor, fire-retardant properties, vapour permeability, shear resistance, conformability, etc. (AWMA, 2011).

No one specific high-specification constant low-pressure support mattress or overlay has been found to be better than another (AWMA, 2011). An alternating redistribution support surface produces programmed cycles of alternating air pressure through air cells in the device. The alternating cycles are usually one in two, that is 50% of the air cells are inflated or deflated at any time for periods of usually 10 minutes or less. Alternating devices are recommended for the care of high-risk individuals or when frequent manual repositioning is problematic (AWMA, 2011).

Factors to consider when selecting a support surface are aligned with patient, environmental and equipment parameters:

- *Patient factors*: risk score, weight, height and body mass index, mobility and comfort preferences;
- *Environmental factors*: shear, friction, pressure, microclimate;

- *Equipment factors*: weight and height limits, pressure-redistribution properties, ease of use and transport, waterproof and bacteria-resistant properties, fire-retardant properties, cleaning and maintenance requirements, local availability and cost.

(AWMA, 2011)

Regular repositioning and selection of an appropriate support surface are crucial elements for the prevention and management of pressure ulcers. The presence of a pressure ulcer on any anatomical location reduces the ability to position the individual on that affected site; thus, they will require more frequent repositioning and possibly a more sophisticated support surface.

> **Practice point**
>
> Foam rings, foam cut-outs, or doughnut-type devices for pressure redistribution should be avoided because they concentrate the pressure to surrounding tissue increasing oedema and venous congestion to the area. They become easily soiled, may act as a reservoir for pathogenic bacteria and they are uncomfortable to sit on and slip so they may inadvertently cause an increase in local pressure (AWMA, 2011).

Management of infection

There are many serious consequences of infected pressure ulcers. The wound will increase in size, produce more exudate, slough and odour and, if unresolved infection, may ultimately lead to septicaemia and death. Pressure ulcers are often colonised by multiple organisms, even though the clinical signs of infection may be absent. These organisms originate mainly from skin flora or from the bowel due to faecal contamination and typically include *Staphylococcus* and *Streptococcus, Proteus mirabilis* and *Escherichia coli*. Pressure ulcers frequently act as a reservoir for multiresistant bacteria.

It is important to maximise the patient's general health to boost host responses as patients are often critically ill and may have already received several courses of antibiotic therapy including maintaining adequate nutrition and correcting electrolyte imbalance.

There is an urgent need to rationalise the use of antibiotics when treating infected pressure ulcers, as it is difficult for antibiotics to reach the wound bed in sufficient therapeutic doses due to the presence of local ischemia and devitalised tissue (AWMA, 2011). Systemic antibiotics are not required for pressure ulcers that exhibit only clinical signs of local infection and should be restricted to those patients with pressure ulceration exhibiting signs of cellulitis, osteomyelitis and bacteraemia (Romanelli and Moore, 2006). These infections should be treated quickly using carefully selected antibiotics of the correct dose and for an appropriate time period (AWMA, 2011).

Superficial infection affects mainly stage II pressure ulcers; in such cases, the application of topical antiseptics has been shown to be of great benefit in controlling bacterial burden and preventing systemic complications, and is becoming a valuable alternative option to the indiscriminate use of systemic antibiotics. However, antiseptics should not routinely be used to clean pressure ulcers and should only be considered when the bacterial load needs to be controlled and then only for a limited period of time until the wound is clean and inflammation reduced (AWMA, 2011).

Deep tissue infection is a frequent complication of stage III and stage IV pressure ulcers, and is characterised by an increase in temperature in the skin surrounding the wound, tenderness and pain. There may also be extended erythema, reaching to the bone and into new areas of breakdown (Sanada et al., 2005). Any pressure ulcer with exposed bone is particularly at risk of osteomyelitis, which should be suspected if clinical signs of infection do not respond to conventional treatment.

Wound dressings: special considerations

Some dressings such as film or hydrocolloid dressings may be used to protect body areas at risk from friction or injury from tape removal, though foam dressings are an option to protect body areas and pressure ulcers at risk of shear injury.

Dressing performance of pressure ulcers is affected by friction and shear forces in areas such as the sacrum and heels where dressings can wrinkle causing additional local pressure, leakage and maceration and fall-off. Hydrocolloid dressings may be used to cover cleaned category/stage II pressure ulcers in body areas where they will not roll or melt but should be used with caution elsewhere. Adhesive dressings should be used carefully, as patients may have fragile, oedematous and macerated skin. Adhesive dressings should be removed with care to reduce skin trauma commonly associated with pressure injury.

Stage III and IV pressure ulcers, subject to their anatomical location, usually present as cavity wounds and produce copious amounts of exudate which can be difficult to manage. These large pressure ulcers require a moisture-retentive, cavity-filling dressing to eliminate the dead space in the wound and facilitate controlled wound closure.

Pressure ulcers are frequently covered in thick, moist, offensive slough and should be debrided to minimise bacterial burden. Dry eschar in pressure ulcers need not be debrided if oedema, erythema, or drainage are not present.

Topical negative pressure (TNP) devices, which utilise foam or gauze dressings to fill the wound defect and the application of suction, are commonly used in the treatment of extensive stage III or IV pressure ulcers. The therapy is reported to increase tissue perfusion, granulation deposition and wound contraction; remove wound fluids, reduce oedema and facilitate epithelialisation, though the latest Cochrane review concluded that there is no valid or reliable evidence that topical negative pressure increases chronic wound healing (Ubbink et al., 2008).

Practice point

Applying dressings to a sacral pressure ulcer can be difficult due to the contour of the body and loose wrinkly skin on the buttocks of elderly patients. It is difficult to make them adhere to the skin due to excessive moisture in this area from sweat, urine and wound exudate, and dressings may be pulled away due to the direct effect of friction and shear forces in patients who are either bed- or chair-bound. The use of skin protection wipes can form a useful barrier to protect the skin and act as a base to increase the adherence of dressings, and are preferable to the use of traditional barrier creams.

Many dressing manufacturers design dressings that are specifically shaped to minimise shear and friction on the sacrum. Most have rounded edges which are tapered to improve conformity, and as a general rule, thinner dressings have less tendency to roll and wrinkle up. When applying a wound dressing to the sacrum, try to position the patient for 15 minutes or longer off the area and make sure that the adhesive dressing is warm (at ambient room temperature) to help it bond to the skin. This can also be improved by placing your warm hands on top of the dressing *in situ*, and pressing gently to ensure the adhesive is in full contact with the skin. If specific sacral dressings are not available, standard dressings should have their square edges rounded off and used in the same way. Remember to use a large enough dressing to maximise adherence, which will be achieved by leaving a margin of at least 5 cm around the wound or broken skin.

Education and support

Education of clinicians, carers and individuals is fundamental for reducing pressure ulcers and optimising their management and healing outcomes. The Registered Nurses' Association of Ontario guideline (2007) proposes that pressure ulcer education programmes for clinicians should contain content outlining

- aetiology and risk factors;
- assessment of risk;
- prevention planning;
- accurate and timely documentation of assessments, management plans and interventions for preventing and managing risk;
- manual handling techniques and facility policies;
- selection, use and maintenance of pressure-redistribution support surfaces;
- assessment and staging;
- principles of wound management including selection of topical products and dressings;
- principles for patient education.

High-risk individuals living independently, especially those with spinal cord or other neurological deficits, should receive regular instruction as to how to conduct self-inspections on a daily or more frequent basis and be advised of processes to be followed for off-loading and reporting identified skin damage.

Education of patients and their families needs to be cognisant of age, cognitive, intellectual, cultural and socio-economic status. Education can be delivered via formal programmes or informal teaching sessions or printed material. However, high-risk populations such as the spinal cord injured or those restricted mobility warrant structured and frequent education to reinforce the importance of prevention.

Criteria for specialist referral

International guidelines (AWMA, 2011) recommend that advice should be quickly obtained from an appropriate specialist if any of the following circumstances apply:

- deterioration of patient's general condition;
- undermining, tunnelling, sinus tracts and/or extensive necrotic tissue;
- clinical signs of a deep-seated infection and/or systemic sepsis;
- exposed bone or tendon in the pressure ulcer;
- evidence of decreased tissue perfusion.

Surgery in the form of flap reconstruction or skin grafting may be required to facilitate complete wound closure, especially amongst compromised individuals or those with extensive ulceration.

Early referral to an occupational therapist, medical bioengineer or seating specialist is recommended for the spinal cord injured or persons with neuromuscular diseases:

- when the pressure ulcer is assessed to be related to, or complicated by, seating or wheelchair issues;
- following flap reconstruction of sacral or ischial tuberosity pressure ulcers;
- when there are posture issues such as scoliosis, kyphosis, obliquity, instability.

Finally, early referral to a physiotherapist can greatly improve mobility and repositioning activities for patients to help prevent further pressure injury occurrence.

Summary

Pressure ulcers are unfortunately common wounds and constitute a drain on health budgets. Moreover, they impact quality of life and healing outcomes for many. Discrepancies in methodologies employed for pressure ulcer prevalence and incidence data collection need to be abolished in order to facilitate useful international benchmarking, as

well as increase awareness of the exact scope of the problem. Clinical practice guidelines outline prevention strategies and best practice management, and it is fundamental that clinicians, consumers and carers are familiar with their content and use them to evaluate their practices. In light of the advances in contemporary knowledge, clinical wound management resources and technology, pressure ulcers should in fact be a relatively uncommon occurrence. Let us look forward to the time when this is indeed the situation.

Useful resources

Clinical guidelines

Australian Wound Management Association. *Clinical Practice Guidelines for the Prediction and Prevention of Pressure Ulcers*. Available at: http://www.awma.com.au/publications/publications.php#clinical

European Pressure Ulcer Advisory Panel and National Pressure Ulcer Advisory Panel. *Prevention and Treatment of Pressure Ulcers: Quick Reference Guide*. Available at: www.npuap.org and www.epuap.org

Registered Nurses Association Ontario (RNAO) *Best Practice Guidelines Risk Assessment and Prevention Pressure Ulcers*. Available at: http://ltctoolkit.rnao.ca/resources/pressure-ulcer

Organisations

European Pressure Ulcer Advisory Panel. Available at: http://www.epuap.org/

National Pressure Ulcer Advisory Panel (American). Available at: http://www.npuap.org/

Further reading

International Review: Pressure ulcer prevention: pressure, shear, friction and microclimate in context. Available at: http://www.woundsinternational.com/clinical-guidelines/international-review-pressure-ulcer-prevention-pressure-shear-friction-and-microclimate-in-context

References

Australian Wound Management Association (AWMA) (2011) *Pan Pacific Clinical Practice Guidelines for Pressure Injury Prevention and Management*. Osborne Park, WA:

Australian Wound Management Association. Available at: http://www.awma.com.au/publications/2012_AWMA_Pan_Pacific_Guidelines.pdf. Last accessed 17 November 2012.

Ayello, E.A., Lyder, C.H. (2008) A new era of pressure ulcer accountability in acute care. *Advances in Skin and Wound Care*, 21, 134–140.

Ayello, E.A., Lyder, C.H. (2009) Initiative-based pressure ulcer care. *Nursing Management*, 40(Suppl.), 16–22.

Baly, M. (1991) *As Miss Nightingale Said . . .* 2nd edn. London: Bailliere Tindall.

Bennett, G., Dealey, C., Posnett, J. (2004) The cost of pressure ulcers in the UK. *Age and Ageing*, 33(3), 230–235.

Black, J., Baharestani, M., Cuddigan J., et al. (2007) National Pressure Ulcer Advisory Panel's pressure ulcer staging system: history of pressure ulcer staging. *Dermatology Nursing*, 19(4), 343–349.

Braden, B., Bergstrom, N. (1988) Braden scale for predicting pressure sore risk. In Agency for Health Care Policy and Research, (1992). Pressure ulcers in adults: Prediction and prevention. *Ostomy/Wound Management*, 38(5), 67–77.

Bridel, J. (1993) The aetiology of pressure sores. *Journal of Wound Care*, 2(4), 230–238.

Burman, P. (1994) Measuring pressure. A guide to the units of measurement used to describe pressure and to the different types of pressure. *Journal of Wound Care*, 3(2), 83–86.

Carville, K. (2007) *Wound Care Manual*. Osborne Park, WA: Silver Chain Foundation.

Clark, M., Romanelli, M., Reger, S.I., Ranganathan, V.K., Black, J., Dealey, C. (2010) Microclimate in context. In: *Pressure Ulcer Prevention: Pressure, Shear, Friction and Microclimate in Context*. London: Wounds International.

European Pressure Ulcer Advisory Panel and National Pressure Ulcer Advisory Panel (2009) *Prevention and Treatment of Pressure Ulcers: Quick Reference Guide*. Washington DC: National Pressure Ulcer Advisory Panel. Available from: www.npuap.org and www.epuap.org. Last accessed 23 February 2012.

Fisher, S., Szymke, T., Apte S., Kosiak, M. (1978) Wheelchair cushion effect on skin temperature. *Archives Physical Medical Rehabilitation*, 59, 68–72.

Gorecki, C., Brown, J.M., Nelson, E.A., et al. (2009) Impact of pressure ulcers on quality of life in older patients: a systematic review. *Journal of the American Geriatrics Society*, 57(7), 1175–1183.

Gorecki, C., Closs, S.J., Nixon, J., Briggs, M. (2011) Patient-reported pressure ulcer pain: a mixed-methods systematic review. *Journal Pain Symptom Management*, 42(3), 443–459.

Graves, N., Birrel, F., Whitby, M. (2005) Modelling the economic losses from pressure ulcers among hospi-talised patients in Australia. *Wound Repair and Regeneration*, 137(5), 462–46.

Gunningberg, L., Donaldson, N., Aydin, C., Idvall, E. (2011) Exploring variation in pressure ulcer prevalence in Sweden and the USA: benchmarking in action. *Journal of Evaluation in Clinical Practice*, ISSN 1365-2753 2011, 1–7.

Hopkins, A., Dealey, C., Bale, S., Defloor, T., Worboys, F. (2006) Patient stories of living with a pressure ulcer. *Journal of Advanced Nursing*, 56(4), 345–353.

James, J., Evans, J.A., Young, T., Clark, M. (2010) Pressure ulcer prevalence across Welsh orthopaedic units and community hospitals: surveys based on the European Pressure Ulcer Advisory Panel minimum data set. *International Wound Journal*, 7, 147–152.

Jolley, D., Wright, R., McGowan, S., et al. (2004) Preventing pressure ulcers with the Australian medical sheepskin: An open-label randomised controlled trail. *Medical Journal of Australia*, 180, 324–327.

Knox, D., Anderson, T., Anderson, P. (1994) Effects of different turn intervals on skin of healthy older adults. *Advances in Wound Care*, 7, 48–56.

Landis, E. (1930) Microcirculation studies of capillary blood pressure in human skin. *Heart*, 15, 209–228.

Lapsey, H.M., Vogels, R. (1996) Cost and prevention of pressure ulcers in an acute teaching hospital. *International Journal of Quality Health Care*, 8(1), 61–66.

Lyder, C.H., Shannon, R., Empleo-Frazier, O., McGehee, D., White, C. (2002) A comprehensive program to prevent pressure ulcers in long-term care: exploring costs and outcomes, *Ostomy/Wound Management*, 48(4), 52–62.

National Pressure Ulcer Advisory Panel (NPUAP) (2007) *Support Surface Standards Initiative*. Available at: http://www.npuap.org/NPUAP_S3I_TD.pdf Last accessed 18 November 2012.

McInnes, E., Cullum, N.A., Bell- Syer, S.E.M., Durnvill, J.C. (2008) Support surfaces for pressure ulcer prevention. cochrane database. *Systemic Reviews*, 4, CD001735.

Norton, D., McLaren, R., Exton-Smith, A. (1962) *An Investigation of Geriatric Nursing Problems in Hospital*. London: National Corporation for the Care of Old People.

Orsted, H., Ohura, T., and Harding, K. (2010) Pressure, shear, friction and microclimate in context. In International Review. Pressure ulcer prevention: Pressure, shear, friction and microclimate in context. London: Wounds International. Available at: http://www.woundsinternational.com/pdf/content_8925.pdf. Last accessed 17 November 2012.

Phillips, L., Buttery, J. (2009) Exploring pressure ulcer prevalence and preventative care. *Nursing Times*, 105, 16.

Pieper, B. (2007) Mechanical forces: pressure, shear, and friction. In: *Acute & Chronic Wounds: Current*

Management Concepts (eds R. Bryant, D. Nix), 3rd edn. Philadelphia, PA: Mosby.

Reger, S.I., Ranganathan, V.K., Orsted, H.L., Ohura, T., Gefen, A. (2010) Shear and friction in context. In: *International review. Pressure ulcer prevention: Pressure, shear, friction and microclimate in context.* London: Wounds International.

Registered Nurses' Association of Ontario (2007) *Assessment and Management of Stage I to IV Pressure Ulcers.* Toronto: RNAO.

Richardson, R. (ed.) (1977) *Nurse Sarah Anne with Florence Nightingale at Scutari.* London: John Murray Publishers Ltd.

Romanelli, M., Moore, Z. (2006) Topical management of Infected Grade III and IV Pressure ulcers. In: *European Wound Management Association (EWMA).* Position document: Management of wound infection. London: MEP Ltd., pp. 11–13.

Sae-Sia, W., Wipke-Davis, D., Williams, D. (2005) Elevated sacral skin temperature (T(s)): a risk factor for pressure ulcer development in hospitalized neurologically impaired Thai patients. *Applied Nursing Research,* 18(1), 29–35.

Sanada, H., Nakagami, G., Romanelli, M. (2005) Identifying criteria for pressure ulcer infection. In: *European Wound Management Association (EWMA).* Position document: Identifying criteria for wound infection. London: MEP Ltd., pp. 10–13.

Shea, J. (1975) Pressure sores: classification and management. *Clinical Orthopaedics and Related Research,* 112, 89–100.

Spilsbury K, Nelson EA, Cullum C, et al. (2007) Pressure ulcers and their treatment and effects on quality of life: hospital inpatient perspectives. *Journal of Advanced Nursing,* 57, 494–504.

Taalajasjo, M., Black, J., Dealey, C., Gefen, A. (2010) Pressure in context. In: *International review. Pressure ulcer prevention: Pressure, shear, friction and microclimate in context.* London: Wounds International.

Thompson, R.J. (1961) Pathological changes in mummies. *Proceedings of the Royal Society of Medicine,* 54, 409.

Ubbink, D.T., Westerbos, S.J., Evans, D., Land, L., Vermeulen, H. (2008) Topical negative pressure for treating chronic wounds. *Cochrane Database of Systematic Reviews,* Issue (3). Art. No.: CD001898. DOI: 10.1002/14651858.CD001898.pub2.

Waterlow, J. (1985) A risk assessment card. *Nursing Times,* 81(48), 49–55.

Wounds International (2010) *International Review. Pressure Ulcer Prevention: Pressure, Shear, Friction, Microclimate in Context. A Consensus Document.* London: Wounds International.

Wound, Ostomy and Continence Nurses Society (WOCN) (2010) *Guideline for Prevention and Management of Pressure Ulcers.* Mount Laurel, NJ: WOCN Society.

9 Diabetic Foot Disease

Jan Apelqvist

Department of Endocrinology, University Hospital of Skåne (SUS), Malmö, and Division for Clinical Sciences, University of Lund, Malmö, Sweden

Overview

- Prevalence of diabetic foot ulceration varies in different geographical areas due to differences in socio-economic conditions, standards of foot care and quality of footwear. Between half and three quarters of all lower extremity amputations are related to diabetes.
- Diabetic foot ulceration should be recognised as a sign of multi-organ disease as co-morbidities such as cardiovascular disease delay healing of diabetic foot wounds.
- Diabetic foot disease is a lifelong condition as patients are always at high risk of developing a new ulcer. It is associated with a high risk of morbidity and mortality.
- Infection in the diabetic foot is a limb-threatening condition. More than 50% of diabetic patients with foot ulcers have signs of infection on admission to hospital.
- Prevention of foot ulceration in patients with diabetes is dependent on identification of risk status, appropriate management of co-morbidities, meticulous foot care and ongoing education of carers and patients.
- Many wound management interventions fail due to lack understanding of the need for effective offloading or non-weight bearing.
- A multidisciplinary approach and long-term follow-up of the management of diabetic foot ulceration results in a substantial decrease in amputation rate.

Introduction

Foot complications in diabetes are costly in human and financial terms worldwide. The prevalence of diabetic foot ulceration varies from country to country due to differences in socio-economic conditions, standards of foot care and quality of footwear. It has been claimed that every 30 seconds, a lower limb is amputated due to diabetes and that 20–40% of total expenditure on diabetes can be attributable to complications related to the diabetic foot (Boulton et al., 2005). Of all amputations in diabetic patients, 85% are preceded by a foot ulcer which subsequently deteriorates due to severe infection or gangrene (Apelqvist and Larsson, 2000; Boulton, 2004; Boulton et al., 2005; IWGDF, 2007).

Wound Healing and Skin Integrity: Principles and Practice, First Edition. Edited by Madeleine Flanagan.
© 2013 John Wiley & Sons, Ltd. Published 2013 by John Wiley & Sons, Ltd.

The complexity of diabetic foot ulcers necessitates an intrinsic knowledge of underlying pathophysiology and a multifactorial approach in which aggressive management of infection and ischaemia is of major importance. The negative consequences of foot ulcers in people with diabetes include not only morbidity but also disability and premature mortality. A multidisciplinary approach including a preventive strategy, patient and staff education and multifactorial treatment of foot ulcers has been reported to reduce amputation rate by more than 50% (IWGDF, 2007; Krishnan et al., 2008; Larsson et al., 2008; Zayed et al., 2009).

Aetiology

A diabetic foot wound is caused by ulceration and destruction of deep tissues associated with neurological abnormalities and various degrees of peripheral vascular disease in the lower limb (Schaper et al., 2003; IWGDF, 2007). A foot ulcer is the general term to describe a full-thickness wound below the ankle in a diabetic patient, irrespective of duration (IWGDF, 2007). Active foot disease may be of recent onset or due to a deteriorating chronic situation and refers to anyone with diabetes who presents with the following:

- a blister or foot wound, however superficial,
- any clinical signs of infection,
- evidence of necrosis or gangrene,
- dislocation or fracture in the foot without significant trauma,
- unexplained foot pain.

Large cohort studies have provided a better understanding of the factors influencing the outcome of foot ulceration (Apelqvist and Larsson, 2000; IWGDF, 2007; Prompers et al., 2007; Prompers et al., 2008; Gershater et al., 2009). Findings from mostly European cohorts show that more than 50% of the diabetic patients with foot ulcers had signs of infection on admission to a hospital-based multidisciplinary foot team. About 50% of these ulcers were neuroischaemic and one-third of patients with foot ulceration had signs of both peripheral artery disease and infection (Prompers et al., 2007, 2008; Gershater et al., 2009). Presence of diabetic foot ulceration is associated with an extensive co-morbidity that increases significantly with severity of foot disease (Apelqvist and Larsson, 2000; IWGDF, 2007; Prompers et al., 2007, 2008; Gershater et al., 2009; Apelqvist et al., 2011).

The most important factors related to development of foot ulcers are peripheral neuropathy, minor foot trauma, foot deformity and decreased tissue perfusion (Apelqvist and Larsson, 2000; Boulton et al., 2005; Boyko et al., 2006; Boulton, 2008). Table 9.1 summarises the contributing factors and clinical indications for diabetic foot ulcers. Diabetic foot ulcers are frequently seen in patients with a combination of two or more risk factors occurring together. Sensory neuropathy is associated with the loss of pain, temperature sensation, pressure awareness and proprioception.

As a consequence, minor trauma that is not felt by the patient can quickly cause skin damage or ulceration. Prospective studies have shown that sensory neuropathy is a major predictor for development of foot ulcers (Abbott et al., 2002; Boulton, 2004, 2008). Motor neuropathy results in atrophy and weakness of the intrinsic muscles of the foot, flexion deformities of the toes and an abnormal walking pattern (Boulton, 2004, 2008; IWGDF, 2007). Autonomic neuropathy results in reduced or absent sweat secretion, causing dry skin, cracks and fissures. Foot deformities, abnormal gait and limited 'joint mobility syndrome' creates a set of conditions that results in altered biomechanical loading of the foot, with increased plantar foot pressures and increased shear forces. The 'stiff foot syndrome' with impaired joint mobility is probably caused by disturbed collagen metabolism, or non-enzymatic glycosylation of proteins in the joint tissue and skin (Boulton, 2004, 2008; IWGDF, 2007). Due to the loss of protective skin sensation, the repetitive trauma of walking is not obvious to the patient and hyperkeratosis (callus) gradually forms and over time a foot ulcer finally develops as seen in Figure 9.1.

Neuropathic bone and joint disease, usually affecting the mid- or hind foot, is sometimes referred to as 'Charcot foot' or neuro-osteoarthropathy with a prevalence of 0.5–1% (Jeffcoate et al., 2005; Trepman et al., 2005). This condition can cause severe deformity and plantar ulceration. The aetiology of osteoarthropathy in the neuropathic diabetic foot is complex and not fully understood, but precipitating trauma is often described in a foot with autonomic and sensori-motor neuropathy. Neuro-osteoarthropathy is an

Table 9.1   Diabetic foot ulceration: contributing factors and clinical indications

Contributing factors	Clinical indications
Sensory neuropathy	Impaired vibration perception (tuning fork 128 MHz)
	Vibratory pressure threshold >25 V
	Impaired protection sensation – monofilaments
	Loss of skin sensation
	Loss of pain, temperature sensation, pressure awareness and proprioception
Motor neuropathy	Muscle atrophy and wasting
	Difficulty in climbing stairs
	Difficulty in lifting/handling small objects
Autonomic neuropathy	Anhidrosis
	Excessive dry, scaly, cracked skin
	Oedema
Biomechanical foot deformity	Osteoarthropathy
	Limited joint mobility
	Stiff foot syndrome
	Bony prominences
	Callus formation
	Previous foot ulcer
	Previous amputation
	Altered walking pattern
Trauma	Ill-fitting shoes/footwear
	Walking barefoot
	Falls/accidents
	Objects inside shoes
Peripheral vascular disease	Absent pedal pulses
	Doppler toe pressures
	Delayed capillary refill
	Claudication
	Gangrene
	Pain at rest
Socio-economic status	Poor access to healthcare
	Low social position
	Social isolation
	Limited knowledge and understanding
	Negligence

acute condition often misdiagnosed as cellulitis or osteomyelitis and presents with a hot, erythematous, swollen foot with or without pain and no ulceration and initially no radiographic findings. A loss of sympathetic tone in the peripheral vessels causes demineralisation of the bones of the foot leading to rapid progression with bone fragmentation and joint destruction especially in neuropathic patients who feel no pain and continue to ambulate. The chronic phase of this condition results in collapse of the mid-foot or ankle leading to the typical 'rocker bottom' deformity followed by plantar ulceration (Figures 9.1 and 9.2), but it should be remembered that the loss of sympathetic tone is just one of the hypothesis behind osteoarthropathy in the diabetic foot (Jeffcoate et al., 2005).

There is limited information about long-term prognosis of diabetic foot ulcers, but available data indicate a probability for developing further ulcers following healing of the first ulcer (Apelqvist et al., 1993; Walsh, 1996; Mantey et al., 1999; Connor and Mahdi, 2004). In preliminary data from a large cohort study, the development of new diabetic foot ulcers was 32% within 2 years of follow-up of which 11% occurred on the same side and site as the initial ulcer (Apelqvist and Larsson, 2000). The mortality rate is substantial in patients with foot ulcers. In a Swedish study, the mortality rate was twice as high among patients with healed foot ulcers and four times as high among patients with a previous amputation compared to an age- and sex-matched population (Apelqvist et al., 1993). Increased mortality among patients with diabetes and foot ulcers has been explained by the presence of concurrent disease such as cardio-cerebrovascular disease and nephropathy. These findings emphasise the need for lifelong observation of the diabetic foot at risk and the importance of preventive foot care.

Psychological impact

Decreased physical, emotional and social function in patients with diabetic foot disease is well known (Carrington et al., 1996; Vileikyte, 2001; Gonzalez et al., 2010). People with foot ulcers and amputations often suffer from depression and have reduced quality of life (Ragnarsson-Tennvall and Apelqvist, 2000; Hjelm et al., 2003; Nabuurs-Franssen et al., 2005; Vileikyte, 2008; Gonzalez et al., 2011). Social isolation, poor education and low socio-economic status place people with diabetes at higher risk of foot problems due to limited access to care and support. (Hjelm et al., 2003; Nabuurs-Franssen et al., 2005; Vileikyte, 2008; Gonzalez et al., 2011). Studies consistently demonstrate that an individual's perception of risk of developing diabetes-related foot complications is based on their own personal symptoms and beliefs about the effectiveness of self-care which can influence their ability to look after their feet and concordance (Ragnarsson-Tennvall and Apelqvist, 2000; Vileikyte, 2001; Hjelm et al., 2003; Gonzalez et al., 2011). Risk of amputation increases when people with diabetes are socially isolated and depressed (Nabuurs-Franssen et al., 2005).

People with diabetes and neuropathy who believe that pain is a reliable symptom of foot ulceration are less likely to seek foot care or follow health advice. Beliefs and expectations about health and illness relating to diabetes and foot ulceration are important and must be taken into account when preventing and managing foot problems (Ragnarsson-Tennvall and Apelqvist, 2000; Vileikyte, 2001, 2008; Hjelm et al., 2003; Nabuurs-Franssen et al., 2005; Gonzalez et al., 2011).

Psychological factors are of utmost importance since most foot ulcers are detected initially by the patient and in 25% of cases, the patient denies the

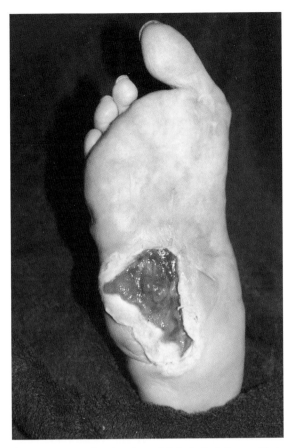

Figure 9.1   Foot showing signs of diabetic foot disease. Photo courtesy of Madeleine Flanagan.

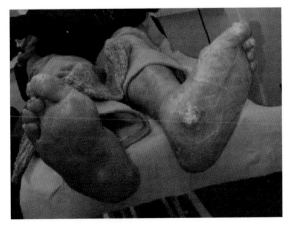

Figure 9.2   Foot showing signs of neuro-osteoarthropathy. Photo courtesy of Richard Leigh.

existence of the ulcer and therefore delays treatment (Apelqvist and Larsson, 2000). Patients with foot ulcers are often considered as non-compliant by healthcare professionals who may not recognise that they have a more negative attitude towards their feet, have limitations in daily living, leisure activities and employment, and have attitudinal differences towards their chronic disease (Hjelm et al., 2003; Nabuurs-Franssen et al., 2005; Vileikyte, 2008; Gonzalez et al., 2011). Major factors influencing an individual's behaviour include limited mobility, reduction in social activities, isolation, increased family tension, increased dependency, gender and have a negative impact on general health.

Principles of diabetic foot ulcer management

Treatment of the diabetic foot requires a multidisciplinary approach because of the complexity of factors related to outcome (IWGDF, 2007). Management includes strategies for treatment of peripheral ischaemia, oedema, pain, infection, metabolic disturbances and malnutrition; aggressive management of concurrent disease; and a coordinated system for support of both patients and carers to implement the treatment strategy (NICE, 2011). The management principles of diabetic foot ulceration are summarised in Table 9.2.

Due to the varying severity of diabetic foot complications, the management of foot ulcers can be divided into four separate categories:

(1) Low risk of foot ulceration;
(2) Increased risk of foot ulceration;
(3) Management of an existing foot ulcer;
(4) Maintenance of the healed foot ulcer.

However, the general principles of managing diabetic foot ulceration are based on the following consensus guidelines (NICE, 2011; IWGDF, 2007):

- All individuals should have emergency access to a specialist foot protection team, including the ability to self-refer and be seen quickly.
- Regular screening for early detection of neuropathy, peripheral vascular disease and foot deformities should occur with frequency depending on individual risk status.

- Every patient presenting with a foot ulcer should be examined for the presence of ischaemia and infection.
- Co-morbidities associated with diabetic foot disease require optimal medical management and regular review.
- Diabetic-foot-related complications should be identified and treated early with appropriate interventions.
- Long-term surveillance and treatment determined by the risk status of the individual should be established.
- Preventative foot-care strategies should be implemented to include ongoing advice and education about foot care and footwear.

Diabetic foot ulceration: assessment considerations

Accurate diagnosis for a patient with an ulcerated foot is essential to facilitate prompt referral and treatment by a multidisciplinary foot team as this has been identified as the most important intervention to prevent amputation (Apelqvist and Larsson, 2000; Schaper et al., 2003; Boulton et al., 2005; IWGDF, 2007). The feet of a diabetic patient should be inspected at every visit to healthcare providers. The International Working Group on the Diabetic Foot (2007) has suggested a simple risk classification with regard to prevention of diabetes-related amputations and foot ulceration (see Table 9.3).

If this strategy is followed it can achieve a 25–40% reduction in the incidence of ulceration or amputation and has been shown to be cost-effective (Ragnarson-Tennvall and Apelqvist, 2001; Ortegon et al., 2004; Boulton et al., 2005).

Practice point

The simplest way to identify a patient's risk status is by taking a history and examination that focuses on the following questions:

(1) Is there any evidence of peripheral neuropathy and loss of sensation?
(2) Is any foot deformity present?
(3) Is there a history of foot ulceration, amputation or Charcot foot?

Table 9.2   Management principles: diabetic foot ulceration

Management principle	Assessment/investigation	Treatment
Improve metabolic control	HbA1c blood test (long-term diabetes control) Self-monitoring of glucose	Insulin treatment often necessary Nutritional support and advice Weight loss
Improve tissue perfusion	Assess extent of tissue damage Non-invasive vascular testing: systolic toe/ankle blood pressure Transcutaneous oxygen pressure Duplex (ultrasound) Invasive vascular testing: angiography, magnetic resonance imaging (MRI), CT angiography CO_2 angiography	Percutaneous transluminal angioplasty (PTA) Subintimal angioplasty Reconstructive vascular surgery Vascular agents Control oedema Hyperbaric oxygen
Identify and treat superficial/deep infection and osteomyelitis	Assess extent of tissue damage ESR, CRP, white blood count, bacterial culture, bone biopsy, X-ray, CT-bone scan, MRI	Antibiotics oral/parenteral Incision/drainage/debridement Surgical removal of bone Amputation
Control oedema	Identify cause of oedema Establish extent of venous insufficiency, neuropathy, hydrostatic oedema, congestive heart failure, nephropathy, malnutrition	External compression therapy Intermittent compression (pumps) Diuretics plus compression Elevation Increase mobility (but remember plantar ulcers limit walking)
Optimise pain control	Identify cause/type/characteristic of pain (ischaemia, infection, inflammation, mechanical pressure, neuropathic pain, etc.) Patient assessment of pain: diary, visual analogue scale, verbal rating scales	Non-pharmacological treatment: immobilisation/offloading, relieve anxiety/fear, relaxation, distraction Pharmacological treatment: analgesic agents local/systemic, anticonvulsants if pain related to neuropathy, antidepressants
Effective offloading	Biomechanical evaluation to evaluate walking capacity/gait pattern	Protective/therapeutic footwear Insoles/orthosis Total contact cast/walkers, crutches, wheelchair, limit ambulation
Prepare wound bed to optimise healing	Assess condition of wound bed: necrosis, slough, exudation, quality of granulation tissue, bioburden Assess condition of surrounding skin: maceration, inflammation	Wound debridement: remove callus/devitalised tissue Control exudate, maintain moist wound healing, control infection If no response use advanced therapies, e.g. NWPT, tissue engineering, monitor carefully
Correct foot deformities	Evaluation of foot deformities	Corrective foot surgery Amputation Physiotherapy
Improve patient's general physical condition	Correct dehydration/malnutrition Treat concurrent disease, e.g. congestive heart failure, metabolic syndrome Monitor smoking habits	Fluid and nutrition replacement therapy Aggressive treatment of intercurrent disease, e.g. antiplatelet drugs, antihypertensive agents, lipid-decreasing agents Cessation of smoking Weight loss Promote exercise

(Continued)

Table 9.2   (*Continued*)

Management principle	Assessment/investigation	Treatment
Provide long-term psychosocial support	Evaluate knowledge/understanding Identify social and economic situation Determine health beliefs, capacity for self-care Assess mood, e.g. anxiety/depression scales QoL assessment	Improve patient/carer education Establish ongoing support and follow-up Improve adherence with treatment Emphasise multidisciplinary team involvement

ESR, erythrocyte sedimentation rate; CRP, C-reactive protein; CT, computed tomography; GCSF, granulocyte colony stimulating factor; MRI, magnetic resonance imaging; NWPT, negative wound pressure therapy.

The answers to these questions help to determine a patient's risk status and guide management decisions about treatment, referral and follow-up. Simple foot screening assessment tools are useful for healthcare professionals to identify those patients that need to be referred to specialist teams. A good example of a quick assessment tool can be downloaded from the Useful Resources section at the end of this chapter (60-Second Diabetic Foot Screen Tool) (Inlow, 2004). This tool has been shown to have content validity and inter-rater reliability in a variety of clinical environments.

Screening for loss of sensation and foot deformities should be performed at least once a year on patients with low risk of foot ulceration. Symptoms of diabetic peripheral neuropathy may include tingling, numbness, burning (especially in the evening), muscle wasting and pain in the toes, feet, legs, hands and arms. Onset is gradual and often is not reported by the patient. The procedure used for a more detailed sensory foot examination can be found at the International Working Group on the Diabetic Foot website listed in the Useful Resources section. Visual inspection of the feet for obvious deformities such as hammer toes, bunions, flat feet, absent pedal pulses, calluses and ulceration should be performed in all diabetic patients and are important predictors of ulceration (Connor and Mahdi, 2004). A history of a previous diabetic foot ulcer puts the patient at an increased risk of future ulceration.

Table 9.3   Risk classification for prevention of diabetes-related foot complications

Presenting features	Risk status	Clinical examination	Podiatry	Orthotic treatment
No ulceration No sensory neuropathy	No additional risk	Once a year	Only if special requirements	Only if special requirements
No ulceration Sensory neuropathy with or without PAD	Low	Every 6 months	Every 6 months	Education of the need for adequately fitted shoes
Previous foot ulcer/amputation Foot deformity Peripheral ischaemia	Moderate	Every 3 months	Regular visits to podiatrist in relation to severity	Fitting of special therapeutic foot wear/insoles
Previous foot ulcer/amputation Foot ulcer osteoarthropathy	High amputation rate increase Mortality rates increase	Typically, every 4–8 weeks, depending on progress	Treatment by Diabetes Foot Team[a]	Specifically designed orthoses, e.g. temporary shoes Total contact cast/walkers

Source: Modified from IWGDF (2007).
[a]Primary or secondary care depending on healthcare setting.

Assessment of vascular status

A diabetic foot ulcer should be considered ischaemic until proven otherwise by extensive clinical examination and non-invasive vascular testing to promptly identify the need for revascularisation. Peripheral vascular disease, in conjunction with minor trauma, may result in painful foot ulcers predominantly ischaemic in origin. However, peripheral vascular disease and neuropathy are frequently present in the same patient (Jeffcoate et al., 2006; Prompers et al., 2007, 2008; Gershater et al., 2009).

No patient should undergo amputation without previous vascular assessment with a view to the possibility of vascular intervention (Apelqvist and Larsson, 2000; IWGDF, 2007; Apelqvist, 2011). Absence of palpable pedal pulses indicates the presence of peripheral vascular disease but cannot discriminate with regard to probability of primary healing (Apelqvist and Larsson, 2000; IWGDF, 2007; Prompers et al., 2007, 2008; Faglia et al., 2009; Gershater et al., 2009).

Ischaemic pain can often be absent and presence of gangrene indicates that severe tissue destruction already has occurred. Because of this, non-invasive vascular testing such as systolic toe/ankle blood pressure, transcutaneous oxygen measurement and ultrasound are recommended for early recognition of neuro-ischaemic or ischaemic ulcers in need of revascularisation (Apelqvist and Larsson, 2000; IWGDF, 2007; Prompers et al., 2007, 2008; Gershater et al., 2009; Apelqvist et al., 2011) to achieve healing. A systolic toe pressure less than 30–45 mmHg, an ankle pressure less than 50–80 mmHg or a transcutaneous oxygen pressure measurement of less than 30 mmHg has been reported to be critical for primary healing of foot ulcers or healing after minor amputation (Dargis et al., 1999; Apelqvist and Larsson, 2000; IWGDF, 2007; Norgren et al., 2007; Mills, 2008; Ihnat and Mills, 2010; Hinchliffe et al., 2011; Apelqvist, 2011). It is important to recognise the problem of falsely increased ankle pressure that is attributable to vascular calcification which is common in patients with diabetes (Norgren et al., 2007; Mills, 2008; Ihnat and Mills, 2010; Apelqvist, 2011; Hinchliffe et al., 2011). An important observation relating to the consequence of peripheral vascular disease is that many diabetic individuals with ischaemia do not have severe rest pain or claudication. This is believed to be related to the loss of sensation due to peripheral sensory neuropathy (Jeffcoate et al., 2006; Prompers et al., 2008; Gershater et al., 2009; Apelqvist et al., 2011).

Assessment of wound infection

The International Working Group on the Diabetic Foot (2007) clinically identifies infection in the diabetic foot wound by the presence of exudate which is often serous or purulent, together with two or more signs or symptoms of inflammation such as redness, induration, pain, tenderness, warmth, necrosis and bone exposure with or without systemic signs such as fever, malaise and hyperglycaemia as seen in Figure 9.3 (Lipsky et al., 2004; Lipsky, 2004).

Symptoms of infection in the diabetic foot are as follows:

- Localised pain and/or tenderness;
- Localised oedema surrounding wound and foot;
- Increased redness and warmth;
- Increased wound exudate;
- Pus discharging from ulcer;
- General discomfort, nausea, loss of appetite;
- Fever and chills;
- Altered walking pattern (limping, immobility).

Infection should be considered whenever local signs, e.g. pain, redness, swelling develop even when they are less pronounced than usual as substantial tissue damage may occur. In almost 50% of patients with diabetes and deep foot infections, local inflammatory signs and symptoms such as

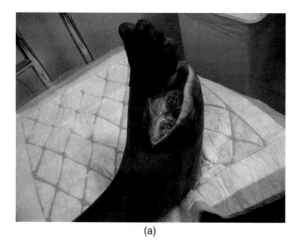

(a)

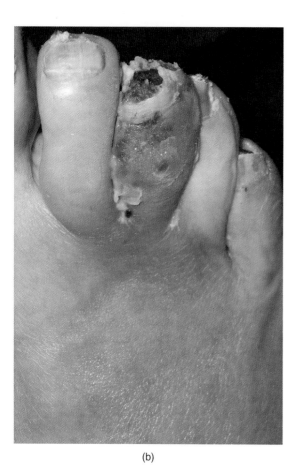

(b)

Figure 9.3   (a,b) Diabetic foot ulcers showing signs of infection. Photos courtesy of (a) Zakiya Ismail Al-Dhahri and (b) Richard Leigh.

increased white blood cell count, erythrocyte sedimentation rate (ESR), C-reactive protein (CRP) concentration, pyrexia and erythema are absent resulting in delayed diagnosis and thus prompt treatment (Lipsky et al., 2004; Lipsky, 2004). This may be due to factors such as an impaired immunoresponse, decreased peripheral vascular insufficiency, peripheral neuropathy and poor metabolic control (Lipsky et al., 2004; Lipsky, 2004). Some patients with diabetic foot infection will have worsening of glycaemic control, but other blood tests are not always easy to interpret. Normal or slightly increased CRP, ESR, white blood counts, body temperature do not exclude the possibility of an infection; however, substantially increased values indicate a high possibility of a deep soft tissue infection such as a abscess.

When infection of a diabetic foot wound is suspected, a microbiological diagnosis will usually assist management. In a superficial infection, acute, Gram-positive cocci are the most common wound pathogen (Lipsky et al., 2004; Lipsky, 2004; IWGDF, 2007). Studies have confirmed that chronic ulcers with deep infection and wounds with necrotic tissue commonly have polymicrobial flora with a combination of Gram-negative, anaerobic and Gram-positive organisms, especially in patients who have received prior antibiotic treatment (Apelqvist and Larsson, 2000; Lipsky et al., 2004; Lipsky, 2004). Studies comparing different antibiotic regimens in the management of skin and soft tissue infection, or infection that involve both soft tissue and bone in diabetic foot ulceration, report no differences between treatment strategies (NICE, 2011). There are substantial limitations in most studies evaluating the efficacy of antimicrobial agents with a high risk of bias. As a consequence, the initial antimicrobial treatment as well as duration of treatment is based on clinical experience rather than a specific evidence base (Apelqvist and Larsson, 2000; Lipsky et al., 2004; Lipsky, 2004).

The extension of soft tissue infection to underlying bone in diabetic foot wounds poses diagnostic and therapeutic challenges (Apelqvist and Larsson, 2000; Lipsky et al., 2004; Lipsky, 2004; Berendt et al., 2008; Butalia et al., 2008). Identification of osteomyelitis is based on detection of the signs and symptoms of infection, although many patients with diabetic foot wounds have no typical local signs. Left untreated, infection becomes chronic and disrupts the local blood supply to the affected bone resulting in eventual death of bone tissue.

Radiological diagnosis is often difficult because changes suggesting osteomyelitis usually take several weeks before they are visible on X-ray. The difficulty in distinguishing between osteomyelitis and osteoarthropathy is well recognised and can be problematic in clinical practice. A bone scan, magnetic resonance imaging (MRI) or CT scan can be of value to determine the existence and extent of deep foot infection but are not always available (Lipsky et al., 2004; Lipsky, 2004; Berendt et al., 2008; Butalia et al., 2008). Blood tests are of limited use but increased ESR, leukocytosis, fever, CRP concentrations, if present, are usually indicative of soft tissue infection (NICE, 2011). In the case of a deep soft tissue infection, abscess or necrotising tendovaginitis, immediate surgery is usually required to save the affected limb (Apelqvist and Larsson, 2000; Lipsky et al., 2004; Lipsky, 2004).

Practice point

What is the best way to detect bone infection in patients with diabetic foot wounds?

The use of microbiological cultures, although common, are often inaccurate as the specimen may not be properly obtained or the patient is on antibiotic treatment and results are not available for 3 or 4 days (NICE, 2011). Assessment of clinical signs of infection in diabetic patients provides limited information for early diagnosis of osteomyelitis, so a quicker, more reliable method is required. Although bone histology is considered to be the most reliable method of diagnosing osteomyelitis (Prompers et al., 2008), it is not frequently used in clinical practice as it is an invasive procedure which puts the patient at risk. However, microbiological cultures are valuable in situations when the patient does not respond to treatment and in clinical environments when information about MRSA and ESBL is mandatory. If an initial X-ray is not conclusive, an MRI can help to identify osteomyelitis in the diabetic foot or if MRI is contraindicated, then white blood cell scanning can be a good alternative (NICE, 2011).

Some studies suggest that the probe to bone (PTB) test is an effective clinical method for detecting bone infection in outpatient populations with a high prevalence of osteomyelitis (Rönnemaa et al., 1997; Ragnarson-Tennvall and Apelqvist, 2001; Prompers et al., 2008). This test is used to detect osteomyelitis using a sterile, blunt probe to palpate bone through the diabetic foot wound and is positive when a hard substance assumed to be bone is detected. However, it must be remembered that use of the PTB test, especially in untrained hands, can itself increase the probability of bone infection. In clinical practice, the presence of exposed bone or probing to bone in a diabetic foot wound increases the probability for osteitis which may be an osteomyelitis. From the scientific perspective, there is no gold standard for the diagnosis of bacterial infection in bone (Berendt et al., 2008 or IWGDF, 2007).

Management of diabetic foot ulcers

It is widely accepted that co-morbidity is strongly related to healing of diabetic foot wounds (Apelqvist and Larsson, 2000; IWGDF, 2007; Prompers et al., 2007, 2008). It is therefore important to recognise that the diabetic foot ulcer is a sign of multi-organ disease rather than an isolated condition and requires management of diabetes and its complications. Aggressive medical treatment with regard to co-morbidity including measures to improve metabolic control, treatment of hypertension and dyslipidaemia and adjuvant treatment with anti-platelet drugs is essential when managing metabolic syndrome and concurrent disease (IWGDF, 2007).

Vascular intervention

Peripheral vascular disease causing arterial insufficiency is the most important factor related to the outcome of diabetic foot ulceration. In large European cohort studies, neuro-ischaemic or ischaemic ulcers accounted for 50–58% of all diabetic foot ulcers admitted to specialist care (Prompers et al., 2007, 2008; Gershater et al., 2009). There is general agreement that surgical treatment is indicated to relieve symptoms of limb-threatening ischaemia including ischaemic pain, ischaemic ulcers and gangrene (Apelqvist and Larsson, 2000; IWGDF, 2007; Norgren et al., 2007; Mills, 2008; Hinchliffe et al., 2011).

Percutaneous transluminal angioplasty (PTA) has a low incidence of complications and is said to produce results comparable to those obtained with vascular surgery in both diabetic and non-diabetic patients (Jacqueminet et al., 2005; Faglia et al., 2009; Ferraresi et al., 2009). However, there are few studies evaluating wound healing and amputation rates after revascularisation in diabetic patients with neuro-ischaemic or ischaemic ulcers as these patients constitute a severe challenge due to the presence of coexistent co-morbidities such as cardio-cerebrovascular disease (IWGDF, 2007; Apelqvist et al., 2011; Hinchliffe et al., 2011). Angiography indicates that intervention is strongly related to the extent of co-morbidity rather than availability of intervention (Gershater et al., 2009; Ihnat and Mills, 2010; Apelqvist, 2011; Hinchliffe et al., 2011).

Bypass surgery and/or subintimal recanalisation should be attempted in patients if PTA is not possible or unsuccessful. A distal bypass reconstruction will often be necessary because of the involvement of vessels in the lower leg (Norgren et al., 2007; Ihnat and Mills, 2010; Apelqvist et al., 2011). Advances in vascular surgery have improved results for these procedures suggesting a decline in amputation rate in ischaemic diabetic feet (Apelqvist and Larsson, 2000; Faglia et al., 2009; Ferraresi et al., 2009).

The benefits of pharmacological treatment to improve perfusion in DFU remain controversial. Treatment to remove peripheral oedema due to congestive heart failure, nephropathy, infection or hydrostatic/neuropathic oedema is mandatory. Drugs such as prostacyclin analogues, buflomedil, ketanserin and urokinase can be used in patients in whom revascularisation is not possible (Apelqvist and Larsson, 2000; Norgren et al., 2007). The use of heparin subcutaneously has shown promising results in a small randomised controlled trial (RCT) of neuro-ischaemic foot ulcers in diabetic patients not available for revascularisation (Kalani et al., 2003). The value of hyperbaric oxygen to treat ischaemic foot ulcers is still controversial but randomised studies with successful results have been published (Abidia et al., 2003; Hinchliffe et al., 2008; Löndahl et al., 2010). Gene therapy using oxygenic growth factors to stimulate development of collateral circulation is under development but still unproven in the clinical setting (Kalani et al., 2003).

Foot surgery and amputation

Some data exist to support the use of surgical techniques to offload a non-infected neuropathic ulcer, including surgical excision of ulcers, arthroplasties, metatarsal head resections and Achilles tendon lengthening. These procedures may be combined with local skin flaps and appear to give good results as long as tissue perfusion is adequate (Mueller et al., 2003; Bus et al., 2008; Cavanagh and Bus, 2010). These surgical techniques seem to contribute to shorter healing times but the healing rate is not higher compared to a non-surgical approach in studies with a longer follow-up, as well as reducing the risk of ulcer recurrence (Mueller et al., 2003). Elective surgery should be considered to correct structural deformities that cannot be accommodated by therapeutic footwear. Common procedures include hammer toe repair, metatarsal osteotomies, plantar exostectomies and Achilles tendon lengthening. Complicated Charcot surgery is also a part of offloading indicated for chronic recurrent ulcerations and joint instability when patients present with unstable or displaced fracture dislocations (IWGDF, 2007; Cavanagh and Bus, 2010).

The major complication for diabetic foot ulcers is lower leg amputation. The indications most commonly cited are gangrene and infection which frequently occur simultaneously. It should be emphasised that a non-healing ulcer in itself should not be considered as an indication for amputation since wound chronicity is a factor that does not necessarily delay healing of an amputation as long as the duration of the ulcer in itself is not considered an indication for amputation (Apelqvist and Larsson, 2000). However, studies have shown that there is an established correlation between duration of neuropathic foot ulceration and probability of healing within 12 weeks (Sheehan et al., 2003). Minor amputations, e.g. those below the ankle should be left open to heal by secondary intention if skin viability is compromised (Larsson et al., 2008; Svensson et al., 2011).

There is still some controversy concerning the benefit of a primary minor amputation versus primary major amputation (below knee) in this patient group (Jeffcoate and van Houtum, 2004; Sheahan et al., 2005; IWGDF, 2007). The advantage of primary major amputation is a lower re-amputation rate and shorter healing time (Svensson et al., 2011). Minor amputations are associated with higher re-amputation rates and as a consequence longer wound healing time. However, in a prospective study, patients with diabetes and foot ulcers with a healed major amputation (at or above the ankle) have a higher mortality rate, equal rate of a future new amputations, an increased rate of future major amputation and a lower potential for rehabilitation compared to an individual with diabetes and foot ulcers and a healed minor amputation (below the ankle) (Larsson et al., 1998). There is a considerable difference regarding economic costs between healing of a minor versus a major amputation from either a short- or long-term perspective due to increased need for home care and social service following a major amputation (Apelqvist and Larsson, 2000; Boulton et al., 2005).

Debridement

The specific aims of debridement in patients with diabetic foot wounds are as follows:

- limit tissue damage to save the leg and life of the patient;
- remove devitalised tissue to optimise wound healing;
- create/produce a foot that can maintain ambulation (Apelqvist and Larsson, 2000; IWGDF, 2007).

Neuropathic ulcers with callus and necrosis should be debrided as soon as possible so that the depth of the ulcer and extent of trauma can be determined. Removal of callus can reduce plantar pressures by as much as 30%, leading to improved wound healing (Cavanagh and Bus, 2010).

In the case of an acute deep foot infection, with or without osteomyelitis, surgical intervention should always be considered because in prospective studies more than 80% of patients required a surgical procedure to achieve healing (Apelqvist and Larsson, 2000; Lipsky et al., 2004; Lipsky, 2004; IWGDF, 2007). In the case of a deep soft tissue infection, or abscess, or necrotising tenovaginitis immediate surgery is usually required (Lipsky et al., 2004; Lipsky, 2004). The presence of active, extensive infection in a diabetic foot wound requires immediate wound debridement regardless of the need for revascularisation. Once the acute infection is under control, the need for revascularisation and evaluation of tissue perfusion should always be considered, together with implementation of a multidisciplinary strategy to optimise healing (Lipsky et al., 2004; Lipsky, 2004; IWGDF, 2007).

The choice of debridement method is dependent on the level of decreased perfusion to the foot, the extent of tissue loss and the expertise of the operator and should focus not only on achieving wound healing but to maintain ambulation. Non-surgical debridement techniques can be used to remove dead tissue when surgery is not an option, and

improve the condition of the wound bed to optimise healing (Edwards, 2002) (see Chapter 6).

Infected diabetic foot ulcers require surgical debridement if possible, in the case of ischaemia, revascularisation should be attempted before debridement; and in foot ulcers with a limited amount of available soft tissue, non-surgical techniques can be helpful to preserve tissue loss and maintain a foot that is ambulative once healed. Surgery is always the quickest way of debridement but results in the most extensive tissue loss. Heel ulcers are especially prone to delayed healing as poor perfusion in the heel fat pad and the danger of debriding into the calcaneus may increase the risk of deep infection.

Infection in diabetic foot wounds

Infection is seldom the direct cause of a foot ulcer. However, once a diabetic foot wound is complicated by infection, the risk for subsequent amputation is greatly increased. In a study by Lavery et al. (Dorresteijn et al., 2010), factors related to development of a wound infection were duration of ulcer >30 days, recurrent ulceration, trauma, probing to bone and co-existent peripheral arterial disease (Lavery et al., 2006). The evidence suggests that the outcome of deep foot infection is related to the extent of tissue involvement, co-morbidity and peripheral vascular disease (Apelqvist and Larsson, 2000; IWGDF, 2007; Prompers et al., 2008; Gershater et al., 2009; Apelqvist et al., 2011). In the EURO-DIALE study, more than 50% of patients with a foot ulcer had received antibiotics prior to admission to a diabetic foot clinic and between 25% and 75% of patients had a wound infection on admission (Prompers et al., 2007, 2008). These findings are cause for concern when multiresistant microbes such as MRSA are so prevalent. An infection in the diabetic foot is a limb-threatening condition and, together with ischaemia, is a direct cause of amputation in 25–50% of diabetic patients (Apelqvist and Larsson, 2000; Lipsky et al., 2004; IWGDF, 2007).

Antibiotic treatment for diabetic foot infection should be based on an understanding of antimicrobial principles and awareness of relevant clinical evidence (Lipsky et al., 2004; Lipsky, 2004). Choice of antibiotic therapy is also governed by national protocols and resource limitations in many parts of the world which poses particular challenges for individuals who live in rural areas. The choice of antibiotic treatment should be based on several factors, the most important of which is the severity of the infection. This also dictates the mode of antibiotic administration, and the need for admission to hospital. Antibiotic therapy should be administered using the drug with the lowest acquisition cost relevant for the clinical circumstances (NICE, 2011). Therapy aimed solely at aerobic Gram-positive cocci may be sufficient for acute mild-to-moderate infections in patients who have not recently received antibiotic therapy (NICE, 2011). Antibiotics should be selected for severe infections that are active against Gram-positive, Gram negative and anaerobic bacteria (Berendt et al., 2008). Mild-to-moderate infections should be treated with oral antibiotics, the intravenous route should be reserved for severe infections (NICE, 2011). In long-standing ulcers or ulcers with delayed healing with ischaemia or necrotic tissue, polymicrobial flora are likely to be present in which the causative agent is unknown. Broad-spectrum antibiotic therapy is not routinely required but is indicated for moderate-to-severe infections. Definitive therapy should be based on both the culture results and sensitivity data and the patient's clinical response to the treatment regimen. Antibiotic therapy should be continued until there is evidence that the infection has resolved, but not necessarily until the wound has healed (Berendt et al., 2008).

Initial treatment should include wound debridement and a tissue sample for culture and sensitivity. The most important step in the control of deep infection is urgent incision and drainage of an abscess and radical debridement of all infected, non-viable necrotic tissue (Lipsky et al., 2004). Wound debridement should be performed first and in the case of ischaemia, revascularisation shortly after (Lipsky et al., 2004; Lipsky, 2004; Ihnat and Mills, 2010). In situations without a limb-threatening infection, the blood supply to the wound or extremity should be optimised before surgical debridement to ensure that potentially viable tissue is not unnecessarily removed (Ihnat and Mills, 2010).

Osteomyelitis

The principle of treating osteomyelitis in the diabetic foot is to eliminate secondary bone infection and prevent development of chronic infection and amputation. The decision to manage osteomyelitis conservatively or surgically is currently debatable and the rationale is unclear (Berendt et al., 2008). Traditionally, the essential treatment of chronic osteomyelitis has always been resection of infected bone and treatment with antibiotics. However, surgical techniques such as ray and metatarsal amputations alter the structure and biomechanics of the foot causing gait problems following surgery and may increase the risk of new ulceration, for example if the second metatarsal head is removed to heal an ulcer, the consequence is increased peak pressure under the third metatarsal head which may result in development of a new ulcer. Current evidence suggests that patients who are thought to need urgent surgery for life- or limb-threatening infection, but are not able to have it, may not routinely need surgical debridement of infected bone and treatment of osteomyelitis may be achieved with antibiotics alone.

Although many experts still believe that resolution of bone infection in diabetic foot wounds is facilitated by appropriate debridement of necrotic tissue, there is increasing evidence that surgical debridement of infected bone is not routinely necessary, especially in the digits (IWGDF, 2007; Berendt et al., 2008). Splinting or cast immobilisation may be required to immobilise the affected bone and soft tissue to minimise further trauma and promote healing. With early referral and prompt treatment, the outcome can be good for osteomyelitis in diabetic foot wounds, although some chronic bone infections can be so resistant to treatment that amputation may be required.

Offloading – non-weight-bearing

An essential part of treatment to achieve healing in diabetic foot ulcers includes effective offloading to achieve non-weight-bearing by using shoes, insoles, casting, other orthoses, crutches or wheelchair. Many wound management interventions have failed due to failing recognition of the need for effective offloading (Bus et al., 2008; Cavanagh and Bus, 2010). The aim of offloading and protection is to maintain ambulation and treat the foot ulcer. In the acute situation, crutches, wheelchair or bed rest might be necessary to achieve this. However, in most situations, an adequately fitting shoe, orthoses or insoles will be sufficient. In cases with plantar ulceration, in which disturbed biomechanic pressures cause deteriorated circulation, techniques to decrease plantar peak pressure is necessary including techniques such as total contact cast (TCC), walkers, removable or non-removable-orthoses, or other devices.

Studies indicate an offloading system has to achieve a threshold of a peak pressure <200 kPa to maintain healing (Owings et al., 2009). This requires shoes provided by an orthopaedic specialist clinic and the patient requires shoes for both indoor and outdoor use. Acceptable techniques used in offloading include soft and shock-absorbing materials, custom moulding, forefoot- or heel-offloading shoes, rocker-bottom shoes, casts, walkers, crutches, wheelchair and surgery (Bus et al., 2008; Cavanagh and Bus, 2010). RCTs have shown that the TCC is more effective than removable devices both with regard to plantar foot ulcer healing and time to heal (Bus et al., 2008; Cavanagh and Bus, 2010). TCCs and other non-removable devices are most effective because they eliminate the problem of non-adherence. Conventional or standard therapeutic footwear is not effective in ulcer healing (Bus et al., 2008; Cavanagh and Bus, 2010). Shoes and insoles that have not been specially adapted for the individual patient's foot have not been proven effective with regard to healing of a diabetic foot ulcer. If footwear cannot achieve or prevent recurrent ulceration, then the patients' activity level must be drastically modified (Bus et al., 2008; Cavanagh and Bus, 2010).

Wound dressings: special considerations

In patients with diabetes mellitus, there is a substantial delay in wound healing which is associated with abnormalities related to hyperglycaemia such as decreased concentrations of growth factors, increased protease activity, abnormalities of the extracellular matrix and reduced fibroblast function (Sibbald and Woo, 2008). Several new treatments related to these abnormalities have been explored in wound healing such as various growth factor products, hyaluronic acid, matrix modulators, skin tissue engineering products, artificial skin and granulocyte colony stimulating factor. Encouraging results have been presented, but at the moment there is no consensus regarding indications for and value of these treatments (IWGDF, 2007; NICE, 2011; Brolmann et al., 2012). The basic principles of dressing choice for diabetic foot ulcers are the same as for other chronic wounds with the exception that foot ulcers are frequently located on weight-bearing areas, lack skin sensation and have an increased risk of infection and ischaemia.

Negative-pressure wound therapy (NPWT) has shown promising results improving the condition of the wound bed in people with diabetes who have cavity ulcers and wounds following forefoot amputation. Two randomised controlled studies have shown that NPWT can reduce wound area and improve wound healing rates at 16 weeks in patients with foot ulcers with adequate circulation compared to controls (Armstrong and Lavery, 2005; Blume et al., 2008; Vikatmaa et al., 2008). However, NPWT therapy has to be performed by healthcare staff with adequate skill and it is essential to apply it to a foot ulcer with adequate tissue perfusion and controlled infection. Hyperbaric oxygen therapy as opposed to a placebo or control treatment has been shown to be effective in reducing amputation rates in patients with diabetic foot ulcers (Brolmann et al., 2012).

Foot care

The provision of appropriate foot care is an essential part of the management of people with diabetes and helps to avoid morbidity due to foot ulceration and amputation. Foot care should be given an equal emphasis in self-care for people with diabetes as the blood glucose control (NICE, 2011). The importance of a suitably trained healthcare professional such as a podiatrist in examination, screening, education and treatment of non-ulcer pathology is well recognised (Schaper et al., 2003; IWGDF, 2007). Correct treatment of callosities, cracked skin, dry skin and nail deformities is essential and requires specific skills. It has been suggested that regular foot care, podiatry and education provided individually by a podiatrist results in significant improvement in knowledge and foot self-care and in the prevalence of minor foot problems such as treatment of severe calluses and nail pathologies (Singh et al., 2005; Cavanagh and Bus, 2006; NICE, 2011). Regular podiatry visits contribute to a careful visual inspection of the feet and helps support patients who experience difficulty in performing self-inspection and self-care. An annual foot inspection and review should be part of ongoing care for people with healed foot ulcers and should be more frequent for those with increased risk of ulceration. These appointments facilitate appropriate foot-care education and foster good self-care practices.

In order to prevent trauma causing ulcers in a non-weight-bearing area, most patients with increased risk of foot ulcers due to neuropathy and foot deformities need to protect their feet by wearing well-fitting shoes (Bus et al., 2008; Cavanagh and Bus, 2010). Since foot deformities are common among patients with diabetes and neuropathy, it is important that there is sufficient space for the toes in shoes. Shoe insoles should reduce foot pressures below the threshold of ulceration. Individuals with diabetes and neuropathy should avoid walking barefoot or with open-toed sandals due to the risk of trauma.

Protective footwear probably prevents plantar ulceration by redistribution and reduction of abnormal pressures (metatarsal heads, great toe and areas of callus formation) and also protects the foot from external trauma (Bus et al., 2008; Cavanagh and Bus, 2010). A number of studies have shown that protective footwear when appropriately worn can prevent re-ulceration in 60–85% of diabetic patients (Bus et al., 2008; Cavanagh and Bus, 2010). Various techniques such as slow motion video, force platforms, pressure distributions which measure ground reaction force, pressure distributions from barefoot walking and pressure measurements made at the foot–shoe interface have been developed to evaluate dynamic changes in plantar pressure when standing and walking, and reduction of loading measured with these techniques has been related to a reduction in the probability of re-ulceration.

Education and support

People with diabetes and increased risk of foot ulcers need to learn to recognise potential foot problems and take appropriate action (Schaper et al., 2003; IWGDF, 2007; Lincoln et al., 2008; Dorresteijn et al., 2010; McInnes et al., 2011). Patient education in preventive foot care, for those who have been identified as 'at risk' of foot ulceration has been described as important in international guidelines (Schaper et al., 2003; IWGDF, 2007; NICE, 2011).

These guidelines emphasise that patient education should include the following:

(1) Daily examination of the feet.
(2) Maintenance of skin hygiene.
(3) How to minimise inadvertent self–harm, e.g. corn removal.
(4) Wearing appropriate footwear.
(5) When to seek advice from heathcare professionals.

Patient education should therefore aim to raise awareness of the link between diabetes, neuropathy and development of foot ulcers; the importance of daily foot inspections; practical self-care actions; choice of appropriate footwear; and the importance of seeking help early in case of any abnormality (Lincoln et al., 2008; Dorresteijn et al., 2010; McInnes et al., 2011). Patients need to be taught the importance of preventative foot care and be encouraged to inspect their feet daily to identify early signs of abnormality and use a mirror to help inspect the plantar aspect of both feet. If the patient is not able to perform this inspection, family or home care services should be encouraged to provide this support.

Practice point

People with diabetes may develop fungal infections and dystrophic changes to the toenails. Surgical-quality nail-cutters should be used to trim and shape thickened, fungus-infected nails. A rotary drum sander can be used by appropriately trained individuals to reduce affected toenails to tissue-paper thinness as an alternative to systemic or local fungicidal agents as the fungus will find it difficult to survive due to the drying effect of the air. Systemic or local fungicidal agents should not be used unless the diagnosis has been confirmed by culture and cytology and in many cases is not warranted.

Recently, there has been substantial interest about patient's beliefs about health and illness and attitudes towards their diabetes (Hjelm et al., 2003; Nabuurs-Franssen et al., 2005; Vileikyte, 2008; Gonzalez et al., 2010). Findings consistently show that people with diabetes and foot ulcers do not always understand the relationship between foot ulceration and chronic disease and frequently underestimate the severity of the situation and consequently do not seek care in the early stages. Frequently, the first recognition of the danger of diabetes causing multiple organ damage is the occurrence of a foot ulcer or gangrene and evidence is growing that it can be traumatic for patients to realise that their foot ulcer is related to their diabetes (Vileikyte, 2008; Gonzalez et al., 2010).

Several studies indicate the importance of education for clinicians regarding early recognition of potential risk relating to the diabetic foot. In one study, delay of treatment of foot ulceration was attributed to patients in 12% of cases and to professionals in 21% of cases (Macfarlane and Jeffcoate, 1997). Another study reported that 29% of patients

Box 9.1   Recommendations for minimum levels of foot-care service (IWGDF, 2007)

Level 1	General practitioner, diabetic nurse and podiatrist
Level 2	Diabetologist, surgeon (general and/or vascular and/or orthopaedic), diabetic nurse and podiatrist
Level 3	Specialised foot centre with multiple disciplines specialised in diabetic foot care

with severe foot ulceration complicated by infection and gangrene delayed presenting to healthcare professionals as a result of underestimation of the severity of tissue damage and lack of recognition of the consequences of ischaemia.

Provision of specialist diabetic foot services

A multidisciplinary approach to the management of diabetic foot disease has been successfully implemented in many different countries with various healthcare delivery systems resulting in a substantial decrease in amputation rate (Krishnan et al., 2008; Zayed et al., 2009). Two comparative studies have shown improved clinical results with multidisciplinary treatment versus standard care in ordinary practise (McCabe et al., 1998; Dargis et al., 1999). Ideally, a specialist foot-care team would consist of a diabetologist, surgeon, podiatrist, orthotist and plaster technician, working in close collaboration with an orthopaedic, podiatric and/or vascular surgeon and a dermatologist (NICE, 2011).

The effective organisation of foot-care pathways is essential to improve the outcome for people with diabetic foot complications and requires guidelines for screening, risk reduction, treatment, education and clinical audit. However, local variations in resources and staffing will determine the way in which care is provided. Box 9.1 highlights the recommendations by the International Working Group on the Diabetic Foot for minimum levels of foot-care service provision. The appropriate use of internationally agreed guidelines and implementation of clinical skills by well-informed multidisciplinary teams can ensure that management of this vulnerable group is optimised (NICE 2011).

Criteria for specialist referral

International guidelines recommend that advice should be quickly obtained from an appropriate specialist if any of the following circumstances apply (IWGDF, 2007; NICE, 2011):

● Worsening serious co-morbidity such as chronic kidney or cardiovascular disease;
● Signs and symptoms of systemic sepsis;
● Clinical signs of a deep-seated infection;
● Evidence of decreased perfusion and limb ischaemia;
● Evidence of Charcot arthropathy.

The combination of ischaemia and infection always necessitates urgent treatment, as 'time is tissue' in these circumstances. Patients should be referred to a multidisciplinary foot-care team as quickly as possible after the detection of serious diabetic foot complications. If possible, these patients should be managed by a consultant member of the team with the appropriate clinical expertise.

Summary

Diabetes-related foot compilations are a tremendous challenge for patients, care-givers and healthcare systems. The diabetic foot should be considered a lifelong condition since after developing an ulcer the patient is always at high risk of developing a new ulcer and the condition is related to substantial co-morbidity with high mortality and future risk of amputation. In an individual with diabetes and foot ulceration the ulcer should be considered as a sign of multi-organ disease and a holistic approach in management and prevention is recommended.

Useful resources

International Working Group on the Diabetic Foot: Available at: www.iwdgf.org
    The International Consensus on the Management and Prevention of the Diabetic Foot
    Translated into 26 languages.
    This site contains specific guidelines relating to DFU including

● Wound and wound bed management
● Treatment of diabetic foot infections

- Diagnosis and treatment of PAD in a diabetic patient with a foot ulcer
- Footwear and offloading

National Institute Clinical Effectiveness guidance:

Available at: www.nice.org.uk/guidance/CG10

- Diabetic foot problems: inpatient management of diabetic foot problems. NICE clinical guidelines.
- Type 2 diabetes – foot care. NICE clinical guideline 10 (2011).

60-Second Diabetic Foot Screen:

Available at: http://cawc.net/images/uploads/Inlow_Tool_2010.pdf

Adapted from Inlow, S. (2004) A 60 second foot exam for people with diabetes. *Wound Care Canada*, 2(2), 10–11. ©CAWC 2010. P1419E.

References

Abbott, C.A., Carrington, A.L., Ashe, H., et al. (2002) The North-West diabetes foot care study: incidence of, and risk factors for, new diabetic foot ulceration in a community-based patient cohort. *Diabetic Medicine*, 19(5), 377–384.

Abidia, A., Laden, G., Kuhan, G., et al. (2003) The role of hyperbaric oxygen therapy in ischemic diabetic lower extremity ulcers: a double-blind randomized-controlled trial. *European Journal of Vascular and Endovascular Surgery*, 25, 513–518.

Apelqvist, J. (2012) The ulcerated leg: when to revascularise. *Diabetes/Metabolism Research and Reviews*, 28 (Suppl 1), 30–35.

Apelqvist, J., Elgzyri, T., Larsson, J., Löndahl, M., Nyberg, P., Thörne, J. (2011) Factors related to outcome of neuroischemic/ischemic foot ulcer in diabetic patients. *Journal of Vascular Surgery*, 53(6), 1582–1588.

Apelqvist, J., Larsson, J. (2000) What is the most effective way to reduce incidence of amputation in the diabetic foot? *Diabetes/Metabolism Research and Reviews*, 16(Suppl. 1), S75–S83.

Apelqvist, J., Larsson, J., Agardh, C.D. (1993) Long term prognosis for diabetic patients with foot ulcer. *Journal of Internal Medicine*, 233, 485–491.

Armstrong, D.G., Lavery, L.A. (2005) Diabetic Foot Study Consortium. Negative pressure wound therapy after partial diabetic foot amputation: a multicentre, randomised controlled trial. *Lancet*, 366, 1704–1710.

Berendt, A.R., Peters, E.J., Bakker, K., et al. (2008) Diabetic foot osteomyelitis: a progress report on diagnosis and a systematic review of treatment. *Diabetes/Metabolism Research and Reviews*, 24(Suppl. 1), S145–S161.

Blume, P.A., Walters, J., Payne, W., Ayala, J., Lantis, J. (2008) Comparisons of negative pressure wound therapy using vacuum assisted closure with advanced moist wound therapy in the treatment of diabetic foot ulcers: a multicenter randomised controlled trial. *Diabetes Care*, 31, 631–636.

Boulton, A.J. (2004) The diabetic foot: from art to science. The 18th Camillo Golgi lecture. *Diabetologia*, 47(8), 1343–1353.

Boulton, A.J. (2008) The diabetic foot: grand overview, epidemiology and pathogenesis. *Diabetes/Metabolism Research and Reviews*, 24(Suppl. 1), S3–S6.

Boulton, A.J., Vileikyte, L., Ragnarson-Tennvall, G., Apelqvist, J. (2005) The global burden of diabetic foot disease. *Lancet*, 366(9498), 1719–1724.

Boyko, E.J., Ahroni, J.H., Cohen, V., Nelson, K., Heagerty, P. (2006) Prediction of diabetic foot ulcer occurrence using commonly available information. The Seattle Diabetic Foot Study. *Diabetes Care*, 29, 1202–1207.

Brollmann, F.E., Ubbink, D.T., Nelson, E.A., et al. (2012) Evidence-based decisions for local and systemic wound care. *British Journal of Surgery*, 99(9), 1172–1183.

Bus, A., Valk, G.D., van Deursen, R.W. et al. (2008) The effectiveness of footwear and offloading interventions to prevent and heal foot ulcers and reduce plantar pressure in diabetes: a systematic review. *Diabetes/Metabolism Research and Reviews*, 24(Suppl. 1), 162–180.

Butalia, S., Palda, V.A., Sargeant, R.J., Detsky, A.S., Mourad, O. (2008) Does this patient with diabetes have osteomyelitis of the lower extremity? *The Journal of the American Medical Association*, 299, 806–813.

Carrington, A.L., Mawdsley, S.K., Morley, M., Kincey, J., Boulton, A.J. (1996) Psychological status of diabetic patients with or without lower limb disability. *Diabetes Research and Clinical Practice*, 32, 19–25.

Cavanagh, P.R., Bus, S.A. (2010) Off-loading the diabetic foot for ulcer prevention and healing. *Journal of Vascular Surgery*, 52(Suppl. 3), 37S–43S.

Connor, H., Mahdi, O.Z. (2004) Repetitive ulceration in neuropathic patients. *Diabetes Metabolic Research Review*, 20(Suppl. 1), 23–28.

Dargis, V., Pantelejeva, O., Jonushaite, A., Boulton, A., Vileikyte, I. (1999) Benefits of a multidisciplinary approach in the management of recurrent diabetic foot ulceration in Lithuania: a prospective study. *Diabetes Care*, 22(9), 1428–1431.

Dorresteijn, J., Kriegsman, D., Assendelft, W., Valk, G. (2010) Patient education for preventing diabetic foot ulceration. *The Cochrane Database of Systematic Reviews*, Issue 5.

Edwards, J. (2002) Debridement of diabetic foot ulcers. *The Cochrane Database of Systematic Reviews [Computer File]*, Issue 4: CD003556.

Faglia, E., Clerici, G., Clerissi, J., et al. (2009) Long-term prognosis of diabetic patients with critical limb ischemia: a population-based cohort study. *Diabetes Care*, 32(5), 822–827.

Ferraresi, R., Centola, M., Ferlini, M., et al. (2009) Long-term outcomes after angioplasty of isolated, below-the-knee arteries in diabetic patients with critical limb ischaemia. *European Journal of Vascular and Endovascular Surgery*, 37(3), 336–342.

Gershater, M.A., Löndahl, M., Nyberg, P., et al. (2009) Complexity of factors related to outcome of neuropathic and neuroischaemic/ischaemic diabetic foot ulcers: a cohort study. *Diabetologia*, 52(3), 398–407.

Gonzalez, J.S., Hardman, M.J., Boulton, A.J., Vileikyte, L. (2011) Coping and depression in diabetic foot ulcer healing: causal influence, mechanistic evidence or none of the above?*Diabetologia*, 54(1), 205–206.

Hinchliffe, R.J., Andros, G., Apelqvist, J., et al. (2011) A systematic review of the effectiveness of revascularisation of the ulcerated foot in patients with diabetes and peripheral arterial disease. *Diabetes/Metabolism Research and Reviews*, 28 (Suppl 1), 179–217.

Hinchliffe, R.J., Valk, G.D., Apelqvist, J., et al. (2008) A systematic review of the effectiveness of interventions to enhance the healing of chronic ulcers of the foot in diabetes. *Diabetes/Metabolism Research and Reviews*, 24(Suppl. 1), 119–144.

Hjelm, K., Nyberg, P., Apelqvist, J. (2003) The influence of beliefs about health and illness on foot care in diabetic subjects with severe foot lesions: a comparison of foreign and Swedish- born individuals. *Clinical Effectiveness in Nursing*, 7(1), 1–14.

Ihnat, D.M., Mills, J.L., Sr. (2010) Current assessment of endovascular therapy for infrainguinal arterial occlusive disease in patients with diabetes. *Journal of Vascular Surgery*, 52(Suppl. 3), 92S–95S.

Inlow, S. (2004) A 60 second foot exam for people with diabetes. *Wound Care Canada*, 2(2), 10–11.

International Working Group on the Diabetic Foot [IWGDF]. (2007) *International Consensus on the Diabetic Foot and Practical Guidelines on the Management and the Prevention of the Diabetic Foot*. Amsterdam, the Netherlands: IWGDF, on CD-ROM. Available at: http://www.iwgdf.org, last accessed on 18 November 2012.

International Working Group on the Diabetic Foot [IWGDF]. (2011) International Consensus Guidelines on the Management and Prevention of the Diabetic Foot. Available at: http://www.iwgdf.org, last accessed on 18 November 2012.

Jacqueminet, S., Hartemann-Heurtier, A., Izzillo, R., et al. (2005) Percutaneous transluminal angioplasty in severe diabetic foot ischemia: outcomes and prognostic factors. *Diabetes and Metabolism*, 31, 370–375.

Jeffcoate, W., Game, F., Cavanagh, P. (2005) The role of proinflammatory cytokines in the cause of neuropathic osteoarthropathy (acute Charcot foot) in diabetes. *Lancet*, 366, 2058–2061.

Jeffcoate, W.J., Chipchase, S.Y., Ince, P., Game, F.L. (2006) Assessing the outcome of the management of diabetic foot ulcers using ulcer-related and person-related measures. *Diabetes Care*, 29, 1784–1787.

Jeffcoate, W.J., van Houtum, W.H. (2004) Amputation as a marker of the quality of foot care in diabetes. *Diabetologia*, 47, 2051–2058.

Kalani, M., Brismar, K., Apelqvist, J., et al. (2003) Effect of Daltiperin on healing of chronic foot ulcers in diabetic patients with peripheral arterial occlusive disease – prospective, randomized, double blind and placebo controlled study. *Diabetes Care*, 6, 2575–2580.

Krishnan, S., Nash, F., Baker, N., Fowler, D., Rayman, G. (2008) Reduction in diabetic amputations over 11 years in a defined U.K. population: benefits of multidisciplinary team work and continuous prospective audit. *Diabetes Care*, 31, 99–101.

Larsson, J., Agardh, C.D., Apelqvist, J., Stenström, A. (1998) Long term prognosis after amputation in diabetic patients. *Clinical Orthopedics and Related Research*, 350, 149–158.

Larsson, J., Eneroth, M., Apelqvist, J., Stenström, A. (2008) Sustained decrease of major amputation in diabetic patients – an analysis of a 20-year period in a defined population (628 amputations in 461 patients). *Acta Orthop*aedica, 79(5), 665–673.

Lavery, L.A., Armstrong, D., Wunderlich, R., Mohler, M., Wendel, C., Lipsky, B. (2006) Risk factors for foot infections in individuals with diabetes. *Diabetes Care*, 29, 1288–1293.

Lincoln, N., Radford, K., Game, F., Jeffcoate, W. (2008) Education for secondary prevention of foot ulcers in people with diabetes: a randomised controlled trial. *Diabetologia*, 51(11), 1954–1961.

Lipsky, B.A. (2004) International consensus group on diagnosing and treating the infected diabetic foot. A report from the international consensus on diagnosing and treating the infected diabetic foot. *Diabetes/Metabolism Research and Reviews*, 20(Suppl. 1), S68–S77.

Lipsky, B., Berent, A.R., Embil, J., de Lalla, F. (2004) Diagnosing and treating diabetic foot infections. *Diabetes/Metabolism Research and Reviews*, 20(Suppl. 1), 56–64.

Löndahl, M., Katzman, P., Nilsson, A., Hammarlund, C. (2010) Hyperbaric oxygen therapy facilitates healing of chronic foot ulcers in patients with diabetes. *Diabetes Care*, 33, 998–1003.

Macfarlane, R.M., Jeffcoate, W.J. (1997) Factors contributing to the presentation of diabetic foot ulcers. *Diabetic Medicine*, 14(10), 867–870.

Mantey, I., Foster, A.V.M., Spencer, S., Edmonds, M.E. (1999) Why do foot ulcers recur in diabetic patients? *Diabetic Medicine*, 16, 245–249.

McCabe, C.J., Stevenson, R.C., Dolan, A.M. (1998) Evaluation of diabetic foot screening and protection programme. *Diabetes Medicine*, 15, 80–84.

McInnes, A., Jeffcoate, W., Vileikyte, L., et al. (2011) Foot care education in patients with diabetes at low risk of complications: a consensus statement. *Diabetic Medicine*, 28(2), 162–167.

Mills, J.L. (2008) Open bypass and endoluminal therapy: complementary techniques for revascularisation in diabetic patients with critical limb ischemia. *Diabetes/Metabolism Research and Reviews*, 24(Suppl. 1), 34–39.

Mueller, M.J., Sinacore, D.R., Hastings, M.K., Strube, M.J., Johnson, J.E. (2003) Effect of Achilles tendon lengthening on neuropatic plantar ulcers. A randomized clinical trial. *Journal of Bone and Joint Surgery. American Volume*, 85-A, 1436–1445.

Nabuurs-Franssen, M.H., Huijberts, M.S., Nieuwenhuijzen Kruseman, A.C., Willems, J., Schaper, N.C. (2005) Health-related quality of life of diabetic foot ulcer patients and their caregivers. *Diabetologia*, 48(9), 1906–1910.

National Institute for Health and Clinical Excellence [NICE]. (2011) Diabetic foot – inpatient management of people with diabetic foot ulcers and infection. Available at: http://guidance.nice.org.uk/CG119, last accessed on 18 November 2012.

Norgren, L., Hiatt, W.R., Dormandy, J.A., Nehler, M.R., Harris, K.A., Fowkes, F.G., TASC II Working Group. (2007) Inter-society consensus for the management of peripheral arterial disease (TASC II). *Journal of Vascular Surgery*, 45(Suppl. 1), S5–S67.

Ortegon, M.M., Redekop, W.K., Niessen, L.W. (2004) Cost-effectiveness of prevention and treatment of the diabetic foot. *Diabetes Care*, 27, 901–907.

Owings, T.M., Apelqvis, J., Stenström, A., et al. (2009) Plantar pressures in diabetic foot ulcer patients who have remained healed. *Diabetic Medicine*, 26(11), 1141.

Prompers, L., Huijberts, M., Apelqvist, J., et al. (2007) High prevalence of ischaemia, infection and serious comorbidity in patients with diabetic foot disease in Europe. Baseline results from the Eurodiale study. *Diabetologia*, 50(1), 18–25.

Prompers, L., Schaper, N., Apelqvist, J., et al. (2008) Prediction of outcome in individuals with diabetic foot ulcers: focus on between individuals with and without peripheral vascular disease. The EURODIALE study. *Diabetologia*, 51, 747–755.

Ragnarsson-Tennvall, G., Apelqvist, J. (2000) Health-related quality of life in patients with diabetes mellitus and foot ulcers. *Journal of Diabetes and its Complications*, 14, 235–241.

Ragnarson-Tennvall, G., Apelqvist, J. (2001) Prevention of diabetes-related foot ulcers and amputations: a cost-utility analysis based on Markov model simulations. *Diabetologia*, 44, 2077–2087.

Rönnemaa, T., Hämäläinen, H., Toikka, T., Liukkonen, I. (1997) Evaluation of the impact of podiatrist care in the primary prevention of foot problems in diabetic subjects. *Diabetes Care*, 20(12), 1833–1837.

Schaper, N.C., Apelqvist, J., Bakker, K. (2003) The international consensus and practical guidelines on the management and prevention of the diabetic foot. *Current Diabetes Reports*, 3(6), 475–479.

Sheahan, M.G., Hamdan, A.D., Veraldi, J.R., et al. (2005) Lower extremity minor amputations: the roles of diabetes mellitus and timing of revascularization. *Journal of Vascular Surgery*, 42, 476–480.

Sheehan, P., Jones, P., Caselli, A., Giurini, J.M., Veves, A. (2003) Percent change in wound area of diabetic foot ulcers over a 4-week period is a robust predictor of complete healing in a 12-week prospective trial. *Diabetes Care*, 26, 1879–1882.

Sibbald, R., Woo, K. (2008) The biology of chronic foot ulcers in persons with diabetes. *Diabetes/Metabolism Research and Reviews*, 24(Suppl. 1), S25–S30.

Singh, N., Armstrong, D.G., Lipsky, B.A. (2005) Preventing foot ulcers in patients with diabetes. *The Journal of the American Medical Association*, 293, 217–228.

Svensson, H., Larsson, J., Apelqvist, J., Eneroth, M. (2011) Minor amputations successful in patients with diabetes mellitus and severe foot ulcers threatening the survival of the foot. *Journal of Wound Care*, 20, 261-2, 264, 266.

Trepman, E., Nihal, A., Pinzur, M. (2005) Charcot neuroarthropathy of the foot and ankle. *Foot and Ankle*, 26, 46–63.

Vikatmaa, P., Juutilainen, V., Kuukasjärvi, P., Malmivaara, A. (2008) Negative pressure wound therapy: a systematic review on effectiveness and safety. *European Journal of Vascular and Endovascular Surgery*, 36, 438–448.

Vileikyte, I. (2001) Diabetic foot ulcers: a quality of life issue. *Diabetes/Metabolism Research and Reviews*, 17, 246–249.

Vileikyte, L. (2008) Psychosocial and behavioral aspects of diabetic foot lesions. *Current Diabetes Reports*, 8(2), 119–125.

Walsh, C.H. (1996) A healed ulcer: what now? *Diabetic Medicine*, 13, 58–60.

Zayed, H., Halawa, M., Maillardet, L., Sidhu, P.S., Edmonds, M., Rashid, H. (2009) Improving limb salvage rate in diabetic patients with critical leg ischaemia using a multidisciplinary approach. *International Journal of Clinical Practice*, 63(6), 855–858.

10 Chronic Ulcers of the Lower Limb

Jeanette Muldoon
Head of Clinical Services, Activa Healthcare, Burton-on-Trent, Staffordshire, UK

Overview

- Leg ulcer prevalence rates vary in different geographical locations (0.45 per 1000 population in the United Kingdom, 0.62 in Australia, 1.0 in Sweden and 1.28 in Poland but are in the region 1.0 per 1000 population).
- Leg ulceration has a profound effect on the quality of life as sufferers encounter pain, leakage, disturbed sleep, impaired mobility and difficulties with everyday activities.
- Leg ulcers cause loss of function and require long-term care resulting in a high financial burden estimated to be more than $1 billion in the United States and £400–£600 million in the United Kingdom per annum.
- There is good evidence that compression bandaging increases healing rates for venous leg ulcers and that multi-component systems seem to be more effective than single-layer systems.
- Healthcare professionals should give clear, unambiguous information to promote treatment adherence in this patient group. A range of adherence-enhancing strategies should be developed to help promote effective self-care for people with leg ulcers.

Introduction

A chronic leg ulcer is a slow healing wound, usually situated on the lower leg and associated with circulatory disorders, mainly of the venous system although there may be other causes. Partsch (2009) states that a leg ulcer is not a disease, but a symptom of a disorder, and usually situated on the leg as humans are 'victims of gravity'. This is an important point as it explains why topical treatments such as wound dressings are often unsuccessful as they fail to address the underlying cause. Sound knowledge of the skin, lymphatics and vascular systems is essential to understand the aetiologies, prevalence and management of leg ulceration.

Epidemiology

Half the Western population have varicose veins, although in two-thirds of cases this is medically insignificant. The remaining third will suffer some form of venous disorder which is progressive (Laing, 1992) with approximately 1% of the population in the United Kingdom suffering from an active leg ulcer at any one time (Weddel, 1966).

Wound Healing and Skin Integrity: Principles and Practice, First Edition. Edited by Madeleine Flanagan.
© 2013 John Wiley & Sons, Ltd. Published 2013 by John Wiley & Sons, Ltd.

In an epidemiological study of 238,000 people in Western Australia, Baker et al. (1991) found that chronic leg ulcer prevalence was 0.62 per 1000 of the population, with venous ulceration accounting for 57% of all patients with a chronic leg ulcer. Of those with venous ulceration, 22% were found to have significant arterial ischaemic disease. More recently, Nelzen (2008) reported that the overall prevalence of venous leg ulceration in Sweden was stable at around 1% of the population whereas point prevalence varied across different countries. Causal factors, reporting methods and variations in practice help to explain the differences in global prevalence rates. In more recent studies more accurate assessment with modern diagnostic methods such as Doppler ultrasound can contribute to variations in data (Nelzen, 2008).

The causes of leg ulceration are multifactorial, approximately 35% of cases have underlying pathologies such as diabetes (11.35%), lymphoedema (42%) and rheumatoid arthritis (26%) (Nelzen, 2008). In this study, uncomplicated venous ulceration accounted for 43% of all ulcers.

Comorbidities and underlying pathologies

Underlying conditions affecting the venous and arterial systems tend to increase in the elderly resulting in leg ulceration. Metabolic disturbances such as diabetes carry an increased risk of infection due to immune deficiency and raised blood glucose levels (McIntosh and Green, 2009). Where peripheral neuropathy exists, loss of sensation could lead to skin and vascular damage if bandages, hosiery and dressings are not carefully checked for pressure injuries. This is particularly important for elderly patients with dry, thinning skin that may easily become damaged. Patients with coexisting congestive heart disease may also present with peripheral oedema, and care must be taken to ensure that only low levels of compression are applied as high-compression bandaging could cause rapid venous return and cardiac overload.

Rheumatoid arthritis and vasculitis

Inflammatory conditions such as rheumatoid arthritis may result in venous disease due to immobility, poor calf pump and ankle function (McRorie,

2000). Rheumatoid arthritis is also commonly associated with pyoderma gangrenosum and vasculitis which cause inflammatory vascular changes. The result is a chronic condition that is difficult to diagnose and painful to treat particularly in the presence of thinning skin (Armitage and Roberts, 2004). Management of venous disease in patients with rheumatoid arthritis is further complicated by the presence of peripheral arterial disease when significant arterial insufficiency may contraindicate the use of compression to manage oedema and venous stasis. However, with specialist assessment, patients can be managed successfully with compression and elevation to aid healing of venous ulcers (McRorie, 2000). Treatment relies on specialist referral where corticosteroids and pain relief forms the mainstay of treatment.

Common causes of leg ulceration:

- Venous
- Lymphovenous
- Diabetic foot ulcers
- Mixed venous arterial
- Pressure ulcers
- Arterial
- Traumatic

Less common causes of leg ulceration:

- Vasculitic causes, e.g. systemic lupus erythematosus, rheumatoid arthritis
- Congenital abnormalities, e.g. Klippel–Trénaunay syndrome, sickle cell disease
- Malignancy
- Lifestyle-induced, e.g. Buerger's disease (smoking-related), or substance abuse
- Pyoderma gangrenosum
- Infection including tropical ulcers
- Psychosocial and self-induced injury
- Trauma

Venous leg ulceration

Venous disorders range from mild thread veins to large areas of ulceration with accompanying lymphatic involvement. Impaired lymphatic function is associated with both venous and chronic venous hypertension and is associated with chronic oedema (Prasad et al., 1990). An international vascular committee in America developed the clinical,

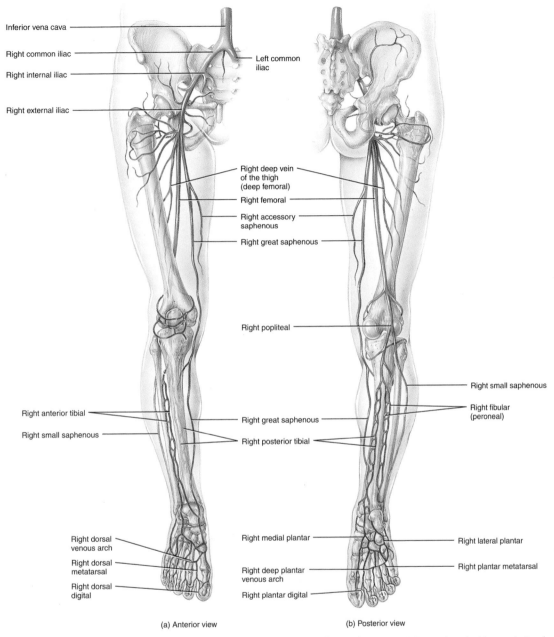

Inferior vena cava

Right common iliac

Right internal iliac

Right external iliac

Left common iliac

Right deep vein of the thigh (deep femoral)

Right femoral

Right accessory saphenous

Right great saphenous

Right popliteal

Right small saphenous

Right fibular (peroneal)

Right anterior tibial

Right great saphenous

Right small saphenous

Right posterior tibial

Right dorsal venous arch

Right medial plantar

Right lateral plantar

Right dorsal metatarsal

Right deep plantar venous arch

Right plantar metatarsal

Right dorsal digital

Right plantar digital

(a) Anterior view

(b) Posterior view

Figure 10.1   The normal venous system in the lower limb. From Tortora and Derrickson (2009). Reproduced with permission from Wiley.

etiological, anatomical pathophysiological (CEAP) classification system to describe the symptoms and severity of venous disorders. This has since been revised and validated and is now widely used in international research (Passman et al., 2011).

The normal venous system consists of deep veins, perforators and superficial veins (Figure 10.1), and blood is prevented from the pooling effects of gravity by non-return valves in the veins.

Unlike arteries which benefit from the continuous pumping action of the heart, the veins rely on the

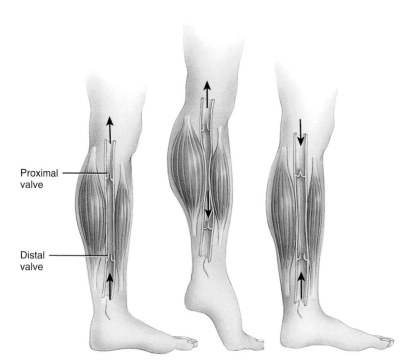

Proximal
valve

Distal
valve

Figure 10.2   The role of the foot pump in venous return. From Tortora and Derrickson (2009). Reproduced with permission from Wiley.

pumping effect of the foot and calf muscles during movement. The role of the foot pump in venous return can be seen in Figure 10.2.

In a healthy individual, venous pressure is 90 mmHg in the deep veins and 25–30 mmHg in the superficial veins when the subject is standing still. On exercise, the pressure in the deep veins falls to 10–20 mmHg, and is called the ambulatory venous pressure (AVP) (Partsch, 2006). This lowering of venous pressure also occurs when the subject is lying in the horizontal position and explains why venous return is facilitated by elevating the legs higher than the heart. Similarly, oedema formation is affected by gravity, giving rise to dependency oedema in the chair-bound patient sitting with their feet on the floor.

Chronic venous insufficiency (CVI) occurs when the venous system fails to facilitate the flow of venous blood from the distal areas in the lower leg into the central venous system (Figure 10.1). CVI has many causes which require thorough assessment in order to select an appropriate level and type of compression. Compression therapy plays a significant role in assisting the blood flow from the large veins in the sole of the foot through the ankle area and up to the calf where it is assisted by the calf muscle which propels the blood towards the upper leg and beyond.

Factors that affect venous return

Increasing age

Numerous studies have shown the impact of age on the prevalence of chronic leg ulceration and chronic oedema. Evans et al. (1999) identified the association between age and the prevalence of CVI in a general population survey, and a more recent UK study by Moffatt et al. (2003) reported a crude prevalence of 823 patients with chronic oedema (1.33/1000, rising to 5.4/1000 in those aged >65 years). Contributory factors may relate to underlying pathologies, general lifestyle, reduced immune response or nutrition.

Deep vein thrombosis

Lindholm (2002) discussed deep vein thrombosis (DVT) as the forgotten factor in leg ulceration, explaining that in 40% of cases, venous leg ulcers are caused by post-thrombotic syndrome (PTS) following DVT. Prandonia et al. (1998) found that 25% of PTS symptoms appeared within 2 years of acute DVT. Eighty-two percent of patients followed up for at least 10 years after a primary thrombosis developed PTS and of these 10% developed venous leg ulcers. A subsequent randomised controlled trial comparing elastic stockings with no compression (Prandonia et al., 2004) demonstrated a reduction in the incidence of PTS by 50% in the group assigned to below-knee compression elastic stockings.

These findings correlate well with those of Partsch (2005) who recommended the use of compression to reduce symptoms associated with PTS and DVT. Traditional treatment of bed rest for DVT has been challenged by Partsch (2005) who found that ambulation and compression led to faster relief of pain and swelling with no risk of the patients developing pulmonary emboli. In a 53-patient randomised controlled trial, 18 patients received strong inelastic compression, 18 wore thigh-length EU Class 11 compression stockings and 17 patients were confined to bed with no compression. In the compression groups, patients were able to walk immediately and after 9 days, pain levels and leg circumference were lower in this group in comparison to the bed-rest group. Ambulation whilst wearing compression is now recommended as the treatment of choice for patients with DVT.

Venous reflux

Backflow of blood occurs as a result of faulty valves which may become less efficient and leaky due to trauma or age. Higher pressure in the deep veins than the superficial veins causes blood to leak from the deep veins via the perforators into the superficial venous system, giving rise to varicose veins. The engorged superficial veins are now at risk of ulceration caused by trauma. A study by Banjo (1987) suggested that an increased number of perforator valves may account for a lower incidence of venous ulceration in a Nigerian population compared to Europeans, although the lower incidence of venous disease could be attributed to more resilient skin, a high-fibre diet and more exercise.

Oedema

As the blood vessels stretch, the walls become more permeable leading to leakage of fluid into the interstitial spaces, and this raises the external pressure that is exerted onto the vessel walls, exacerbating the problem of venous hypertension.

Increased pelvic congestion

Obesity, pregnancy and the presence of pelvic obstructive tumours can reduce the physical flow of venous blood as it enters the pelvic area from the upper legs, leading to pooling of blood and oedema formation in the legs. Lane et al. (2009) found that obesity was linked with popliteal vein compression syndrome (PVCS) leading to venous disease symptoms. Obesity as a risk factor for venous disease was also cited by Rabe et al. (2004) and is a growing problem worldwide.

Muscle wasting

The calf muscle is instrumental in assisting the action of the venous system in blood flow within the lower leg, confirmed in a study by Padberg et al. (2004) who demonstrated that exercise increases blood flow through the veins by stimulating the calf pump as seen in figure 10.2.

Immobility

Lack of movement is undoubtedly a contributory factor in the formation in oedema in the lower limb as demonstrated in gravitational oedema or 'armchair legs' commonly seen in patients who sit with their legs dependent for long periods of time (Green and Mason, 2006). As the weight of the oedematous limb inhibits movement, oedema increases giving rise to the oedema–immobility–oedema cycle (Muldoon, 2011) as seen in Figure 10.3. This depicts the vicious cycle of prolonged oedema leading to lack of immobility which in turn encourages oedema formation by the action of gravity.

Exercise and movement have another role in activating the thoracic/respiratory pump which helps to stimulate blood and lymph flow (Mortimer and Levick, 2004; Abadi et al., 2007). Compression that is insufficient to reverse venous hypertension and improve blood flow will have a similar effect in prolonging or encouraging peripheral oedema, which in turn will affect the flow of blood from the foot.

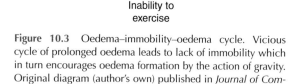

Figure 10.3 Oedema–immobility–oedema cycle. Vicious cycle of prolonged oedema leads to lack of immobility which in turn encourages oedema formation by the action of gravity. Original diagram (author's own) published in *Journal of Community Nursing* (Muldoon, 2011).

Arterial ulceration

Arterial ulcers occur when vessel narrowing restricts the flow of arterial blood from the heart to the lower limb. Narrowing can be caused by atherosclerosis, making the vessels less elastic and able to respond to the pumping action of the heart. Resulting ischaemia is most evident in the most distal parts of the limb, and if perfusion is not regained, tissue loss will occur. As arterial blood flow is compromised, it is imperative that this flow is not further restricted by compression therapy. Patients with suspected arterial disease should always be referred to the vascular team for diagnosis and treatment.

Mixed venous arterial ulcers

Venous and arterial disease often coexist making treatment decisions about compression therapy difficult. It is common for clinicians to under compress a limb with 'reduced compression' in order to avoid applying compression where an arterial component may be suspected. This may leave the venous system without the compression necessary to reduce venous hypertension. Where possible, patients should be referred to the specialist vascular practitioners who have the ability and experience to safely manage them with compression (Mosti, 2012; Neil and Turnbull, 2012).

Rarer leg ulcer aetiologies

Congenital causes of ulceration such as sickle cell disease and thalassaemia may be race-related. A common cause of leg ulcers in tropical Africa, the Caribbean, the Middle East and the Indian subcontinent is sickle cell disease, a genetic haemolytic disorder resulting in painful joint movement (Sickle Cell Society, 2008). Classically, sickle cell ulcers are circular, with raised, punched-out margins and may be deep (Trent et al., 2004). These ulcers are very painful and referral to a pain specialist is often necessary. The risk of infection is high, they are often associated with cellulitis, and recurrence is common. It is important to identify sickle cell disease so that the patient's management can be overseen by a specialist haematology department.

Conservative treatment consists of systemic medication prescribed by haematologists and blood transfusions. If the ulcer heals, the blood transfusions or exchange transfusions should be slowly withdrawn over a 3–6-month period. If there is no healing in 6 months, transfusions should be stopped. The ulcer should be managed with moist wound dressings, modified compression applied by a specialist and overnight high leg elevation which can drastically improve healing rates (Moffatt, 2008). Patients with non-healing wounds may be referred to a plastic or a vascular surgeon for skin grafting although recurrence is high (Trent and Kisner, 2004).

Tropical ulcers

Tropical ulcers are widely prevalent in developing countries and are not confined to tropical regions. They present as deep, painful lesions usually on the lower legs of unknown aetiology leading to misdiagnosis in most cases. They have a clearly defined edge and are often sloughy and surrounded by hyperpigmentation which can last many months. Consideration of where the sufferer lives or a travel history is the main source for diagnosis (MacDonald, 2003). The aetiology of tropical ulcers is uncertain. Infection is most likely to be the main cause which explains why well-nourished and well-shod travellers to tropical and remote regions may succumb to ulceration which is difficult to heal. The exact cause is thought to be a combined infection by *Fusobacterium ulcerans* (anaerobic bacterium) plus other bacteria which may be present in stagnant water. They enter the skin via minor traumatic wounds and are thought to release toxins that cause a necrotic reaction in dermal tissue leading to ulceration. Inaccessibility to effective treatments, good nutrition and education may have a role in exacerbating this condition. Treatment should involve moist wound healing and antibiotic therapy adjusted after the causative organism has been identified.

Psychological impact

Complications such as pain associated with cellulitis, and 'stretched' skin coupled with embarrassment and inconvenience can lead to isolation and feelings of helplessness (Green, 2008). Non-healing of open chronic leg ulceration can also cause sufferers to feel depressed (Williams et al., 2004). Brown (2005) and Charles (2010) in separate studies explored the concept of the so-called social ulcer which refers to the assumption that some health professionals have that patients prolong their ulcers as a means of maintaining social contact and support. They found no evidence to support this assumption as the majority of leg ulcer sufferers encountered were fiercely independent and were desperate to heal their ulcers. Many patients are described as non-concordant as bulky bandages are not always well tolerated.

The pain from leg ulcers can be intermittent (and may be linked to dressing change or bandage application) or persistent and usually gets worse as the day progresses (Nemeth et al., 2004). Pain may be worse at night, which can cause problems sleeping. Pain also restricts mobility which in turn can lead to social isolation, depression and feelings of hopelessness and affects adherence with treatment (Persoon et al., 2004) (see Chapter 5).

Principles of managing leg ulcers

The general principles of managing leg ulceration are as follows:

(1) Identify likely causation of leg ulcer by obtaining a thorough history and examination.
(2) Perform a bilateral lower-leg assessment of all patients with leg ulcers to determine extent of arterial disease.

(3) Develop an individual management plan that takes into account the degree of arterial and venous involvement.
(4) Establish the cause and extent of oedema which will influence subsequent management.
(5) Optimise local wound conditions, debridement, infection control, moisture balance. Consider adjunctive therapies if ulcer is not healing at the expected rate.
(6) Manage patient's pain and optimise mobility.
(7) Provide ongoing education to improve adherence to treatment and minimise ulcer recurrence.
(8) Frequently reassess vascular status to monitor for any changes.

The general principles of leg ulcer management need to be adapted to effectively manage patients with different types of ulcers. The specific principles of managing venous, mixed and arterial ulceration are summarised in Table 10.1.

Leg ulceration: assessment considerations

Accurate diagnosis is essential to decide on safe and effective treatment of leg ulcers, and should include specific wound, skin, vascular, oedema, pain and mobility assessment. All patients presenting with leg ulceration should have calculations of ankle brachial pressure index (ABPI) and Doppler sounds assessed during initial examination. In some countries, this may be a nurse-led procedure and may be performed in a primary care setting such as a community clinic or within the patient's own home.

Regular reassessment of vascular status should occur every 3 months to monitor treatment efficacy (Royal College of Nursing [RCN], 2006; Registered Nurses' Association of Ontario [RNAO], 2008; Scottish Intercollegiate Guidelines Network [SIGN], 2010). It is important to note that vascular assessment, in particular the simple measurement of ankle brachial pressure (ABP), should not be used in isolation without a detailed patient assessment when selecting treatment, as false positives may be obtained in certain diseases such as diabetes mellitus, atherosclerotic disease, rheumatoid arthritis and systemic vasculitis due to calcification of the blood vessels.

Table 10.1   Specific principles of managing venous, mixed and arterial ulceration

	Venous leg ulcer	Mixed leg ulcer	Arterial leg ulcer
Assessment	Identify cause of chronic venous insufficiency and implement appropriate medical management	Identify vascular component and underlying pathology to determine if safe to compress limbs as some arterial disease is present	Identify vascular component and underlying pathology and implement appropriate medical management
Compression	Management of co-existing oedema with compression therapy and leg elevation is essential; compression therapy should be applied to control venous oedema; the level and type of compression will vary according to patient tolerance	Determine if venous or arterial disease is dominant and extent of ischaemia as this determines if compression is indicated; apply modified compression to treat venous component if ABI >0.6; compression should only be prescribed and monitored by specialists	Do not apply high-compression bandaging if arterial disease is present (ABI <0.9); requires no compression or very low levels of compression depending on disease severity; compression should only be prescribed and monitored by specialists
Surgical intervention	Consider surgical management if superficial vein disease present		Refer for revascularization if ABI <0.6, and refer urgently if ABI <0.5
Education	Educate patient to understand need for lifelong compression hosiery; reinforce message frequently	Educate patient to be extra vigilant about deterioration of arterial component, e.g. worsening pain	Educate patient to avoid further tissue damage, e.g. tight socks, badly fitting shoes
Mobility	Optimise patient mobility and exercise to improve venous return	Optimise patient mobility and exercise to improve venous return within limitations of ischaemic pain	Optimise patient mobility and exercise within limitations of ischaemic pain

---

Practice point

Sufficient time of at least 1 hour should be allocated to obtain a detailed history and examination of a patient with a leg ulcer presenting for the first time. The patient should be examined in a well lit room and be able to lie down in a supine position with legs extended if possible.

When taking a history of a patient presenting with leg ulceration the following specific areas should be discussed:

- familial history of venous disease;
- familial history of cardiac/arterial disease;
- past history of DVT;
- past history of trauma to the leg including iatrogenic causes from bandages or hosiery;
- immobility including occupational hazards, e.g. prolonged standing/sitting;
- lifestyle factors, e.g. obesity, smoking, drug injection;
- infection;

- malignancy;
- congenital abnormalities of the venous, arterial or lymphatic system including the presence of oedema.

Skin assessment

Both legs should be examined for signs of venous and/or arterial disease which may be identified during a thorough assessment of the skin. Over time, venous hypertension causes a variety of skin changes which if treated early may prevent the progression to open ulceration. It is important to understand what these skin changes are and what they look like and to use the relevant terms to describe them so that documentation is precise and appropriate treatment instigated.

Ankle flare refers to small purplish thread veins in the ankle region indicating early signs of venous insufficiency but this does not necessarily lead to skin breakdown and ulceration. As venous return diminishes and veins become congested and more permeable, red blood cells leak into the

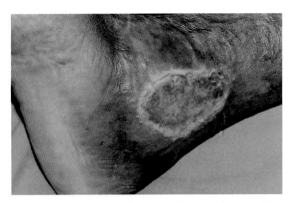

Figure 10.4 Venous leg ulcer: lipodermatosclerosis. Photo courtesy of Madeleine Flanagan.

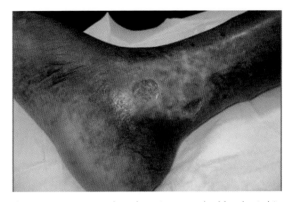

Figure 10.5 Venous leg ulceration: atrophe blanche (white areas) on black skin. Photo courtesy of Madeleine Flanagan.

surrounding tissue resulting in hyperpigmentation (brown staining on the skin) which is called lipodermatosclerosis (LDS) (Figure 10.4).

The gradual build up of haemosiderin deposits in the subcutaneous tissue makes them feel hard and 'woody', described as induration which is only detected by palpation. LDS is a condition that affects the skin around the ankles and lower limbs of individuals with long-standing venous disease and is a gradual process in which the skin becomes brown, smooth, tight and painful. LDS is caused by abnormally high venous pressure in the subcutaneous veins in the lower leg. LDS is indicative of venous disease and is an important warning sign but once established causes permanent and irreversible damage so early identification is important to help prevent progression to a painful, chronic, leg ulcer.

Atrophie blanche is another painful cutaneous symptom of venous disease and is characterised by the absence of pigmentation in the skin. It is often found in the same areas as hyperpigmentation resulting in irregular patches of dark and light skin as seen in Figure 10.5.

Chronic wound fluid left in contact with the skin may result in waterlogged tissue that is prone to infection and easily damaged. Protein-rich exudate particularly associated with venous leg ulcers is a painful irritant that causes maceration and excoriation and breakdown of skin integrity. Skin damage arising from wound exudate can be differentiated from other types of damage as it will always be found distal to the wound and may be worse if retained for longer periods underneath compression bandages.

Varicose eczema causes pruritis which can be very uncomfortable, and leads to scratching and further skin damage. Varicose eczema may be misdiagnosed as cellulitis leading to inappropriate prescription of antibiotics. In venous disease, layers of loose, dry, scaly skin develop and become hardened to form hyperkeratosis which, if left *in situ* can delay healing. Contact dermatitis caused by preservatives, adhesives or allergens are common in leg ulcer patients who may develop sensitivities to topical preparations (see Chapter 13).

Cellulitis is an acute episode of infection affecting large areas of the skin and subcutaneous tissues, and is potentially life-threatening if left untreated (Wingfield, 2009). Cellulitis may recur leading to systemic infection with fever requiring antibiotic treatment, pain management, bed rest and close monitoring (see Chapter 11). The Lymphoedema Framework (2006) recommends that compression should not be discontinued for long periods of time as worsening oedema increases the risk of cellulitis.

Tissue grading

Tissue grading is used by lymphoedema practitioners to assess the extent of oedema before swelling becomes apparent by limb circumference increase. The International Society for Lymphology Staging System (ISL, 2003) can be found in Box 11.1.

Changes in tissue density are also a good indication of successful treatment with compression and massage. These indicators are now being used more widely by non-lymphoedema practitioners who may be responsible for treating patients with lymphovenous oedema in the community (see Chapter 11).

Vascular assessment for arterial disease

The most basic form of vascular assessment is palpation of pulses in the foot. The peroneal pulse is located on the inner (anterior) aspect of the foot, the post-tibial pulse behind the malleolus and the most easily palpated is the dorsal pulse on the top aspect of the foot. It is now widely accepted that pedal pulses alone are insufficient to make an accurate clinical assessment of arterial blood flow to determine if compression therapy can be safely used (Moffatt et al., 2004; SIGN, 2010).

Arterial blood flow should be routinely assessed using a Doppler ultrasound by obtaining an ABPI in both legs at the initial visit. This is the ratio of the ankle to brachial systolic pressure and can be measured using a sphygmomanometer and hand-held Doppler device. More detailed information about how to carry out this procedure can be found in the Useful Resources section at the end of this chap-ter. The use of a hand-held Doppler to determine ABPI requires appropriate skills training due to the complexity of interpretation and reproducibility of results (Vowden, 2012).

Although the ABPI test result is described as an index, the calculation is recorded as a ratio which is usually 1.0 if there is no evidence of arterial insufficiency. A resting ABPI cut-point of 0.9 has been shown in several clinical studies to be highly sensitive and specific for peripheral arterial disease (positive predictive value of 95% and negative predictive value of 99%), and, in practice, an ABPI of <0.9 is considered to be abnormal (SIGN, 2010). There is a general agreement that compression therapy may be safely applied in patients with an ABPI greater than 0.8 in conjunction with a detailed patient history. At an ABPI of 0.6–0.8, compression should only be applied by a specialist practitioner following a more thorough vascular assessment. An ABPI of below 0.6 indicates that compression is contraindicated (RNAO, 2008; WUWHS, 2008; SIGN, 2010). The clinical implications of ABPI results are summarised in Table 10.2.

Care must be taken while interpreting ABPI results in isolation as patients with heavily calcified vessels, such as some patients with diabetes and

Table 10.2   Clinical implications of ABPI results

>1.3	1.0–1.3	0.8–1.0	0.5–0.8	<0.5
Possible false high reading due to calcification arteries	Normal range – no arterial disease	At risk of arterial disease but still with normal range	Mixed aetiology some venous and arterial component (predominantly venous)	Arterial component is predominant
Refer to specialist for further tests	Patient may be managed by non-specialists	Patient may be managed by non-specialists	Refer to specialist	Urgent referral
Do not apply compression	Compression bandages may be applied	Compression applied only under specialist supervision	Compression only applied by specialists; Inelastic or IPC advised with caution	No compression; symptom control
Repeat ABPI	Reassess ABPI every 6 mo depending on risk of PVD, e.g. increased age smoking, diabetes, etc.	Reassess ABPI every 3 mo depending on risk of PVD	Reassess ABPI every 3 mo depending on risk of PVD	May need to reassess ABPI more frequently
Do not apply until vascular status determined	Any compression is safe if the patient history indicates safety to compress	ABPI >0.8 Class 2 (European) hosiery	Consider Class 1 (European), if patient can tolerate	Avoid compression, manage symptoms

Source: Adapted from WUWHS (2008).

advanced chronic renal failure, may have misleadingly high results. Similarly, normal values have been found to be misleading as well where history-taking led to further investigations (Mosti, 2012). For values above 1.5, the vessels are likely to be incompressible, and the ABPI result cannot be relied on to guide clinical decisions.

Patients with an ABPI of below 0.7 or above 1.3 should be referred for more specialist vascular assessment, e.g. colour duplex scanning which can be used to accurately identify vessel obstruction.

Practice point

How can I effectively assess distal limb perfusion in a patient with incompressible blood vessels such as patients with diabetes or renal failure?

In this situation, systemic pressure is no longer a good predictor of leg ulcer healing as calcified blood vessels give a false high reading as the sphygmomanometer cuff will fail to compress the artery. Very dense or hyperkeratotic tissue may also be difficult to penetrate with a normal probe, so specialist Doppler probes of 4 MHz may be more reliable.

Simpler, alternative methods of assessment such as pulse oximetry are now being used more commonly to assess patient's suitability for compression therapy. Pulse oximetry measures pulsatile flow and oxygen saturation in the tissues, and can be performed whilst bandages and hosiery are in place. Sensors are placed on the toes and fingers to measure the toe finger oxygen index (TOFI) when the blood pressure cuff is inflated and released on the limb.

Where these methods are not available, pedal pulses and good history-taking, accompanied by close monitoring of the patient whilst compression is being worn, is essential, and the patient should always be referred to a specialist if there is any doubt about the arterial status.

Limb circumference measurement

Limb circumference measurements have a dual function in assessing oedema and for the selection of the appropriate compression bandaging and hosiery. Most generalist practitioners take measurements at the ankle, mid-calf and just below the knee but these measurements subject to error if measurements are taken under tension or at different points at each assessment. This may be overcome by the use of a spring-loaded tape measure and by marking measurement points along the limb.

Pain assessment

Pain in leg ulcer patients may be caused by many interrelated factors and may be due to inflammatory processes related to the skin or wound such as eczema, maceration, infection or oedema or as a consequence of treatment, e.g. compression therapy.

In addition, comorbidities may contribute to increased pain, particularly in the elderly and can cause confounding variables during assessment. Leg ulcer pain may be exacerbated by a diverse range of coexistent diseases including diabetic neuropathy, osteoarthritis, rheumatoid disease, pyoderma gangrenosum, leprosy, depression and anxiety. Pain assessment is a critical part of leg ulcer management and can help indicate causation (McMullen, 2004). Heavy, aching pain is associated with increased venous flow when the lower leg becomes swollen, whilst sudden, gripping pain on exercise may indicate intermittent claudication due to reduced arterial perfusion. Neuropathic pain is characteristically described as burning, tingling, or stabbing or shooting pains. The persistent pain frequently experienced by people with venous leg ulcers is frequently described as feeling 'red raw, burning and like having acid thrown onto the skin' (Nemeth et al., 2004).

Mobility assessment

Restricted ankle mobility caused by pain, arthritis or ulceration may affect the ability to exercise which is essential for lymph flow and venous return, whilst unresolved oedema or bulky bandages are contributory factors that are often overlooked as a cause of restricted joint movement. Patient mobility in the form of movement and exercise is therefore important in the management of venous and lymphovenous disease. Assessing patient mobility can be subjective and the Leg Clubs® in the United Kingdom which provide community-based treatment, health promotion and ongoing care for people with leg ulcers are finding the use of a more objective patient mobility assessment tool very helpful. Box 10.1 shows an example of an ambulatory assessment chart.

Box 10.1   Ambulatory assessment chart

Ambulatory assessment chart	Circle number
• Immobile: unable to move unaided either in bed or chair; cannot take own weight, even with assistance	7
• Assisted mobility: needing physical assistance from another person/s to walk or move; can transfer with assistance	6
• Restricted/limited mobility: able to transfer with assistance; can walk a few steps but limited by physical or psychological problems, e.g. shortness of breath, pain, failing sight, fear of falling, agoraphobia	5
• Poor mobility: poor walking pattern, shuffling gait, decreased stride-length, poor posture, muscle weakness or deformity	4
• Independent with equipment: able with specific (daily living) equipment to achieve independence	3
• Independent with supervision: physically able to take own weight but needs supervision and/or prompting to ensure correct use of equipment, walking pattern or orientation	2
• Independent mobility: able to walk, transfer, lie down/get up, ability to exercise within their limitations	1

Source: Lindsay et al. (2003).

Management of chronic oedema in leg ulcers

Persistent chronic oedema and venous ulceration can present problems such as poor healing and increased immobility which in turn lead to the risk of gravitational oedema perpetuation and non-healing. Sedentary lifestyle and dietary habits are contributory factors not just in weight gain but also in the ability to exercise. Similarly, oedema formation is affected by gravity in less mobile people, giving rise to dependency oedema in the chair-bound patient.

Compression therapy

High compression remains the cornerstone for reducing venous hypertension by exerting pressure higher than the pressure in the veins (Partsch, 2006 and is most commonly available as compression bandages (inelastic and elastic, single- and multi-layer), compression hosiery and intermittent pneumatic compression (WUWHS, 2008).

In countries with remote areas that are not easily accessible, compression garments that may be applied with little training by patients or their relatives may be preferable to bandages. Simi-

larly, financial constraints in poorer countries may necessitate the use of reusable, locally produced bandages (Ryan, 2007). However, there are still many countries where the majority of patients with venous leg ulcers are still not diagnosed and compression therapy is not widely available (MacDonald and Geyer, 2010). In these countries, evidence is emerging to demonstrate that the use of any type of compression is better than no compression and improves ulcer healing rates.

New therapies, such as low-dose ultrasound, are being investigated to manage the hard-to-heal ulcer.

The aims of compression therapy are therefore to:

• reverse venous hypertension;
• reduce and control oedema;
• control excessive exudate and odour;
• prevent recurrence of infection;
• promote wound healing;
• reduce pain and improve patient comfort;
• improve skin condition.

Effective compression is identified by an improvement in oedema and exudate production from the ulcer which may happen quickly. Clinical guidelines recommend that reassessment within 12 weeks is essential to monitor treatment efficacy and that if no improvement is seen then the patient

Clinical factors	Patient factors	Organisational factors
• Comorbidities, e.g. renal status, cardiac overload • Arterial status • Exudate level • Infection, e.g. cellulitis • Skin fragility • Amount of oedema • Shape of leg • Pain • Mobility	• Health beliefs • Patient preference • Education and support • Motivation, adherence with treatment • Lifestyle choices, e.g. frequent travel, swimming	• Availability of multidisciplinary team • Resource availability • Access to specialist services and training • Experience, knowledge, skills and attitude of individual clinicians

Figure 10.6   Factors influencing choice of compression therapy.

is referred to an appropriate specialist (RCN, 2006; RNAO, 2008; SIGN, 2010).

The factors influencing choice of compression therapy are shown in Figure 10.6.

Compression bandaging

There is a strong body of evidence to support the use of high compression versus low compression but there is less evidence of effect comparing multi and single component bandage systems (Brolmann et al., 20012). Although many bandage systems are based on pressures of 40 mmHg which was originally suggested by Stemmer in 1969 to be the optimal pressure required for effective graduated compression, this has not been empirically proven. Indeed a study by Partsch (2006) found that intermittent pressures of >50 mmHg were required to improve severe venous incompetence. He does state however, that lower levels of compression at 40 mmHg as achieved with elastic stockings may be suitable for preventing or reducing mild oedema. The International Compression Club (ICC) recommends that bandage manufacturers should state the pressures achieved with and the mode of action of their bandage systems as compression should be considered as a treatment requiring accurate dosage as advised by Mosti (2012). Long-stretch elastic bandages deliver sustained compression over a 24-hour period whereas short-stretch inelastic bandages have alternating high therapeutic working and lower tolerable resting pressures.

Partsch (2006) demonstrated the importance of these alternating pressures in stimulating venous return by mimicking the contractile action of the veins when they are squeezed by the muscle pumps which is called the stiffness index. The lymphatic vessels also respond to variations in pressure which cause a massaging effect on the lymphatics by creating pressure peaks (Mortimer and Levick, 2004; Partsch, 2007). This explains why bandage systems that produce a high stiffness index are recommended for the reduction of oedema (European Wound Management Association, 2005; Lymphoedema Framework, 2006). This recommendation is supported by a 90-subject randomised controlled trial (Badger et al., 2000) that demonstrated that compression bandaging with inelastic bandages following maintenance with compression hosiery was twice as effective as compression hosiery alone. Similarly, Mosti et al. (2008) discussed the effectiveness of high working pressures coupled with the tolerability of the lower resting pressures in a study comparing elastic and inelastic compression in clinical practice, and concluded that a lower resting pressure with an inelastic system was more comfortable for patients, particularly at night. The differences between different types of compression therapy are summarised in Table 10.3.

Compression hosiery

Compression bandaging may not always be suitable due to unavailability of trained people to apply them. They may not always be preferred by patients, and layered hosiery kits provide an ideal solution and effective treatment where the

Table 10.3   Differences between different types of compression therapy

Compression hosiery	Elastic bandages	Inelastic bandages	Multilayered bandages
Two-layer hosiery kits	Single layers or multilayered applied over padding	Short-stretch bandages applied over padding	Bandage kits such as the four-layer bandage system, padding layer, crepe, two compression layers
Cumulative pressure of ±40 mmHg	Constant 40 mmHg pressure over 24 h	Intermittent high working, lower resting pressures	Cumulative pressure of 40 mmHg
May be self or carer applied	Applied at mid stretch with 50% overlap by trained person	Applied at full stretch with 50% overlap by trained person	Both compression layers applied at mid stretch, first compression in a figure of 8, second layer in a spiral with 50% overlap by trained person
Washable and reusable non-cohesive	Non-cohesive are washable: cohesive bandages are not washable and reusable	May be cohesive or non-cohesive: cohesive bandages are not washable and reusable	Single use: cohesive bandages are not washable or reusable
Not suitable for large or heavily exuding ulcers or where shaping is required with significant oedema	Not recommended for significant oedema[a] or patients with suspected mild-to-moderate arterial disease	Recommended for significant oedema[a] and for patients with mild-to-moderate arterial disease	Not recommended for significant oedema[a]
	May also be used with zinc paste bandages	May also be used with zinc paste bandages to form Unna Boot	

[a]Significant oedema is indicated where there are skin folds, grossly misshapen limbs or fibrotic skin changes.

leg ulcer is small with minimal exudate and the limb is not grossly swollen or misshapen as seen in Figure 10.7.

Compression hosiery kits and compression stockings may be more suitable for able patients with small, uncomplicated ulcer who wish to take control of their own care, care by less skilled staff or where compression bandaging may not be tolerated.

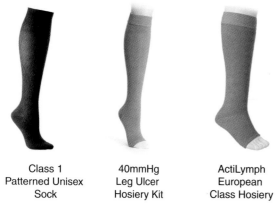

Class 1	40mmHg	ActiLymph
Patterned Unisex	Leg Ulcer	European
Sock	Hosiery Kit	Class Hosiery

Figure 10.7   Compression hosiery. With kind permission from Activa Healthcare.

Wound dressings: special considerations

Wound dressings are usually unable to control the volume and flow of chronic wound fluid produced by leg ulcers and are therefore considered less important in their overall management. Compression therapy is currently the most effective method of controlling oedema and fluid formation associated with venous leg ulcers and is the mainstay of treatment (WUWHS, 2008; O'Meara et al., 2009). Table 10.4 describes factors influencing the production of exudate in leg ulcers.

However, the occlusion created by compression therapy may affect the fluid-handling properties of absorbent dressings by altering the moisture vapour transmission rate (MVTR).

Table 10.4   Factors influencing the production of exudate in leg ulcers

Patient factors	Treatment factors
Position of the limb	Type of wound dressing
Skin/wound infection	Absorbency occlusion
Degree of chronicity	Frequency of dressing change
Vascularity	Compression
Underlying conditions, e.g. oedema	Debridement

Wound management for leg ulcers therefore requires a different approach to other chronic wounds due to adjunct compression therapy, peri-wound complications and increased risk of contact dermatitis:

- Dressings that rely on absorption and moisture vapour transmission to manage exudate may not be effective due to reduced evaporation caused by occlusion and the effects of localised pressure as a result of compression therapy.
- Hyperkeratosis associated with leg ulceration reduces the efficacy of topical pain-relieving dressings, steroids or antimicrobial agents by creating an impenetrable barrier on the surface of the skin and should be removed.
- Some local wound treatments, e.g. larvae do not survive well under the pressure of compression bandaging and may necessitate a 'compression holiday' that may delay healing.
- Application of topical agents is not always possible and monitoring the progress of healing is challenging when the treatment regime requires the limb to be bandaged for 5–7 days.
- Adhesive dressings should be used with caution under compression therapy as they may cause skin stripping due to increased adherence caused by the effects of localised pressure and increased temperature.
- Patients with chronic leg ulcers are susceptible to sensitivities to preservatives found in topical preparations. A thinner epidermis and increased vascular permeability caused by oedema exacerbates the risk of tissue trauma and may cause further skin irritation.

Prevention of ulcer recurrence

Once the ulcer has healed, compression hosiery plays a key part in the prevention of recurrence. Vandongen and Stacey (2000) reported that recurrence rates at 6 months could be reduced from 46% to 21% by wearing Class 3 compression stockings compared with not wearing stockings. Bentley (2001) advises that lower compression garments may be prescribed to achieve concordance which could also be encouraged by patient education and a clinic environment.

Factors to consider when selecting compression hosiery are as follows:

- presence and level of oedema which determines the stiffness of the garment;
- severity of venous disease which indicates the class of compression;
- presence of cardiac oedema/significant arterial disease which would present a risk factor contraindicating the use of high compression;
- varicosities or swelling extending into the thigh when full-length garments should be prescribed;
- compression hosiery is not suitable for large, exuding wounds, although a leg ulcer hosiery kit could be used for some open wounds;
- patient or carer's ability to apply and remove the garment; below-knee garments are easier to apply and aids are available to assist application;
- limb circumference and size of foot: larger feet benefit from open-toed garments which provide the right level of compression at the ankle without causing discomfort, e.g. crowding toes; open-toed styles are usually selected where infection might be suspected to facilitate observation of the feet;
- if the patient is unable to remove hosiery at night, open-toed stockings are safer and more hygienic;
- patient preference should be considered as garments are worn for life and concordance is essential.

Classification of compression hosiery varies in different countries. Please refer to local guidelines for further information as this is beyond the scope of this chapter.

Higher levels of compression do not necessarily indicate a stiffer garment. British Standard hosiery is more elastic, better suited to legs with no oedema and in some cases may be easier to apply. European Standard garments are stiffer and may be circular knit or flat knit, making them more suitable for limbs which are oedematous or prone to oedema in order to contain the swelling.

Education and support

As compression hosiery is worn for life to prevent recurrence, aesthetics and patient preference should be considered to encourage concordance. Reminders of previous ulceration may be enough to convince reluctant patients to wear their compression garments.

Advice should be given about skin care, prevention of trauma, monitoring of oedema and care of the compression garments. Patients should be shown examples of compression hosiery and encouraged to take an active role in hosiery selection. Some clinics delegate this task to older healthcare assistants who may better relate to elderly patients.

Provision of specialist services

Models of service delivery and provision of care for leg ulcer patients vary from country to country but it is well recognised that effective management of people with leg ulcers requires an integrated, multidisciplinary team approach (RCN, 2006; RNAO, 2008; SIGN, 2010). In the United Kingdom and Australia the introduction of Leg Clubs® which are based on the concept of a club atmosphere rather than a clinic has shown that this environment is conducive to concordance and healing. Audit data over a 6-year period demonstrated a 16% transfer of care from active treatment to a well leg programme (Clark, 2010).

In some countries, lymphoedema specialists with a background in physiotherapy, dermatology manual lymphatic drainage or nursing now work closely with leg ulcer teams to provide care for chronic oedema patients in the community. Partnerships exist in some clinical settings that include vascular, dermatology, physiotherapy, nursing and podiatry clinicians combined with engineers, research scientists and industrial partners. A good example of this type of collaboration is the ICC which incorporates these disciplines to provide education, research and development to advance compression therapy internationally.

Reimbursement and local policies are key influencers in clinical practice with international variations in service provision. Compression in different countries varies according to tradition, reimbursement, provision of care and training, e.g. in France only long-stretch bandages are reimbursable; in the United Kingdom, elastic, four-layer bandages and inelastic systems are used; clinicians in the United States still favour Unna Boot systems; whilst in mainland Europe, inelastic bandages or short stretch have a long history of successful management. Local preferences and infection control policies may favour the use of single-use non-washable bandage systems, whilst developing countries may only be able to afford locally produced, washable bandages that have to be used more than once.

The selection and application of compression therapy is a complex skill requiring training and regular updating to achieve and maintain competence. Generally speaking there is a significant lack of appropriately skilled practitioners in hospital and community settings to effectively treat people with venous ulcers and lymphoedema which is compounded by a lack of international competencies for leg ulcer management (Anderson, 2010). Yet international guidelines all agree that training and education for those involved in the care of this patient group is crucial (RCN, 2006; RNAO, 2008; WUWHS, 2008; SIGN, 2010).

The burden of care for leg ulcer management is mainly in the community. In some countries like the United Kingdom, community nursing services (visiting people in their own homes and provision of specialist community leg ulcer clinics) are well established and have proven to provide cost-effective treatment (Thurlby and Griffiths, 2002). However, in some areas there is minimal community support for people with leg ulcers. In the future, services for people with leg ulcers should be developed linking community nursing services to specialist dermatology, vascular and wound management services.

Criteria for specialist referral

Clinical guidelines recommend that reassessment of leg ulcers should be conducted at 12 weeks to establish progress (RCN, 2006; RNAO, 2008; SIGN, 2010). Best practice has demonstrated that oedema reduction should be apparent after 1–2 weeks and leg ulcer healing rates of over 70% at 12 weeks are achievable (EWMA, 2005, Moffatt et al., 2010).

Patients who have the following criteria should be referred to the appropriate specialist at an early stage (RCN, 2006; RNAO, 2008; SIGN, 2010):

- diagnostic uncertainty;
- atypical distribution of ulcers;
- ulcers of non-venous aetiology, e.g. diabetes, rheumatoid arthritis/vasculitis;

- reduced ABPI (<0.8);
- increased ABPI (>0.3);
- suspicion of malignancy;
- suspected contact dermatitis;
- cellulitis;
- rapid deterioration of ulcers;
- non-healing ulcer(s) (failure to progress or heal after 12 weeks of active treatment).

Referral criteria should be agreed locally and information disseminated widely and made available for inclusion in local clinical guidelines.

Summary

Compression therapy is essential and the most effective way of treating venous leg ulcers but poses a number of challenges as it is not always available, requires a high level of knowledge and practical skills to apply and motivation from the patient. Interdisciplinary collaboration has led to improved research, sharing of expertise and comprehensive treatment outcomes for leg ulcer patients where in the past, treatment may have been delayed. Assessment and reassessment within agreed timelines are essential for timely management of patients with leg ulcers to ensure that they are treated effectively or referred appropriately to specialist services. Availability of resources, education and training, and patient advice are key elements in providing care for this client group and will help to alleviate suffering associated with chronic leg ulceration.

Useful resources

Clinical guidelines

Scottish Intercollegiate Guidelines Network (SIGN) (2010) Management of chronic venous leg ulcers. A National Clinical Guideline. 120. Available at: http://www.sign.ac.uk/pdf/sign120.pdf

Aberdeen (2009) *Skills for Practice: Management of Chronic Oedema in the Community*. Wounds UK, Available at: http://www.woundsinternational.com/pdf/content_206.pdf

Registered Nurses' Association of Ontario (RNAO) (2008) *Nursing Best Practice Guideline. Assessment and Management of Venous Leg Ulcers*. Registered Nursing Association of Ontario, Supplement. Available at: http://rnao.ca/bpg/guidelines/assessment-and-management-venous-leg-ulcers. Last accessed 18 November 2012

Health Education Fact Sheet: Taking Care of Your Legs Registered Nurses' Association of Ontario (RNAO). Available at: http://rnao.ca/sites/rnao-ca/files/Taking_Care_of_Your_Legs.pdf. Last accessed 18 November 2012.

EWMA Position Document: Understanding Compression Therapy (2003). London: MEP Ltd. Available at: http://ewma.org

Best Practice Statement: Compression Hosiery. Available at: www.wounds-uk.com. Last accessed 19 November 2012

Useful websites

International Compression Club. Available at: http://www.icc-compressionclub.com/

European Venous Forum. Available at: http://www.europeanvenousforum.org/links.htm

American Venous Forum. Available at: http://veinforum.org/

The Lindsay Leg Club Foundation. Available at: http://www.legclub.org/

Further reading

Technical Guide: How to Obtain the Resting ABPI in Leg Ulcer Management. Available at: http://www.wounds-uk.com/pdf/content_9368.pdf

References

Abadi, S., Nelson, E.A., Dehghani, A. (2007) Venous ulceration and the measurement of movement: a review. *Journal of Wound Care*, 16(9), 396–402.

Anderson, I. (2010) Costs can be cut by providing high quality training in leg ulcer care. *Nursing Times*, 106(35), 8. Available at: NursingTimes.net, retrieved on August 2011.

Armitage, M., Roberts, J. (2004) Caring for patients with leg ulcers and an underlying vasculitic condition. *British Journal of Community Nursing*, 9(Suppl 12) S16–S22.

Badger, C.M.A., Peacock, J.L., Mortimer, P.S. (2000) A randomized, controlled, parallel group clinical trial comparing multilayer bandaging followed by hosiery versus hosiery alone in the treatment of patients with lymphedema of the limb. *Cancer*, 88, 2832–2837.

Baker, S.R., Stacey, M.C., Jopp-McKay, A.G., Hoskin, S.E., Thompson, P.J. (1991) Epidemiology of chronic venous ulcers. *British Journal of Surgery*, 78, 864–867.

Banjo, A.O. (1987) Comparative study of the distribution of venous valves in the lower extremities of black Africans and Caucasians. *The Anatomical Record*, 217, 407–412.

Bentley, J. (2001) Preventing unnecessary suffering: an audit of a leg ulcer clinic. *British Journal of Community Nursing*, 6(3), 136–144.

Brolmann, F.E., Ubbink, D.T., Nelson, E.A., Munte, K., van der Horst, C.M.A.M. (2012) Evidence-based decisions for systemic wound care. *British Journal of Surgery*, 99, 1172–1183.

Brown, A. (2005) Chronic venous leg ulcers, part 1: do they affect a patient's social life? *British Journal Nursing*, 14(17), 894–898.

Charles, H. (2010) The influence of social support on leg ulcer healing. *British Journal of Community Nursing*, 15(12), 14–21.

Clark, M. (2010) The Lindsay leg club model. *EWMA Journal*, 10(3), 38–40.

European Wound Management Association (EWMA) (2005) *Position Statement: "Identification of Wound Infection"*. London: MEP Ltd.

Evans, C.J., Fowkes, F.G., Ruckley, C.V., Lee, A.J. (1999) Prevalence of varicose veins and chronic venous insufficiency in men and women in the general population: Edinburgh Vein Study. *Journal of Epidemiology and Community Health*, 53, 149–153.

Green, T. (2008) Understanding body image in patients with chronic oedema. *Chronic Oedema Supplement British Journal of Community Nursing*, 13(10), S15–S18.

Green, T., Mason, W. (2006) Chronic oedema, identification and referral pathways. *The Lymphoedema Supplement British Journal of Community Nursing*, 11 (Suppl 4), S8–S16.

Laing, W. (1992) *Chronic Venous Diseases of the Leg*. Whitehall, London: Office of Health Economics.

Lane, R.J., Cuzzilla, M.L., Harris, R.A., Phillips, M.N. (2009) Popliteal vein compression syndrome: obesity, venous disease and the popliteal connection. *Phlebology*, 25, 201–207.

Lindholm, C. (2002) DVT: the forgotten factor in leg ulcer prevention. *Journal of Wound Care*, 11(1), 5.

Lindsay, E.T., Muldoon, J., Hampton, S. (2003) Short stretch compression bandages and the foot pump: their relationship to restricted mobility. *Journal of Wound Care*, 12(5), 185–188.

Lymphoedema Framework (2006) *Best Practice for the Management of Lymphoedema. International Consensus*. London: MEP Ltd.

MacDonald, P. (2003) Tropical ulcers: a condition still hidden from the Western world. *Journal of Wound Care*, 12(3), 85–89.

Macdonald, J., Geyer, M. (2010) *Wounds and Lymphoedema Management*. Geneva: WHO–Global Initiative for Wound and Lymphoedema Care.

McIntosh, C., Green, T. (2009) An overview of lower limb lymphoedema and diabetes. *Journal of Lymphoedema*, 4(1), 49–58.

McMullen, M. (2004) The relationship between pain and leg ulcers: a critical review. *British Journal of Nursing*, 13, S30–S36.

McRorie, E.R. (2000) The assessment and management of leg ulcers in rheumatoid arthritis. *Journal of Wound Care*, 9(6), 289–292.

Moffatt, C. (2008) Using compression in complicated situations. *Wounds UK*, 4(4), 84–94.

Moffatt, C.J., Doherty, D.C., Smithdale, R., Franks, P.J. (2010) Clinical predictors of leg ulcer healing. *British Journal of Dermatology*, 162, 51–58.

Moffatt, C.J., Franks, P.J., Doherty, D.C., Martin, R., Blewett, R., Ross, F. (2004) Prevalence of leg ulceration in a London population. *Quarterly Journal of Medicine*, 97(7), 431–437.

Moffatt, C.J., Franks, P.J., Doherty, D.C., et al. (2003) Lymphoedema and underestimated health problem. *Quarterly Journal of Medicine*, 96(10), 731–738.

Mortimer, P.S., Levick, J.R. (2004) Chronic peripheral oedema: the critical role of the lymphatic system. *Clinical Medicine*, 4(5), 448–453.

Mosti, G., Mattaliano, V., Partsch, H. (2008) Inelastic compression increases venous ejection fraction more than elastic bandages in patients with superficial venous reflux. *Phlebology*, 23, 287–294.

Mosti, G. (2012) Elastic stockings versus inelastic bandages for ulcer healing is a fair comparison. *Phlebology*, 27, 1–4.

Muldoon, J. (2011) Assessment and monitoring of oedema. *Journal of Wound Care*, 25(6), 26–28.

Neil, K., Turnbull, K. (2012) Use of specialist knowledge and experience to manage patients with mixed aetiology leg ulcers. *Journal of Wound Care*, 21(4), 168–174.

Nelzen, O. (2008) Prevalence of venous leg ulcer: the importance of the data collection method. *Phlebolymphology*, 15(4), 143–150.

Nemeth, K.A., Harrison, M.B., Graham, I.D., Burke, S. (2004) Understanding venous leg ulcer pain: results of a longitudinal study. *Ostomy Wound Management*, 50, 34–46.

O'Meara, S., Cullum, N.A., Nelson, E.A. (2009) Compression for venous leg ulcers. *The Cochrane Database of Systematic Reviews*, CD000265.

Padberg, F.T., Johnston, M.V., Sisto, S.A. (2004) Structured exercise improves calf muscle pump function in chronic venous insufficiency: a randomized trial. *Society of Vascular Surgery*, 39(1), 79–87.

Partsch, H. (2005) Ambulation and compression after deep vein thrombosis: dispelling myths. *Seminars in Vascular Surgery*, 18(3), 148–152.

Partsch, H. (2006) Compression therapy of venous ulcers. Haemodynamic effects depend on interface stiffness. *EWMA Journal*, 6(2), 16–20.

Partsch, H. (2007) Assessing the effectiveness of multi-layer inelastic bandaging. *Journal of Lymphoedema*, 2(2), 55–61.

Partsch, H. (2009) Why are most ulcers located on the leg? *Phlebology*, 24(4), 143–144.

Passman, M., McLafferty, R., Iafrati, M., et al. (2011) Validation of venous clinical severity score. *Journal of Vascular Surgery*, 54 (Suppl 6), 2S–9S.

Persoon, A., Heinen, M.M., van de Rooij, M.J., van de Kerkhof, P.C., van, A.T. (2004) Leg ulcers: a review of their impact on daily life. *Journal of Clinical Nursing*, 13, 341–354.

Prandonia, P., Frulla, M., Sartor, D., Concolato, A., Girolami, A. (2005) Venous abnormalities and the post-thrombotic syndrome. *Journal of Thrombosis and Haemostasis*, 3(2), 401–402.

Prandonia, P., Lensing, A.W., Prins, M.R. (1998) Long-term outcomes after deep venous thrombosis of the lower extremities. *Vascular Medicine*, 3, 57–60.

Prasad, A., Ali-Khan, A., Mortimer, P.S. (1990) Leg ulcers and oedema: a study exploring the prevalence, aetiology and possible significance of oedema in leg ulcers. *Phlebology*, 5, 181–187.

Registered Nurses' Association of Ontario (RNAO) (2008) *Nursing Best Practice Guideline. Assessment and Management of Venous Leg Ulcers*. Registered Nursing Association of Ontario, Supplement. Available at: http://rnao.ca/bpg/guidelines/assessment-and-management-venous-leg-ulcers. Last accessed 18 November 2012

Royal College of Nursing (RCN) (2006) *Clinical Practice Guidelines for the Nursing Management of Patients with Venous Leg Ulcers*, 2nd edn. RCN Institute, Centre for Evidence Based Nursing, University of York.

Sickle Cell Society (2008) *Standards for the Clinical Care of Adults with Sickle Cell Disease in the UK*. London: Sickle Cell Society.

Scottish Intercollegiate Guidelines Network (SIGN) (2010) Management of chronic venous leg ulcers. A National Clinical Guideline. Edinburgh, Scotland: SIGN publication, no.20. Available at: http://www.sign.ac.uk/pdf/sign120.pdf

Stemmer, R. (1969) Ambulatory elastocompressive treatment of the lower extremities particularly with elastic stockings, *Der Kassernarzt*, 9, 1–8.

Thurlby, K., Griffiths, P. (2002) Community leg ulcer clinics vs home visits: which is more effective? *British Journal of Community Nursing*, 2, 260–264.

Tortora, G.J., Derrickson, B.H. (2009) *Essentials of Anatomy and Physiology*, 8th edn. John Wiley & Son.

Trent, J. T., Kirsner, R.S. (2004) Leg ulcers in sickle cell disease. *Advances in Skin & Wound Care*, 17(8), 410–416.

Vandongen, Y., Stacey, M. (2000) Graduated compression elastic stockings to reduce lipodermatosclerosis and ulcer recurrence. *Phlebology*, 15, 33–37.

Vowden, P. (2012) Understanding ankle brachial pressure index to treat venous ulceration. *Wounds UK*, 8(1), 10–15.

Weddel, J.M. (1966) Varicose veins pilot survey. *British Medical Journal*, 2, 591–595.

Williams, A., Moffatt, C., Franks, P. (2004) A phenomenological study of the lived experiences of people with lymphoedema. *International Journal of Palliative Nursing*, 10(6), 279–285.

Wingfield, C. (2009) Chronic oedema and the importance of skin care. *Wound Essentials*, 4(26), 34.

World Union of Wound Healing Societies (WUWHS) (2008) *Principles of Best Practice: Compression in Venous Leg Ulcers. A Consensus Document*. London: MEP Ltd.

11 Lymphoedema

David Keast

Aging, Rehabilitation and Geriatric Care Research Centre, Lawson Health Research Institute, and St. Joseph's Parkwood Hospital, London, Ontario, Canada

Overview

- Lymphoedema is more common than realised; most clinicians have little experience of this complex condition and its associated problems which delays diagnosis and leads to inappropriate management.
- The general public have a limited knowledge and understanding of lymphoedema which leads to difficulties ensuring concordance with treatment.
- There is an urgent need for the development of specialist lymphoedema services based on multidisciplinary team expertise and involvement.
- There is a lack of evidence-based guidance to direct the clinical management of lymphoedema and chronic oedema.

Introduction

Lymphoedema is currently recognised globally as an important cause of skin breakdown and because of its association with cancer treatment, it is becoming a growing concern (Sheffield et al., 2004). In developed countries, the incidence of secondary lymphoedema following cancer treatment has been reported in up to 63% of women following breast cancer surgery and up to 70% of men after prostate cancer treatment. The *International Lymphoedema Framework Annual Report* in 2008 estimated that 48% of chronic oedema/lymphoedema in England and Scotland was secondary to malignancy and 52% was related to other causes.

The most common cause of secondary lymphoedema worldwide is lymphatic filariasis (LF) (Sheffield et al., 2004). An estimated 1.3 billion people around the world are at risk of LF infection, and more than 120 million are infected. Countries where LF is found are mostly in the tropical and subtropical regions of the world. They also are among the world's poorest countries, as LF is closely linked to poor sanitation and poor housing quality. The growing obesity epidemic has resulted in increasing numbers of patients with secondary lymphoedema due to morbid obesity. Lymphoedema produces significant physical and psychological morbidity. Increased limb size may interfere with mobility and affect body image (Consensus Document of

Wound Healing and Skin Integrity: Principles and Practice, First Edition. Edited by Madeleine Flanagan.
© 2013 John Wiley & Sons, Ltd. Published 2013 by John Wiley & Sons, Ltd.

Box 11.1   Causes of secondary lymphoedema

- Tissue damage through trauma or surgery
- Malignant disease
- Chronic venous disease
- Infection – bacterial or parasitic
- Inflammatory conditions of skin or systemic inflammatory conditions
- Endocrine disorders – myxoedema
- Immobility and dependency from any cause, including conditions leading to paralysis
- Self-harm

Source: Lymphoedema Framework (2006).

the International Society of Lymphology, 2009; Ridner, 2009), create pain and discomfort for the patient, and increase susceptibility to acute infections such as cellulitis or erysipelas (Mayrovitz, 2009; Gethin et al., 2012). Yet, lymphoedema is poorly recognised, undertreated and inadequately resourced.

Lymphoedema is defined as an abnormal swelling of a limb and/or the related quadrant of the trunk due to the accumulation of protein-rich fluid in the tissue spaces of the skin (Lawenda et al., 2009). Clinically, lymphoedema may be defined as chronic oedema lasting more than 3 months which is minimally responsive to overnight leg elevation or diuretics and is accompanied by skin changes such as thickened skin, hyperkeratosis and papillomatosis (Kubik and Kretz, 2006). Primary lymphoedema is related to congenital absence or malformation of lymphatics, and may appear at birth or later in life. Secondary lymphoedema results from damage to lymphatics. Common causes of secondary lymphoedema are shown in Box 11.1.

Pathophysiology

The lymphatic system consists of lymph vessels, lymph nodes, the spleen, the thymus, the tonsils and Peyer's patches in the gut. In addition to its role of transporting lymph fluid, it has a major role in the functioning of the immune system. Within the capillary bed of the skin are lymphatic capillaries (Figure 11.1) that connect to vertical precollectors. These drain into a common lymphatic collector that merges into a single lymph vessel (Kubik and Kretz, 2006).

The lymphatic capillaries have anchoring filaments, and the cells of the lymphatic capillary wall are able to separate creating a lumen through which fluid, protein and macromolecules can flow into the lymphatic capillary. Smooth muscle in the lymphangion contracts once distended, to propel lymph forward though the valves in a peristaltic manner. Normal lymph propulsion is aided by adjacent arterial pulsations, muscle contractions, body movements, respiration and skin distention (Sheffield et al., 2004).

Lymphatic fluid (also known as lymph) primarily consists of water and protein filtrate. Lymph also contains macromolecules which do not cross the semipermeable membrane of capillary walls into the arteriovenous system. These may include lipids, waste products of metabolism, matrix metalloproteases (MMPs), cytokines, polysaccharides and fibronectin, which are transported by the lymphatic system into the venous system. Normal functioning depends on a balance between the load and transport capacity of this system. The load consists of the fluid volume including lymphatic proteins, cells, lipids and hyaluronan (Zuther, 2005), whereas the transport capacity is the maximum quantity of volume that can be functionally transported in a given period of time. The functional reserve is the difference between transport capacity and lymphatic load. The lymphatic system becomes overworked when load exceeds maximum transport capacity, resulting in insufficiency or failure (Lawenda et al., 2009).

Lymphatic failure is best discussed in the context of overall tissue fluid dynamics. The cells sit within an extracellular matrix and are bathed in a constant flow of tissue fluid which nourishes and supports them as well as carry away waste products of metabolism. Approximately 20 L of fluid per day filters out of the capillary bed into the extracellular matrix. The capillary bed reabsorbs 17 L of that fluid with the remaining 3 L being reabsorbed and transported by the lymphatic system as seen in Figure 11.2.

Fluid moves under the influence of the push of hydrostatic pressure, within the capillaries and in the extracellular compartment, and the pull of osmotic force, where fluid moves across a semipermeable membrane from areas of low concentration of dissolved proteins to a region of higher

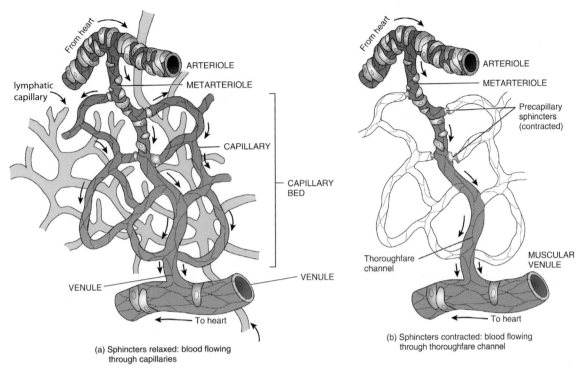

Figure 11.1   Relationship between lymphatics and the capillary bed. Adapted from Tortora and Derrickson (2009). Reproduced with permission from Wiley.

concentration. These are known as Starling Forces. When filtration and reabsorption are in balance, no excess fluid accumulates in the extracellular matrix.

There are three methods by which the lymphatic system may fail:

(1) dynamic insufficiency (high-output insufficiency);
(2) mechanical insufficiency (low-output failure);
(3) a combination of the two.

When the lymphatic system becomes overwhelmed, the tissue spaces become saturated with proteinaceous fluid. This is observed clinically as oedema. If left untreated, the presence of macromolecules, such as growth factors, proteases and proinflammatory molecules, may lead to chronic inflammation and hardening of the skin (MacLaren, 2001; Foldi, 2005; Lawenda et al., 2009). Clinically, this may be seen as acute lipodermatosclerosis or as stasis dermatitis. Additionally, the accumulation of cellular debris blocks the lymphatic vessels and

impedes transportation of macrophages and lymphocytes. Thus, limbs affected by lymphoedema are more prone to infection (Lawenda et al., 2009).

Examples of high-output failure when the normal transport capacity of an intact lymphatic system is overwhelmed by excessive burden of blood capillary filtrate include hepatic cirrhosis (ascites), nephrotic syndrome and chronic venous insufficiency of the leg (Consensus Document of the International Society of Lymphology, 2009). These causes of oedema should be identified and medically managed. Situations in which high-output failure is long-standing, functional deterioration of the lymphatic system is inevitable, and results in a reduction of overall transport capacity and lymphatic failure. Low-output failure may relate to tissue damage through trauma or surgery, external obstruction by obesity or malignant tumours of the lymph vessels or immobility and dependency of the limb. Recurrent infection, thermal burns and repeated allergic reactions are known as 'safety valve insufficiencies' of the lymphatic system, are considered a mixed

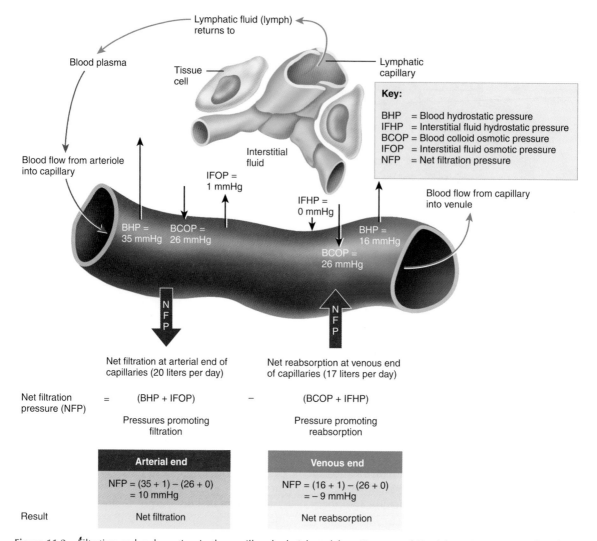

Figure 11.2 Filtration and reabsorption in the capillary bed. Adapted from Tortora and Derrickson (2009). Reproduced with permission from Wiley.

form of oedema/lymphoedema and are particularly difficult to treat (Consensus Document of the International Society of Lymphology, 2009).

Risk factors

The true epidemiology of risk factors for the development and progression of lymphoedema is at the moment uncertain. There may be a considerable delay between the causative event and the onset of lymphoedema which can further complicate the identification of risk factors.

Common risk factors may include

- surgery (interfering with or removing lymph nodes and vessels, e.g. lymph node dissection, breast surgery, varicose vein surgery);
- trauma in 'at-risk' regions, e.g. BP measurement, injections;
- radiotherapy near lymph nodes, e.g. mammary glands, pelvis;
- scar formation, e.g. fibrosis/radiodermatitis;
- recurrent soft tissue infections;
- chemotherapy;
- obesity, poor nutrition;

- congenital predisposition;
- chronic skin disorders and inflammation;
- hypertension;
- lymphatic filariasis (living or visiting endemic area);
- intrapelvic or intra-abdominal tumours;
- thrombophlebitis and chronic venous insufficiency;
- concurrent illnesses, e.g. phlebitis, hyperthyroidism, kidney or cardiac disease;
- cancer, e.g. melanoma, gynaecological cancer, head and neck cancer; immobilisation and prolonged limb dependency.

Simply put, any damage to the system has permanent negative effects on transport capacity of the traumatised region, therefore increasing the risk of lymphoedema in that region.

Psychological impact

Lymphoedema, like all other chronic medical conditions which may cause functional impairment, is often associated with poor self-esteem, altered body image, loneliness, isolation, depression and anxiety (Gethin et al., 2012). Family, social and sexual relationships are impacted. Persons living with lymphoedema may have poor understanding of their disease and cognitive impairment or poor coping strategies which may interfere with adherence to care plans. Living conditions, financial status including availability of benefits to cover aspects of treatment, social support, employment and the effect of the condition on employment all need to be explored.

Psychosocial support is an integral component of any lymphoedema treatment (International Society of Lymphology, 2009). This support enhances concordance, encourages self-management and maximises quality of life. Planning and implementation of psychosocial care strategies are crucial to help patients and their family/caretakers to have a positive impact on their lymphoedema and achieve maximal quality of life. Some general intervention strategies include the provision of information and support, improvement of communication between caretakers and patient, increased patient involvement in care and encouragement of family/caretaker involvement.

Current best practice

National Lymphoedema Frameworks have been developed in nine countries. They are a collaboration of stakeholder groups including academics, health professionals, patients, and industry and community organisations to promote research, best practice guidelines and lymphoedema clinical development worldwide.

Current principles of practice for lymphoedema services as taken from the *Best Practice for the Management of Lymphoedema*, international consensus document (Lymphoedema Framework, 2006) are as follows:

Standard 1: Identification of people at risk of or with lymphoedema
Systems to identify people at risk of or with lymphoedema, regardless of cause, will be implemented and monitored to ensure that patients receive high-quality education and lifelong care.

Standard 2: Empowerment of people at risk of or with lymphoedema
Individual plans of care that foster self-management will be developed in partnership with patients at risk of or with lymphoedema (involving relatives and carers where appropriate), in an agreed format and language.

Standard 3: Provision of lymphoedema services that deliver high-quality clinical care that is subject to continuous improvement and integrates community, hospital- and hospice-based services
All people at risk of or with lymphoedema will have access to trained healthcare professionals, including lymphoedema specialists, who will work to agreed standards for comprehensive ongoing assessment, planning, education, advice, treatment and monitoring. Care will be of a high standard and subject to continuous quality improvement.

Standard 4: Provision of high-quality clinical care for people with cellulitis/erysipelas
Agreed protocols for the rapid and effective treatment of cellulitis/erysipelas, including prevention of recurrent episodes, will be implemented and monitored by healthcare professionals who have completed recognised training in this subject.

Standard 5: Provision of compression garments for people with lymphoedema
Agreed protocols for assessment of and the provision of compression garments for people with

lymphoedema, or where warranted, those at risk of lymphoedema, will be implemented and monitored.

Standard 6: Provision of multiagency health and social care

Following comprehensive assessment, any patient at risk of or with lymphoedema who requires multiagency support will have access to and receive care appropriate to their needs from health and social services.

Prevention strategies: risk factor management

Patients at risk should be identified and monitored for early signs or symptoms of lymphoedema.

Patients should be advised of the following self-care strategies:

Skin

Skin should be protected from trauma and should be kept soft and supple (Rich, 2007). The affected areas should be kept clean, dry and moisturised with hypoallergenic emollients. Nails and cuticles should be properly maintained. Additional signs of possible infection such as rash, itching, increased skin temperature or flu-like symptoms should be monitored and reported (Zuther, 2005).

Lifestyle

Maintaining a healthy weight has been shown to be helpful (Forum, National Obesity, 2004). Exercise is recommended and should be gradually built up in both duration and intensity (Johansson et al., 2005; Bicego et al., 2006). Frequent rest periods should be taken during activity to allow for limb recovery as well as monitoring the affected area during and after activity for changes in size, shape, texture, soreness and similar symptoms (Moseley et al., 2005; Ahmed et al., 2006).

Avoid limb constriction

Patients at risk should wear loose-fitting jewellery and clothing and avoid having blood pressure taken on at-risk extremity.

Compression garments

If no contradictions exist, compression garments should be worn in order to prevent accumulation of oedema in the at-risk limb. They should be well-fitting and supportive, and worn particularly for strenuous activities such as weight-bearing exercise and prolonged standing. Compression bandages are more appropriate for patients with open wounds (Marston and Vowden, 2003).

Avoid extremes of temperature

Extreme cold can be associated with skin chapping and rebound swelling, leading to increased flow of unnecessary fluid to the area. Similarly, prolonged exposure to heat should also be avoided, particularly for periods greater than 15 minutes and temperatures above 39°C should be avoided (Rich, 2007).

Additional practices specific to lower extremity lymphoedema

Individuals at risk for lower extremity lymphoedema should avoid prolonged sitting, standing or crossed legs (National Lymphedema Advisory, 2011). Well-fitted footwear and compression hosiery, if not contraindicated, should be worn, particularly for strenuous activities.

Lymphoedema: assessment considerations

All major diagnostic assessments of lymphoedema should be performed by a healthcare professional experienced in the management of this condition (Table 11.1). General assessment should include a medical assessment to screen for risk factors (and to distinguish from other conditions), laboratory investigations, optional specialised investigations, limb volume assessment, skin condition, pain, psychosocial issues, nutrition and mobility.

Differentiation of lymphoedema from other forms of oedema includes examination of other systemic forms of oedema: cardiac failure, renal failure and other protein-losing conditions as well as local problems such as deep vein thrombosis, chronic venous insufficiency, and cyclical oedema (Warren et al., 2007).

Table 11.1   Investigations to determine causation of lymphoedema

General investigations	
Routine blood tests	Full blood count, renal function tests, liver function tests, thyroid function tests, serum albumin, total protein, erythrocyte sedimentation rate (ESR), C-reactive protein (CRP) and fasting glucose
	A filarial antigen test should also be obtained if patient has lived in or travelled to a filariasis-prone area
Vascular assessment	Ankle brachial pressure index (ABPI)
	Toe brachial pressure index (TBPI) is useful when ABPI measurement is not possible or too painful
Duplex Doppler	Excludes DVT in unilateral lower limb swelling
Specialist investigations	
Genetic testing	Identifies specific types of primary lymphoedema originating from hereditary syndromes
Isotope lymphography	Nuclear isotopes are injected to visualise the lymphatic network to detect abnormalities of the lymphatic system
CT/MRI scans	May help to detect the typical honeycomb pattern produced by lymphoedema to differentiate it from lipoedema; also useful if an obstructing tumour is suspected

Table 11.2 indicates how lymphoedema should be distinguished from lipoedema which is a subcutaneous accumulation of fat. These differences can be difficult to distinguish in clinical practice. Figure 11.3 shows a patient with lymphoedema and Figure 11.4 a patient with lipoedema.

Practice point

A thorough history and examination in combination with appropriate investigations is required to assure appropriate diagnosis. To diagnose primary lymphoedema, the causes of secondary lymphoedema must first be ruled out.

Questions focusing on the following areas are helpful during history-taking:

- Ask about age of onset, as this helps differentiate primary from secondary lymphoedema, because early onset is more likely to be due to an inherited condition.
- Ask patients if they have chronic venous insufficiency, thyroid dysfunction, arthritis or hypertension, because it is important to distinguish lymphoedema from other forms of oedema.
- Ask about past surgery and postoperative complications to establish if surgery was for cancer and if any lymph nodes were removed, as secondary lymphoedema usually results from an event such as radiotherapy or surgery.

Table 11.2   Comparison of lymphoedema and lipoedema

	Lymphoedema	Lipoedema
Location	May involve limbs and trunk	Commonly lower limb only
Gender	Both	Predominantly female
Stemmer's sign	Positive	Usually negative
Foot/hand involvement	Yes	Stops at ankle or wrist
Pain	Possible	Prominent feature especially to touch
Cause	Disordered lymph transport	Unknown; excessive subcutaneous fat deposition
Oestrogen dependency	No	Yes
Lymphoscintigraphy	Abnormal lymphatics	Normal
MRI	Honeycomb pattern	Fat tissue with absent oedema

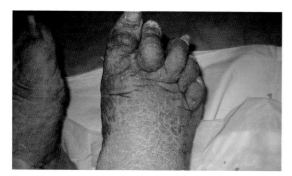

Figure 11.3   Lymphoedema. Photo courtesy of David Keast.

- Ask about any trauma to the legs, abdomen or genital region, as scarring may have damaged the lymphatic system.
- Ask about residence in or visits to Third World countries due to the risk of filariasis.
- Ask about speed of onset of swelling, as rapid onset may indicate tumour infiltration or blockage of a major lymphatic pathway.

Lymphoedema is often mistaken for acute deep vein thrombosis, post-thrombotic syndrome, congestive heart failure or chronic venous insufficiency, which delays treatment and impacts on outcome.

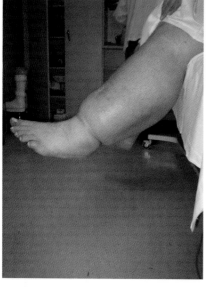

Figure 11.4   Lipoedema. Photo courtesy of David Keast.

Clinically, lymphoedema is defined as chronic oedema which:

- has been present for more than 3 months;
- is minimally responsive to leg elevation or diuretics;
- and has the presence of one or more secondary skin changes such as a positive Stemmer's sign, elephantiasis, skin folds, hyperkeratosis or papillomatosis.

Moffatt et al. (2003)

Limb volume assessment

The extent of swelling, duration, location and the presence or absence of lymphadenopathy should be documented. Limb volume is used to determine the severity of the lymphoedema and to prescribe appropriate management and treatment (Lymphoedema Framework, 2006). Swelling can be either unilateral or bilateral. In unilateral swelling, both limbs are measured and the difference in volume between the affected and unaffected limb is measured in millilitres or as a percentage (Lymphoedema Framework, 2006). The gold standard for calculating limb volume is using water displacement, also known as plethysmography, but it is only reliable for the hands and feet. Circumferential measurements are more commonly used, since they are a simple, easily accessible method, and are reliable if a standard protocol is in place (Lymphoedema Framework, 2006). The limb is marked off in standardised 4 cm intervals and the circumference measured. Volume is calculated using the formula volume $=$ circumference$^2/\pi$. Additional problems with the measurement of limb volume occur in cases with severe thickening of the tissues, such as hyperkeratosis or elephantiasis. The proportion of volumetric change will be due to multiple factors including excess fluid. In unilateral swelling, if excess limb volume is >20%, intensive therapy is indicated. If excess limb volume is <20%, maintenance therapy may be considered. In cases of lymphoedema of the neck, breast, trunk or genitalia, digital photography is recommended as a subjective record to monitor oedema.

Assessment of skin condition

Skin should be examined for dryness, fragility, dark-brown pigmentation, abnormal temperature

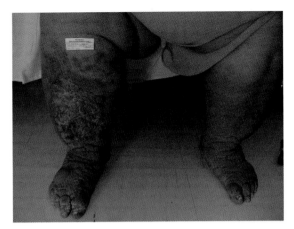

Figure 11.5 Stage III lymphoedema showing skin folds and hyperkeratosis. Photo courtesy of David Keast.

and general dermatitis. Skin changes, such as hyperkeratosis (scaling), skin folds (Figure 11.5), lymphangiectasia (the dilation of lymph vessels that may appear as blister-like protuberances on the skin), lymphorrhoea (lymph leakage on the skin surface) which predisposes patients to cellulitis, papillomatosis (warty growths consisting of dilated lymphatics and fibrous tissue) that look like cobblestones (Figure 11.6) and lipodermatosclerosis (thickening and hardening of the subcutaneous tissues with brown discolouration of the skin) should be carefully documented. Finally, note any wounds on the skin which may be hidden in skin folds and hard to detect, as this also predisposes patients to cellulitis.

Practice point

Lymphoedema commonly affects the extremities, with clinical signs occurring in the skin and subcutis. Limbs

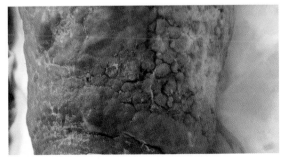

Figure 11.6 Stage III lymphoedema showing papillomatosis. Photo courtesy of David Keast.

can be easily checked for Stemmer's sign, which is the inability to pinch up a fold of tissue at the base of the second digit of the hand or foot. A positive Stemmer's sign is indicative of the presence of lymphoedema and may be detected before any more permanent skin changes have occurred (Mortimer, 2000). Since the skin and subcutaneous tissues are affected the most by lymphoedema, regular monitoring using the Stemmer's sign is a quick way of evaluating treatment efficacy.

Pain assessment

Pain should be assessed at every visit. Unmanaged pain may interfere with adherence to planned care. There are many different causes of pain in patients with lymphoedema, including inflammation, infection, tissue distention/distortion, nerve entrapment or neuropathy, as well as degenerative joint disease. Effective pain management requires assessment of cause, nature, frequency, timing, site, severity and impact of the pain on activities of daily living.

Nutrition (obesity assessment)

Although the role of diet in lymphoedema is not a critically established factor, obesity is, particularly after breast cancer treatment (Lymphoedema Framework, 2006). The frequency of coexistence of obesity and lymphoedema indicates that it could be a contributing factor, perhaps via the reduction of mobility (Ryan, 2002). Guidelines recommend that body mass index (BMI) be less than 25, and that patients with BMI of 30 or greater should be offered additional dietary guidance (Ryan, 2002; Forum, National Obesity, 2004). The reduction of caloric intake in combination with a supervised exercise programme has been found to be particularly valuable in reducing limb bulk of obese patients suffering from lymphoedema (International Society of Lymphology, 2009).

Functional assessment

Observing the mobility and functionality of a patient is crucial to developing an appropriate plan for lymphoedema management as well as determining the need to seek additional guidance. Assessment of particularly challenging areas (head,

Table 11.3   Staging of lymphoedema

ISL STAGE 0	Sub-clinical stage where swelling is not evident despite lymphatic damage
	May exist for months before swelling becomes evident
	No swelling visible or palpable
	Skin has normal appearance
ISL STAGE I: Mild lymphoedema	Early onset due to an accumulation of tissue fluid that subsides with limb elevation
	Oedema present (normally pitting) but no fibrosis
	Swelling reduces overnight after bed rest
	Skin has normal appearance
ISL STAGE II: Moderate lymphoedema	Accumulation of protein-rich fluid and oedema
	Pitting becomes progressively worse and fibrosis is present.
	Elevation overnight in bed rarely reduces swelling
	Early skin changes
ISL LATE STAGE II: Moderate to severe lymphoedema	Pitting oedema may be present but tissue fibrosis more pronounced and limb/affected body part becomes misshapen/skin folds may develop and are generally larger and heavier
	Skin changes evident (hyperpigmentation), may develop skin folds
ISL STAGE III: Complex lymphoedema	Tissues are hard and fibrotic and pitting is absent
	Fibrosis/sclerosis can be extensive
	Gross skin changes evident: hyperkeratosis, papillomas, lymphorrhoea

Source: Adapted from *Best Practice Framework Document*, Lymphoedema Framework Project (2006).

neck, trunk, genitalia), however, should be undertaken by a specialist. Developing treatment plans to increase general function, to improve range of motion of joints or to improve mobility should be addressed in consultation with appropriate therapy providers such as physiotherapists and occupational therapists.

Staging lymphoedema

Several staging systems exist for lymphoedema but currently no international consensus exists. The most commonly used staging system is that proposed by the International Society of Lymphology (2009) which is shown in Table 11.3.

Treatment strategies

The most common and widely accepted method of treatment is complete decongestive therapy, also known as combined, complex or comprehensive decongestive therapy (CDT). Widely known as the 'gold standard' of treatment for lymphoedema (Lasinski, 2002; Thomas et al., 2007; International Society of Lymphology, 2009; Mayrovitz, 2009), this treatment consists of two phases. In the initial *reductive or intensive phase*, the main goals are volume reduction of the affected area and skin improvement. The second phase is called the *maintenance phase* and is an ongoing self-management phase to make sure the gains of phase I are maintained in long term (Johnstone et al., 2006). The effects and intents of this treatment are to decrease swelling, increase lymph drainage from the congested areas, reduce skin fibrosis and improve skin condition. All of these improvements thus result in an enhanced functional status of the patient, relief of discomfort and improved quality of life, as well as reduced risk of cellulites. A third but distinct phase of treatment, *Palliative*, should be also considered. This phase applies to those with lymphoedema at the end of life or to those for whom patient or system factors may interfere with standard treatment.

Transition management

Transition management is required for a 1–3-month period post-intensive therapy, before progressing into long-term management. The transition period is required to both maximise the oedema-reducing effects of the intensive therapy via stabilisation of the fluctuations in swelling such as rebound swelling related to the transfer from compression bandages to hosiery (Lymphoedema Framework, 2006). It is also a period during which long-term maintenance strategies are evaluated and education on self-management is encouraged.

The choice of treatment during this time is individual to the patient. It may or may not include compression garments or bandages, manual lymphatic drainage (MLD) or intermittent pneumatic compression (IPC). Transition management programmes should be put in place by a specialist practitioner and consequently shared with community staff.

Since one of the main aspects of success in long-term care of lymphoedema is self-management (Johnstone et al., 2006), promoting the active engagement of patients in their self-care plans is a primary goal of the transition phase. A period of transition management for upper and lower limb lymphoedema is usually recommended for individuals for whom there is difficulty maintaining limb shape and managing skin condition as well as rebound swelling. For these individuals, the transition phase requires weekly reassessment until stability in swelling and shape is achieved. Occasionally, patients may require the transition phase as a 'reality check' that they are not yet ready for long-term management and require further intensive therapy.

Long-term management

Long-term management is the goal of all treatments for lymphoedema. Its purpose is to enhance the function of the lymphatic system, limiting further deterioration of lymphatics and swelling as well as gaining long-term control. Lymphoedema is a chronic condition for which there is no cure, but consistent and appropriate management can minimise subsequent side effects of this condition. Like the transition phase, long-term management requires commitment to daily skin care, exercise/

movement, compression, limb elevation and self-monitoring. Compression garments are most commonly involved, but there are exceptional cases which require long-term use of compression bandaging. Certain cases of lower limb lymphoedema may be deemed unsuitable for compression hosiery for a number of reasons. Severe arterial disease, swellings uncontainable by compression hosiery, fragile skin or skin ulceration, inability to apply or tolerate hosiery as well as psychosocial issues or palliative needs are all indications for long-term use of compression bandaging. In these cases, a washable and reusable system which can be applied by patients or informal caregivers should be considered.

Manual lymphatic drainage

MLD is a specialised light massage technique that stimulates superficial lymphatic vessels to remove excess interstitial fluid (Williams et al., 2002; Pilch et al., 2009). It is a manual, light skin technique learned by lymphoedema therapists designed to improve fluid removal from congested areas and into lymph vessels and lymph nodes that are functioning. Patients and caregivers can also be taught a form of MLD often called simple lymphatic drainage (SLD).

Exercise

Appropriate exercise enables the patient to resume activity while minimising the risk of exacerbation of swelling. Compression garments or bandages must be worn during exercise (except aqua therapy) to counterbalance the build-up of interstitial fluid (National Lymphoma Network, 2011). Generally, exercise improves muscular strength, cardiovascular function, psychological well-being and functional capacity. Gentle resistance exercise stimulates the muscle pump and increases lymph flow. Aerobic exercise increases intra-abdominal pressure which facilitates pumping of the thoracic duct (Miller, 1998; Cohen et al., 2001)

Managing the skin in lymphoedema

Lymphoedema patients are susceptible to a number of skin problems. Deep folds of the skin that result from extensive swelling are a regular environment for bacterial and fungal infections. Chronic inflammation of the skin tissues causes the deposition of fibrin and collagen, resulting in skin thickening and firming (National Lymphoma Network, 2011). The increase in skin thickening also results in decreased lymph flow. Skin should be cared for to improve and preserve the barrier function via washing with natural and pH-neutral soaps (see Chapter 2). Patients should ensure that skin folds are clean and dry. Emollients may be used to reestablish the skin's protective lipid layer. Skin also needs to be monitored for cuts, insect bites or similar abrasions that might be susceptible to infection or affected by sensory neuropathy. Patients should be taught good skin hygiene because if skin changes are left untreated they can escalate in severity (Lawenda et al., 2009).

Approaches to special skin problems in lymphoedema are described below:

- Skin sacs and lobes

    After successful management of extreme lymphoedema, the remaining empty sacs of skin may hinder continued therapy. A lobe is an excess quantity of tissue (similar to a skin sac) that remains when successful therapy has reduced the volume of an oedematous area. Both of these may be corrected surgically in order to avoid unnecessary skin infections (National Lymphedema Network, 2011).
- Fibrosclerotic areas

    Fibrosclerotic tissue describes an affected area of skin in which inflammatory proteins of the lymph, including fibrin, have built up and caused the tissues of the skin to harden. Fibrosclerotic areas will remodel over time with appropriate compression therapy.
- Fistulas

    Lymphatic fistulas may occur when the lymphatic system is damaged, during radiation therapy or as a complication of surgery. Fistulas may also appear on the skin. Anastomotic breakdown following surgical procedures, cancer and radiotherapy are frequently reported causes (Cheville and Gergich, 2004). Fistulas are potential indications for surgical intervention. Conservative fistula management is best done by experienced practitioners such as enterostomal therapists.

Management of infection

Lymph stasis-related infections such as cellulitis/lymphangitis or erysipelas are characterised by pain, high fever and even possibly septic shock. Skin infections are primarily caused by Group A β-haemolytic Streptococcus bacteria and less commonly, Staphylococcus bacteria. Cellulitis describes the inflammation and infection of connective tissue between neighbouring tissues and organs, commonly resulting from bacterial infection, and can be located in the toes, dorsum and plantar surfaces of the feet and lower leg and is generally reddish in appearance (Kelechi, 2007). Lymphangitis refers to an infection of the lymph vessels. Infections that travel to the lymphatic system indicate worsening of a skin infection and also put the patient at risk of sepsis, which is life-threatening. Lymphangitis must be distinguished from superficial thrombophlebitis which is an inflamed superficial vein as a result of a blood clot (Dugdale, 2011).

Erysipelas refers to infections of the superficial epidermis, resulting in visible swelling. An erysipelas skin lesion has a raised border and is sharply demarcated from normal skin. Affected skin is painful, oedematous and indurated. Many clinicians use the terms erysipelas and cellulitis interchangeably, and since the treatment is essentially the same, the difference is primarily of academic interest. Figure 11.7 summarises the management of cellulitis in patient with lymphoedema.

Amoxicillin or amoxicillin/clavulinic acid is usually the first-line treatment for acute therapy. Clindamycin is a second-line agent and for those allergic to penicillin. Prophylaxis is recommended for people with two or more episodes per year. Low-dose erythromycin or clindamycin may be used for prophylaxis (Le Frock et al., 2004). However, local protocols should determine which antibiotics may be prescribed. For further guidance refer to the *Best Practice for the Management of Lymphoedema* (Lymphoedema Framework, 2006).

Fungal infections are common in oedematous weeping limbs especially between the toes. These infections may also provide a portal of entry for bacteria and increase the risk of cellulites. Treatment should be aimed at prevention through meticulous skin hygiene and management of oedema and drainage.

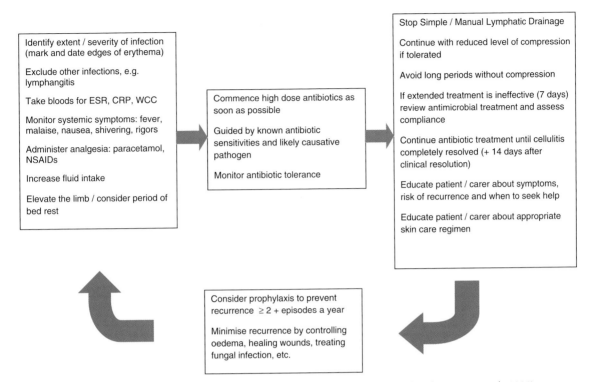

Figure 11.7   Management of cellulitis in patients with lymphodema (CREST, 2005; Lymphoedema Framework, 2006).

Practice point

Topical antifungals such as 1% terbinafine cream may be used but may not be sufficiently penetrating to rid thickened or keratinous tissues of the infection. If there is no response to 6 weeks of treatment including meticulous skin care, referral should be made to a dermatologist for treatment with an oral antifungal. Bacteria can also cause infection in areas in which the skin has been severely compromised, and a topical antibiotic may be used in conjunction with the antifungal treatment as the skin is intact (Kelechi, 2007).

Compression therapy

Compression is the most common and useful treatment of lymphoedema. It works to restore limb shape to the affected area, reduces skin changes, provides support to overstretched skin, eliminates lymphorrhoea and softens subcutaneous tissues (Lymphoedema Framework, 2006). It can be provided by means of bandaging, both elastic and inelastic, as well as compression hosiery. The type of compression provided is indicated based on the patient's needs. Intensive therapy required for individuals with severe oedema and significant skin disorders require inelastic bandaging initially but may eventually transition into compression hosiery for long-term care.

The contraindications for compression are

- severe arterial insufficiency (ankle brachial pressure index <0.5);
- uncontrolled heart failure;
- severe peripheral neuropathy.

Patients with cellulitis or erysipelas can tolerate compression therapy with bandages, but at reduced pressure depending on individual tolerance. Compression garments can be used once the patient is in the maintenance stage of therapy. Compression garments may be contradicted in arterial insufficiency, acute cardiac failure, peripheral neuropathy, extreme shape distortion, very deep skin folds, lymphorrhoea or similar weeping skin conditions and extensive ulceration. Those cases require compression bandaging for treatment.

Multilayer lymphoedema bandaging

Compression bandaging refers to specific technique using multilayer components. The components may include a bandage lining (tubular), digit bandages, under-bandage padding (polyester, cotton or foam), multiple layers of either non-stretch or short-stretch bandages. With inelastic bandages resting pressure is low but with activity the sub-bandage pressure increases. High working pressures assist in creating a pump-like action via the differential pressures, as skeletal muscles alternately relax and contract. As oedema is reduced, the secondary changes begin to resolve. Certain areas, such as head and neck, are not amenable to high-compression bandaging. Low-compression garments or bandages may be employed by trained therapists but these patients commonly require alternative treatments. In all other cases, bandages are better options for treatment of lymphoedema, particularly for persons with grossly misshapen limbs or areas unsuitable for compression garments. Trunk and genital bandaging are best done by specialist lymphoedema therapists.

Bandaging techniques

Bandaging of limbs and digits should be performed by a trained healthcare practitioner. When wrapped properly, the applied pressures to the limbs produce a massaging effect that stimulates lymph flow. There are multiple techniques for applying compression bandages. For an illustrated description of bandaging, the *Best Practice for the Management of Lymphoedema* document is recommended (Lymphoedema Framework, 2006).

Intermittent pneumatic compression

IPC uses pump garments with multiple chambers and sequential pressure delivery determined individually for the patient's diagnosis and pattern of lymphoedema (Pilch et al., 2009). IPC is not used as a solitary treatment for lymphoedema and patients should maintain oedema control with a compression garment or bandaging between treatments (International Society of Lymphology, 2009; Pilch et al., 2009). In addition to the usual contraindications for compression, contraindications to IPC include the following: untreated non-pitting chronic lymphoedema, pulmonary embolism, thrombophlebitis, acute skin inflammation, pulmonary oedema, active metastatic disease, oedema at the root of the affected limb or truncal oedema. There is no international consensus on the use of IPC and it should be used only by specialist practitioners.

Compression stockings/garments

Compression garments may be used for the initial treatment of lymphoedema and for the maintenance phase of treatment for higher stages. In order to use compression garments successfully, one must have good dexterity, intact resilient skin, no or minimal shape distortion and no or minimal pitting oedema. The ability to tolerate and manage hosiery as well as the ability to monitor skin condition and engage in prevention strategies is also important. The use of compression garments by the patient requires more consideration and research than limb bandaging, due to the fixed nature of the garment. Limb shape is an important factor while choosing a garment. Ready-to-wear manufactured garments are easily suited for individuals with minimal or no shape distortion, but can be more difficult to fit precisely. Custom-made garments are better as they do not roll, curl or twist, providing a better fit, and can be made with additional aids for ease of application, such as zippers. Compression garments should be fitted by appropriately trained practitioners and their prescription requires a comprehensive assessment of patient condition.

Other therapies

Elevation of a lymphoedematous limb often reduces swelling, particularly in Stage I or early Stage II lymphoedema. If elevation successfully reduces swelling, the effect should be maintained by wearing a low-stretch elastic stocking or sleeve when the limb is not elevated (International Society of Lymphology, 2009). Breathing exercises are recommended to help clear the central lymphatics prior to interventions that promote lymph drainage from the periphery. A recent clinical study demonstrated that a combination of exercise and deep-breathing significantly reduced the volume of the lymphoedematous limb (Lymphoedema Framework, 2006). Breathing exercises are not harmful, are inexpensive and may be beneficial. As with any chronic condition there are a variety of therapies that are reported as being successful for the management of lymphoedema including hyperbaric oxygen, laser therapy, lymphoedema taping, but there is a current lack of substantial evidence to support their use. Further research is required to establish the benefits of these treatments and the optimal regimen.

Surgical intervention

Debulking surgery removes excess subcutaneous tissue associated with the affected area. Risks include poor wound healing, nerve damage or loss, significant scarring, destruction of the remaining lymphatic vessels in affected area, loss of limb function, return of swelling, poor cosmetic results and decrease in quality of life. Compression garments are still necessary and must be worn lifelong due to lymphatic scarring and insufficiency (National Lymphedema Network, 2011). Liposuction is the removal of fatty tissue deposits in the affected area and is similar to but not the same as cosmetic liposuction. Lifelong compression is still required to prevent recurrence. Liposuction is considered only if the limb has not responded to standard conservation therapy but is not indicated when pitting oedema is present. Risks include bleeding, infection, skin loss, abnormal sensation (numbness, tingling) and lymphoedema returning (National Lymphedema Network, 2011).

Microsurgical techniques have been developed to move lymph vessels to congested areas and improve lymphatic drainage. This surgery involves connection of lymph vessels and veins, nodes and veins or vessels to vessels. Reductions in limb volume have been observed and preliminary studies have been done (National Lymphedema Network, 2011). Bypass operations aim to restore lymphatic function through lymphovenous anastomoses and lymphatic or venous vessel grafting, and may also involve lymph node transplantation. Anastomosis of lymph vessels to the venous system may be attempted in patients with proximal lymphatic obstruction and patent distal lymphatics and produces better results at earlier stages of lymphostatic disease.

Pharmacological management

There is no evidence that diuretics encourage lymph drainage although theoretically by reducing blood volume, capillary filtration should be reduced together with lymph formation. Diuretics are therefore not consistently recommended (National Lymphedema Network, 2011), and have limited use during the initial treatment phase of CDT and should be reserved for patients with specific co-morbid conditions or complications (International Society of Lymphology, 2009). They may be helpful in cases of effusions in body cavities (ascites, hydrothorax) and with protein-losing enteropathy (International Society of Lymphology, 2009). Patients with peripheral lymphoedema from malignant lymphatic blockage may also benefit from a short course of diuretics.

Benzopyrones are based on a variety of naturally occurring substances such as flavonoids and oxerutins. They are reported to hydrolyse tissue proteins and facilitate absorption and have been used as adjunct therapy in primary and secondary lymphoedema treatment including filariasis. Some data indicate that they may stabilise swelling by reducing microvascular filtration, but high doses have been linked to liver toxicity so they are not meant to be used as an alternative or substitute for CDT (International Society of Lymphology, 2009).

Education and support

Educating patients living with lymphoedema is crucial at every step of the treatment process, but mostly when patients begin home-maintenance programmes, where adherence is crucial to the prevention of reoccurrence (Lawenda et al., 2009). Education should include the importance of skin care, exercise, weight reduction and self-monitoring for complications. Patients may also be trained about use of an inelastic adjustable compression device, SLD or compression garments.

It is known that consistent adherence of patients to their self-care programme has significant correlation with better outcomes (National Lymphodema Network, 2012). At the time of follow-up, patients reporting self-adherence presented with continued loss of swelling versus patients reporting non-adherence showed increasing oedema (Johnstone et al., 2006). Emphasis on and instruction in skin care, SLD, signs and symptoms of infection, proper fit and care of garments as well as possible modification to lifestyle and activity levels to reduce risks are important in the initial stages of diagnosis and treatment (National Lymphedema Advisory, 2011). As the condition continues, use of compression garments and limb elevation, and avoidance of extreme temperatures should also be emphasised (National Lymphoma Network, 2011). Some studies suggest that pretreatment lymphoedema education could be very useful to patients and practitioners as an easy way to improve outcomes, increase adherence and prevent additional trauma (Ridner, 2006). Patient and caregiver education needs to be provided through multifaceted approaches which are consistent with level of education and learning styles. Education needs to be reinforced at every follow-up visit. Regularly scheduled follow-up visits are required to monitor self-management and to ensure compression garments are still effective.

Provision of specialist services

The diagnosis, assessment and treatment of chronic oedema/lymphoedema require an integrated approach involving multiple disciplines. Patients require thorough medical assessment, skilled nursing services and health practitioners skilled at bandaging and MLD. They may require assessment by a dietician and assistance in coping with psychosocial issues from a social worker. Surgical services may be required. Care needs to be coordinated from hospital to clinic to home. Patients should be able to move seamlessly from one area of service to another. Sadly, in much of the world this does not exist, and lymphoedema clinicians have a major role in advocating for integrated care. A practical template to help development of specialist lymphoedema services is available (see Useful Resources section), and can be used by the multidisciplinary team in areas where lymphoedema services are inadequate (Lymphoedema Framework, 2007).

Criteria for specialist referral

International guidelines recommend that advice should be quickly obtained from an appropriate specialist if any of the following circumstances apply (Lymphoedema Framework, 2006; International Society of Lymphology, 2009):

- swelling of unknown origin;
- midline lymphoedema, e.g. head, neck, trunk, breast, genitalia;
- primary lymphoedema;
- sudden increase in pain or swelling of lymphoedematous site;
- severe foot distortion;
- severe papillomatosis or other chronic skin condition;
- recurrent cellulitis/erysipelas;
- failure to respond to standard treatment in 3 months;
- unresolved psychological issues, e.g. depression within 3 months.

Summary

Lymphoedema is a hidden epidemic. It is under-recognised and undertreated worldwide. It is a chronic condition, and is best managed using chronic disease models which focus on self-management, with professional support for assessment, treatment recommendations and monitoring. The cornerstone of treatment is appropriate compression therapy to manage oedema. It requires a partnership between healthcare systems, health professionals, persons living with lymphoedema and their families or caregivers.

Useful resources

Lymphoedema Framework Best Practice for the Management of Lymphoedema International Consensus document (2006). Available at: International Lymphoedema Framework website: http://www.lympho.org

The Management of Lymphoedema in Advanced Cancer and Oedema at the End of Life (2010) Available at: http://www.lympho.org

Lymphoedema Framework (2007) *Template for Management: Developing a Lymphoedema Service*. London: MEP Ltd. Available at: http://www.lympho.org

Aberdeen (2009) *Skills for Practice: Management of Chronic Oedema in the Community. Wounds UK*. Available at: http://www.woundsinternational.com/clinical-guidelines.

Useful websites

British Lymphology Society. Available at: http://www.lymphoedema.org

Lymphoedema Network (Europe).

Lymhovenous Canada. Available at: http://www.lymphovenous-canada.ca

Lymphodema Association of Australia. Available at: http://www.lymphoedema.org.au

Lymphedema Association of Ontario. Available at: http://www.lymphontario.ca

References

Ahmed, R.L., Thomas W, Yee, D. (2006) Randomized controlled trial of weight training and lymphedema in breast cancer survivors. *Journal of Clinical Oncology*, 24(18), 2765–2772.

Bicego, D., Brown B, Ruddick, M, Storey, D., Wong, C., Harris S.R. (2006) Exercise for women with or at risk for breast cancer-related lymphedema. *Physical Therapy*, 86(18), 1398–1405.

Cheville, A., Gergich, N. (2004) Wound care practice. In: *Lymphedema: Implications for Wound Care.* (eds A.P.S. Smith, C.E. Fife, P.J Sheffield), pp. 285–303. Flagstaff, AZ: Best Publishing Company.

Cohen, S.R., Payne, D.K., Tunkel, R.S. (2001) Lymphedema: strategies for management. *Cancer*, 15(92, Suppl 4), 980–987.

Clinical Resource Efficiency Support Team (CREST) (2005) *Guidelines on the Management of Cellulitis in Adults.* Belfast: CREST.

Diagnosis and Treatment of Peripheral Lymphedema. (2009) Consensus document of the International Society of Lymphology. *Lymphology*, 42(2), 51–60.

Dugdale, D.C. (2011) *National Centre for Biotechnology Information, US National Library of Medicine. A.D.A.M. Medical Encyclopedia,* Available at: http://www.ncbi.nlm.nih.gov/pubmedhealth/PMH0004551, retrieved on September 21, 2011.

Foldi, M. (2005) *The Science of Lymphoedema Bandaging.* European Wound Management Association (EWMA). Focus Document: Lymphoedema Bandaging in Practice.

Gethin, G., Byrne, D., Tierney, S., Strapp, H., Cowman, S. (2012) Prevalence of lymphoedema and quality of life among patients attending a hospital-based wound management and vascular clinic. *International Wound Journal*, 9(2), 120–125.

Guidelines on Management of Adult Obesity and Overweight in Primary Care. (2004) Forum, National Obesity. Available at: www.nationalobesityforum.org.uk. Last accessed 18 November 2012.

Lymphoedema Framework (2006) *Best Practice for the Management of Lymphoedema.* International consensus. London: MEP Ltd. Available at: http://www.woundsinternational.com. Last accessed 18 November 2012.

Lymphoedema Framework (2007) *Template for Management: Developing a Lymphoedema Service.* London: MEP Ltd.

Johansson, K., Tibe, K., Weibull, A. (2005) Low intensity resistance exercise for breast cancer patients with arm lymphedema with or without a compression sleeve. *Lymphology*, 4(38), 167–180.

Johnstone, P.A., Hawkins, K., Hood, S. (2006) Role of patient-adherance in the maitenance of results after manipulative therapy for lymphedema. *Journal for the Society of Integrated Oncology*, 4 (3), 125–129.

Kelechi, T. J. (2007) Management of common foot problems. In: *Wound Care: A Collaborative Practice Manual for Health Professionals* (eds C. Sussman, B. Bates-Jensen)., 3rd ed. Baltimore: Lippincott Williams & Wilkins.

Kubik, S., Kretz, O. (2006) Anatomy of the lymphatic system. In: *Foldi's Textbook of Lymphology,* (eds M. Foldi, E. Foldi), pp. 1–50. Munich: Elsevier.

Lasinski, B. (2002) Comprehensive lymphedema management: results of a five-year follow-up. *Lymphology*, 35(Suppl), 301–305.

Lawenda, B.D., Mondry, T.E., Johnstone, P.A.S. (2009) Lymphedema: a primer on the identification and management of a chronic condition in oncologic treatment. *CA: A Cancer Journal For Clinicians*, 59(1), 8–24.

Le Frock, J.L., Mader, J.T. (2004) Skin, skin structure, and muscle infections. In: *Wound Care Practice* (eds P.J. Sheffield, A.P.S. Smith, C.E. Fife). Flagstaff, AZ: Best Publishing Company.

MacLaren, J. (2001) Skin changes in lymphoedema: pathophysiology and management options. *International Journal of Palliative Nursing*, 7(8), 381–384.

Marston, W., Vowden, K. (2003) *Understanding Compression Therapy: A Guide to Safe Practice.* London: MEP Ltd.

Mayrovitz, H.N. (2009) The standard care for lymphedema: current concepts and physiological considerations. *Lymphatic Research and Biology*, 7(2), 101–108.

Miller, L.T. (1998) Exercise in the management of breast cancer-related lymphoedema. *Innovations in Breast Cancer Care*, 4(3), 101–106.

Moffatt, P.J., Franks, D.C., Doherty, A.F., et al. (2003) Lymphoedema: an underestimated health problem. *Quarterly Journal of Medicine*, 96, 731–738.

Mortimer, P.S. (2000) Swollen lower limb-2: lymphedema. *BMJ: British Medical Association*, 320(7248), 1527.

Moseley, A.L., Piller, N.B., Carati, C.J. (2005) The effect of gentle arm exercise and deep breathing on secondary arm lymphedema. *Cancer Control*, 38(3), 136–145.

National Lymphoma Network (2011) Position Statement of the National Lymphoma Network: *The Diagnosis and Treatment of Lymphedema.*

National Lymphodema Advisory (2011) Committee, Position Papers. Available at: http://www.lymphnet.org/pdfDocs/nlntreatment.pdf, retrieved on October 20, 2011.

National Lymphodema Network. (2012) Lymphedema risk-reduction practices. s.l. Available at: http://www.lymphnet.org/pdfDocs/nlnriskreduction.pdf. Last accessed 18 November 2012.

Pilch, U., Wozniewski, M., Szuba, A. (2009) Influence of compression cycle time and the number of sleeve chambers on upper extremity lymphedema volume reduction during intermittent pneumatic compression. *Lymphology*, 42(1), 26–35.

Rich, A. (2007) How to care for uncomplicated skin and keep it free of complications. *British Journal of Community Nursing*, 12(4), S6–S9.

Ridner, S.H. (2009) The psycho-social impact of lymphedema. *Lymphatic Research and Biology*, 7(2), 109–112.

Ridner, S.H. (2006) Pretreatment lymphedema education and identified education resources in breast cancer patients. *Patient Education and Counseling*, 61(1), 72–79.

Ryan, T.J. (2002) Risk factors for the swollen ankle and their management at low cost: not forgetting lymphedema. *International Journal of Lower Extremity Wounds*, 1(3), 202–208.

Sheffield, P.J., Smith, A.P.S., Fife, C.E. (2004) *Wound Care Practice*. Flagstaff, AZ: Best Publishing Company.

Tortora, G.J., Derrickson, B.H. (2009) *Essentials of Anatomy and Physiology*, 8th edn. John Wiley & Son.

Thomas, R.C., Hawkins, K., Kirkpatrick, S.H., Mondry, T.E., Gabram-Mendola, S., Johnstone, P.A. (2007) Reduction of lymphedema using complete decongestive therapy: roles of prior radiation therapy and extent of axillary dissection. *Journal of the Society for Integrative Oncology*, 3(5), 87–91.

Warren, A.G., Brorson, H., Borud, L.J., Slavin, S.A. (2007) Lymphedema: a comprehensive review. *Annals of Plastic Surgery*, 59(4), 464–472.

Williams, A.F., Vadgama, A., Franks, P.J., Mortimer, P.S. (2002) A randomized controlled crossover study of manual lymphatic drainage therapy in women with breast cancer related lymphoedema. *European Journal of Cancer Care*, 11(4), 254–261.

Zuther, J.E. (2005) *Lymphedema Management: The Comprehensive Guide for Practitioners*. New York: Thieme Medical Publishers.

12 Malignant Wounds

Wayne Naylor
Palliative Care Council of New Zealand, Wellington, New Zealand

---

Overview

- Limited information exists about prevalence and incidence of malignant wounds, but they develop in approximately 5% of people with cancer.
- Malignant wounds are difficult to treat as they are an active malignancy that can only be healed if the tumour responds to anticancer treatment.
- The aim of malignant wound management is symptom control and maintenance or improvement of quality of life.
- Palliative anticancer therapies should always be explored in the management of malignant wounds. Alongside wound management strategies, people with malignant wounds also require psychological and social support to cope with the impact of the wound and related cancer diagnosis.
- Malignant wounds require a holistic approach provided by a multidisciplinary team.

Introduction

Malignant wounds may also be called fungating wounds or malignant cutaneous wounds. The term 'malignant' refers to the underlying malignant cancer that gives rise to the wound, while 'fungating' generally describes the proliferative growth pattern seen in many malignant wounds, which results in a fungal or cauliflower like appearance of wound tissues.

Malignant wounds occur more frequently in older adults and usually develop in the last 6 months of life (Ivetić and Lyne, 1990; Haisfield-Wolfe and Rund, 1997); they are rare in children.

While a malignant wound may arise anywhere on the body, the most frequent site is the female breast, with other common sites being the neck, head, chest, extremities and genitals (Thomas, 1992; Wilkes et al., 2001; Maida et al., 2009; Probst et al., 2009). Female breast cancer is the most common cause of a malignant wound, but most solid tumours and some haematological malignancies can give rise to a malignant wounds; for example, cancers of the head and neck, kidney, lung, ovary, colon, penis, bladder and lymphomas.

A small number of people with malignant wounds will achieve wound healing with cancer therapy, such as radiotherapy, chemotherapy or

---

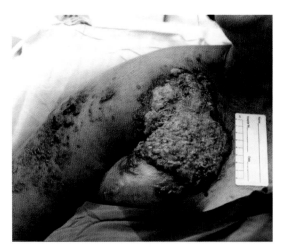

Figure 12.1   Fungating breast cancer wound with extensive spread. Photo courtesy of Wayne Naylor.

surgery. In most cases, however, the wound continues to deteriorate, and treatment is therefore aimed at symptom control and maintaining or improving quality of life.

Malignant wounds: aetiology

Malignant wounds are a complication of cancer and their development can be directly attributed to the activity of a malignant tumour. Thus, a malignant wound may develop from:

- invasion of the skin by an underlying locally advanced primary or recurrent cancer (Figure 12.1);

- a primary skin cancer (in particular, an untreated or recurrent squamous cell carcinoma or malignant melanoma);
- metastatic spread from a distant tumour (Figure 12.1);
- implantation or 'seeding' during surgery;
- malignant transformation in a long-standing chronic wound (usually an aggressive squamous cell carcinoma) (Malheiro et al. 2001).

In general, a malignant wound indicates a poor prognosis, with most patients dying within 6 months of developing cutaneous metastases (Saeed et al., 2004; Fyrmpas et al., 2006; Wu et al., 2006).

Early skin infiltration often presents as discrete, non-tender skin nodules, which enlarge as the underlying tumour grows, until they reach a size where skin capillaries and lymph vessels are disrupted (Pearson and Mortimer, 2004). This impairs skin perfusion causing tissue hypoxia and necrosis. Abnormal clotting and disorganised microcirculation within the tumour further compromise tissue viability. The tumour may also invade and destroy deeper structures, which can result in fistula formation within the wound.

The resulting wound may be a shallow or deep crater-like ulcer, or it may present as a raised nodular lesion. In many cases there is a combination of proliferative growth and central necrosis. The wound shown in Figure 12.2a is a good example of this combined presentation, with proliferative growth around the edges and deep necrotic ulceration in the centre. The accompanying CT scan of this wound (Figure 12.2b) clearly shows both

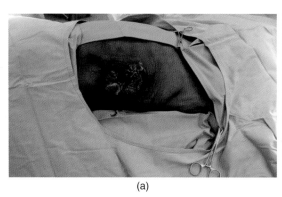

(a)

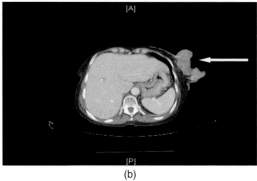

(b)

Figure 12.2   (a) Malignant wound caused by breast cancer that demonstrates proliferative growth at the margins with central necrosis and ulceration. (b) A CT scan of the patient in (a) clearly illustrating the elevated edges of the wound (proliferative growth), the central necrotic area (arrow) and the enhancing area of breast tumour. (Copyright © 2010, Dr Abbas A.R. Mohamed, reproduced with permission.)

these aspects of the wound. It also illustrates how the 'wound' is entirely formed of tumour (enhancing area). This is why malignant wounds are so difficult to treat; they are in fact an active malignancy that can only be healed if the tumour responds to anticancer treatment.

The occurrence of malignant wounds is not recorded in cancer registries, and only a few studies have attempted to determine the frequency with which they occur. From current literature (Haisfield-Wolfe and Rund, 1997; Maida et al., 2008; Alexander, 2009; Probst et al., 2009) it appears that

- around 5% of people with cancer develop malignant wounds;
- the incidence is higher (10–14%) in those with metastatic cancer;
- 2–13% of people who present with a malignant wound may never have had cancer diagnosed;
- the incidence of malignant wounds may be higher in developing countries where awareness of cancer and access to treatment is limited (Mohamed et al., 2010).

In 2008, there were an estimated 12.7 million new cancer cases worldwide, with over 60% in developing countries (Jemal et al., 2011). Based on an estimated 5% prevalence rate, this could mean that globally there were 635,000 people living with a malignant wound.

Psychological impact

Malignant wounds can have a profound impact on the patient, their family and healthcare professionals. These wounds are an outward and very obvious sign of advanced and life-limiting cancer, which itself is an extremely difficult diagnosis to deal with. Although there is relatively little research on the impact of malignant wounds, the evidence that is available points to a significant psychological and social burden associated with these complex wounds (Lund-Nielsen et al., 2005; Lazelle-Ali, 2007; Alexander, 2010; Dolbeult et al., 2010).

Common psychological issues are usually related to the symptoms and appearance of the wound and the underlying diagnosis, and can include

- body image alteration;
- denial;
- depression;
- embarrassment;
- fear;
- guilt;
- lack of self-respect/self-esteem;
- problems with sexual expression;
- revulsion/disgust;
- shame.

Social factors may also influence wound-related symptoms and problems, but can also arise due to issues of access to treatment, financial pressures and the need for complex and time-consuming personal care. These issues may include social isolation, lack of support and resources, communication difficulties and restrictions due to dressing changes. It is important that these concerns are considered as part of a holistic management plan.

Malignant wounds often have an offensive odour and heavy exudate. Uncontrolled wound malodour can have a devastating effect on the patient, and is particularly difficult for the family and/or caregivers to cope with, including healthcare professionals (Probst et al., 2009; Alexander, 2010). Patients may feel embarrassed or disgusted by the smell, and the social stigma, and the guilt and shame associated with a malodorous wound may lead to depression, social isolation and relationship problems (Lund-Nielsen et al., 2005; Lo et al., 2008; Piggin and Jones, 2009; Dolbeult et al., 2010). Exudate leakage from wound dressings and saturated or stained clothing and bedding is a common problem, which often results in embarrassment, depression and social isolation (Davis, 1995; Lund-Nielsen et al., 2005). The appearance and location of a malignant wound can have a profound effect on body image; for example, an exuding, malodorous breast wound will deeply affect femininity, causing women to avoid physical closeness and sexual activity (Lund-Nielsen et al., 2005). The subsequent effects on self-esteem and sexual expression can lead to significant relationship problems (Haisfield-Wolfe and Rund, 1997; Grocott, 1999; Young, 2005).

Therefore, formal or informal counselling will be helpful, along with spiritual care according to the patient's beliefs. The patient and their family should have appropriate social support, as this will decrease stress and anxiety. A great deal of this supportive care can be provided by a specialist palliative care service, so their involvement should be encouraged if available and the patient agrees.

Principles of palliative wound management

The word palliate means to 'make less severe without removing the cause' (Oxford University Press, 2011), or in the case of palliative care, to give temporary relief from the symptoms of a disease but not aiming to cure the disease. This approach seems incongruous in relation to wound management, as the aim of care is usually to heal the wound. However, for most malignant wounds healing is very difficult or impossible to achieve. In these instances, the principles of a palliative approach can prove useful (McDonald and Lesage, 2006; Alvarez et al., 2007).

The principles of palliative wound management aim to

- prevent and relieve suffering through early identification, assessment and treatment of pain and associated problems;
- ensure a 'whole-of-patient' approach to address physical, psychological, social and spiritual needs;
- facilitate the identification of patient's and family's wishes;
- ensure a collaborative multidisciplinary approach.

(World Health Organization, 2002)

There are particular patient characteristics that can indicate a palliative approach is more appropriate, these include

- an underlying disease process that cannot be corrected;
- the disease is in its end stages;
- healing of the wound is not a priority of care;
- treatment demands on the patient are too great;
- the patient is in the end-of-life phase (e.g. hours or days to live).

These features mean that the patient has little or no healing potential. For these people, wound management should be guided by realistic and achievable goals of care, and the simplest management strategy that achieves these goals should be used. This may mean that basic dressing products are used, but it does not mean that patient care should be compromised; a palliative approach is *not* an excuse for poor wound care.

Malignant wounds: assessment considerations

Because the effects of a malignant wound extend beyond the actual wound itself, a holistic approach to patient assessment is essential. This should include gathering information on the patient's psychological response to their wound and the effect of the wound on their family and social life.

The symptoms related to malignant wounds are not unique, but tend to be extreme and occur in combination, making management much more challenging (see example in Figure 12.3). The most frequently reported wound-related symptoms in

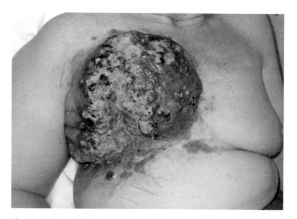

Figure 12.3   A large malignant wound caused by an untreated breast cancer. Photo courtesy of Wayne Naylor.

people with malignant wounds are malodour, heavy exudate, pain, bleeding and skin irritation (Maida et al., 2009). Understanding the causes of these symptoms is important, as this underpins the management strategies and also helps anticipate the potential needs of the patient.

The extensive necrosis gave rise to extreme malodour along with heavy exudate, pain and skin irritation. New tumour nodules can be seen arising in the skin around the wound.

It is important to remember that the main goal of treatment is to improve the patient's quality of life, so assessment must involve ascertaining the patient's own concerns and priorities. These, combined with the clinical concerns of healthcare professionals, should form the basis of a patient-focused management plan. In these circumstances, the wound management plan will need to be dynamic to respond to changes in skin integrity, wound status and the patient's wishes. Frequent reassessment of the wound is vital, as changes in wound appearance over time are an important indicator of cancer treatment response.

The essential parameters to include when assessing a malignant wound are listed in Table 12.1.

Table 12.1   Wound assessment parameters and rationale for malignant wounds

Assessment parameter	Rationale in malignant wounds
Duration	• Wound development in relation to cancer diagnosis • May highlight psychological and social issues
Previous treatments	• Information on what dressing products have and have not worked in the past • Include cancer treatments, as this will inform treatment approach
Location	• Assess potential for complications such as blood vessel erosion • Inform method of dressing fixation and need for consideration of cosmetic appearance • May indicate potential for psychological/social problems if in a sensitive/private area of the body
Size, depth and shape	• Selection of appropriate size and shape dressing(s) to fit irregular-shaped wound • Monitor improvement or deterioration in response to cancer treatment
Type of tissue present	• Selection of appropriate type of dressing(s) • Contribution to wound malodour (necrotic tissue) • Monitor response to cancer treatment (note: an increase in necrotic tissue may be due to tumour necrosis)
Amount and nature of exudate	• Selection of appropriate type of dressing(s) • Increasing exudate may be a sign of infection
Presence and level of malodour	• May indicate infection • Will inform type of treatment required for malodour • Monitor effectiveness of treatment for malodour • Can cause distress for patient and family
Episodes of bleeding	• Identify risk for serious bleed • Selection of appropriate dressing/topical treatment for bleeding • Prepare carers in advance
Nature and type of pain	• May indicate infection • Appropriate selection of analgesia for type of pain, including topical • Assessment of effectiveness of analgesia • Pain related to dressing procedures may indicate need for alternative dressing(s)
Signs of wound infection	• Need for topical and/or systemic antibiotic therapy • May be masked in chronic wound or immunosuppressed patients
Condition of surrounding skin	• Development of new tumour nodules • Assess for itching/irritation in skin • Identify excoriation/maceration from exudate • Identify skin stripping from adhesives

Given that people with malignant wounds can suffer from a number of psychological and social problems, it is essential to remember that their care involves the whole person and not just the wound. This will require, first, a comprehensive assessment to establish psychological and social problems, and then a multidisciplinary team approach to address any issues. It will be important to involve the patient and their family in any decisions about care, and open and honest communication will ensure everyone is aware of decisions and goals.

Management of malignant wounds

A significant issue in terms of managing malignant wounds is the relatively small amount of high-quality research-based evidence that is available to guide practice (Adderley and Smith, 2007; Alexander, 2009). Current practice is therefore based primarily on expert opinion and the translation of evidence from other chronic wounds. There is an urgent need for more clinical research aimed at determining the most effective methods of symptom control for malignant wounds.

Cancer therapy options

As noted earlier, malignant wounds are a direct consequence of cancer eroding through or infiltrating the skin. As such, palliative anticancer therapies should always be explored in the management of malignant wounds. When considering such an intervention, it is important to remember that there must be a positive benefit to the patient, in relation to control of the cancer and wound-related symptoms, but with minimal side effects.

External beam radiotherapy is the most commonly used palliative treatment, and will usually reduce the size of the wound, reduce symptoms of high exudate and bleeding and alleviate pain (Hoskin, 2004). Single agent or low-dose chemotherapy may be effective in relieving symptoms, but the response may be minimal in recurrent or advanced disease. Hormonal manipulation can also be an effective method of symptom control, but only if the primary tumour is hormone sensitive, for example oestrogen-receptor-positive breast cancer (National Cancer Institute, 2011).

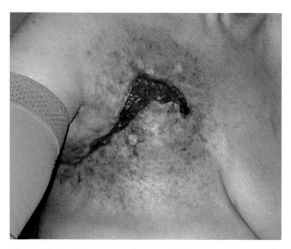

Figure 12.4   The same patient as in Figure 12.3, 8 months after initial presentation, following treatment with intravenous chemotherapy and external beam radiotherapy to the breast. Photo courtesy of Wayne Naylor.

Surgical resection of the wound is also a potential palliative treatment, but one that is possibly underutilised in the management of malignant wounds. There are a number of associated risks that limit the usefulness of this method, such as bleeding and underlying malignant disease. However, in selected cases excision of the wound 'en masse' followed by repair using plastic surgical techniques could potentially be a useful method of symptom control (Offer et al., 2000; Mohamed et al., 2010). This type of palliative surgery can dramatically improve the patient's cosmetic appearance, as well as providing an extended symptom-free period.

Figure 12.4 shows the same patient shown in Figure 12.3 following intravenous chemotherapy and external beam radiation therapy. While the final result of treatment is impressive, this patient died soon after from metastatic breast cancer.

Pain

Wound-related pain may be due to nerve and blood vessel damage by infiltrating tumour, or exposure of dermal nerve endings from superficial ulceration. Patients often complain of superficial stinging or a persistent deeper ache due to painful ulceration (Grocott, 1999). Nerve damage can cause neuropathic pain, which may be characterised by burning pain with intermittent sharp shooting or stabbing pains. Wound care procedures such as debridement, inappropriate cleansing technique or the dressings adhering to the wound bed may also contribute to wound pain.

Pain can never be fully controlled unless treatment is preceded by an accurate and in-depth assessment to identify the location, duration, intensity, quality, onset and impact on activities of daily living (Price et al., 2007). This will enable a proactive approach to preventing wound pain by prescribing and administering suitable analgesia and initiating appropriate wound care practices.

Analgesia should be prescribed following the guidelines for the control of cancer pain proposed by the World Health Organization, and specialist advice is helpful in this regard. These guidelines provide a stepwise and proven approach to pain management in cancer patients (World Health Organization, 1996). In addition, 'as-required' analgesics should be prescribed for use prior to wound care procedures. Appropriate wound care practices include gentle cleansing by irrigation and using non-adherent dressings. Less frequent dressing changes will also help by reducing the need for painful wound care episodes.

There is a growing body of evidence to support the use of topical opioids for pain in chronic wounds, although continuing research is required (LeBon et al., 2009). This approach is based on the presence of opioid receptors on peripheral nerves, which can be activated to block nerve impulses by the application of opioid drugs directly to the wound surface (Back and Finlay, 1995; Stein, 1995; Krajnik et al., 1999; Twillman et al., 1999; Grocott, 2007). This method of opioid administration may offer an alternative treatment for patients whose pain is not responsive to conventional analgesia. Topically applied lignocaine in a carrier gel or paste may also be effective in controlling wound pain (Alvarez et al., 2007).

Practice point

A topical morphine preparation can be made by mixing morphine for injection with a wound hydrogel to a concentration of approximately 0.1% w/w (about 1 mg of morphine to 1 g of hydrogel). It should be applied directly to the wound surface once or twice daily. Metronidazole gel has also been used as a carrier for morphine to provide combined pain and odour control (Flock et al., 2000; Grocott, 2000).

Malodour

The often putrid odour associated with a malignant wound is considered the most distressing symptom for patients and can be a significant problem for family and caregivers as well. Healthcare practitioners also find wound malodour a very difficult problem to deal with (Alexander, 2010). The odour is commonly strong, unpleasant and persistent, and can trigger gagging and vomiting reflexes (Van Toller, 1994).

Malodour is predominantly a by-product of bacterial activity in the hypoxic, devitalised tissue present within the wound. In particular, anaerobic bacteria of the *Bacteroides* and *Clostridium* species are involved (Thomas et al., 1998a; Hack, 2003; Draper, 2005). These bacteria break down amino acids in necrotic tissue, resulting in the production of the organic chemicals putrescine and cadaverine, which are primarily responsible for the foul odour of putrefying flesh associated with malignant wounds (Thomas et al., 1998a). Aerobic bacterial species, such as *Proteus*, *Klebsiella* and *Pseudomonas*, may also be present but tend to produce less toxic by-products. Stale exudate in dressings and fistula effluent can also be a source of malodour.

The three key approaches to successful malodour management are

- removing the medium for bacterial growth (moist necrotic tissue);
- killing the bacteria responsible for odour production;
- containing or masking the odour.

Debridement of necrotic tissue from the wound will deprive odour-causing bacteria of a growth medium. However, the risk of bleeding and pain means that surgical or sharp debridement must be performed with extreme caution by practitioners who have been properly trained and only loose tissue carefully removed. Autolytic debridement is the preferred method, but there is a potential for increased levels of exudate through the use of fluid-donating dressing products, such as hydrogels, and from tissue breakdown (Grocott, 2007).

In order to kill bacteria an antibiotic or antiseptic is required. The most common treatment for malignant wound malodour is metronidazole, an antibiotic that is active against the anaerobic bacteria responsible for odour production (Bower et al., 1992; Finlay et al., 1996). Metronidazole may be given systemically, at a dose of 200–400 mg three times a day. This method of administration is particularly suitable for wounds that have invaded a body cavity where topical application is difficult, or where there are systemic signs of infection, such as general malaise, fever and/or rigors (Draper, 2005). There is a risk of gastrointestinal side effects with systemic therapy, and it has been suggested that systemic use in poorly vascularised necrotic wounds may result in an inadequate dose reaching the wound (Thomas et al., 1998a).

Practice point

Topical metronidazole may be a more effective delivery method than oral metronidazole and easier for patients who may have difficulty in swallowing. Usually a 0.75–0.8% gel is applied directly to the wound surface once or twice daily and is effective in odour control within 2–5 days (Finlay et al., 1996; Bale et al., 2004). Because the topical gel can be expensive, some clinicians have used crushed metronidazole tablets or oral suspension mixed with a wound gel as an alternative. Note that the use of these medicines in this way is not a licensed indication, and so they must be dispensed on a named patient basis only and according to local policy on the use of medicines off-licence.

Activated charcoal dressings are commonly used to control wound malodour. These dressings contain a layer of charcoal cloth that attracts and binds the molecules responsible for wound odour (Hampton, 2006). Activated charcoal dressings are available as a simple secondary cloth dressing or may incorporate other dressing materials, such as foam, alginate or hydrofibre. In general, activated charcoal dressings work best when kept dry and when a complete seal is maintained over the wound by the dressings. Some dressings are also impregnated with silver for its bactericidal effect. The highly bactericidal nature of silver may have some effect on malodour by killing the causative bacteria in wound exudate, or in the wound tissues if silver is released into the wound environment from the dressing. However, there is limited evidence for the use of silver dressings in malignant wounds and cost may be prohibitive due to the frequency of dressing changes.

Other methods of odour control that may be effective but have limited supporting evidence include sugar paste or sterile honey, both of which are highly bactericidal and encourage wound debridement (Hampton, 2006). Silver- or iodine-impregnated dressings may also be effective, as they kill a wide range of odour-causing bacteria, however cost can be an issue. Some essential oils may help disguise odour (Mercier and Knevitt, 2005), and daily dressing changes and disposal of soiled dressings will prevent odour from stale exudate.

Exudate

Heavy exudate is a common problem with malignant wounds, and is most likely due to excess leakage of fluid from blood vessels as a result of a disorganised and highly permeable tumour local blood supply. Tumour cells may also secrete vascular permeability factor, which exacerbates leakage of fluid from blood vessels (Haisfield-Wolfe and Rund, 1997). In addition, inflammation associated with heavy bacterial colonisation or infection, and tissue breakdown by bacterial proteases also contribute to exudate production. If the wound is complicated by a fistula, it could result in the discharge of high volumes of corrosive or malodorous effluent. Tumour necrosis as a consequence of cancer therapy, particularly with radiotherapy, can also cause an increase in exudate.

Management of malignant wounds requires a balance between exudate absorption or containment, and maintenance of a moist wound environment to encourage potential healing and prevent dressing adherence and wound desiccation (drying out). Lesions that are dry should be covered by a dry dressing to protect them from trauma and prevent further deterioration.

Dressings suitable for moderate-to-high exudate include alginate and hydrofibre dressings, foams and silicone-coated non-adherent wound contact layers with a secondary absorbent pad (Grocott, 1999). For very heavy exudate, a highly absorbent incontinence pad can be used as a secondary dressing. These usually have a superabsorbent core and waterproof backing, making them ideal for containing large volumes of exudate. For wounds with a small opening or which contain a fistula, a drainable stoma appliance, such as a urostomy bag, or specially designed wound manager bag, may be appropriate.

In general, the use of topical negative pressure therapy (TNP) is not recommended for malignant wounds due to the risk that increased blood flow to the area will encourage growth of the malignancy, and may increase the chances of metastatic spread of the cancer. However, in cases where symptoms of exudate and odour are proving difficult to control and the patient is near the end of life, TNP may be used effectively to contain symptoms and improve quality of life. Caution is advised if bleeding is present in the wound and wound pain should be carefully monitored.

With highly exudating wounds, the patient's skin is at risk of breakdown due to maceration and/or the corrosive effects of exudate. Skin can easily be protected using an alcohol-free skin barrier film, or by cutting a thin hydrocolloid sheet to fit around the wound. These strategies will also protect the skin from stripping by self-adhesive dressings and tapes.

Itching and skin irritation

Itching and skin irritation may occur when tumour nodules develop within the skin. Stretching of the skin irritates nerve endings causing a biochemical reaction leading to local inflammation, which causes irritation and itching. Wound exudate or fistula effluent can also cause skin excoriation and maceration, which may be irritating or painful, and skin stripping by adhesive tapes or dressings may exacerbate skin irritation.

Applying hydrogel or sheets can produce a cooling effect on itching skin. The hydrogel may be covered with a semipermeable film to prevent dehydration. Transcutaneous electrical nerve stimulation (TENS) has also been reported as being effective in relieving itching (Grocott, 2007).

Practice point

Aqueous cream with menthol is a simple, cost-effective, topical application that has a cooling and soothing effect while also moisturising the skin. This cream can be easily made by a pharmacy and applied to itchy areas two to three times a day, or as necessary (Naylor et al., 2001).

Infection

Due to the chronic nature of malignant wounds and possible compromised immune system, malignant wounds may not display classic signs of infection. Instead, a sudden increase in wound symptoms, such as pain, exudate and malodour, may be the first indicators of wound infection. Generally, a wound swab will be unhelpful due to high microorganism contamination of malignant wounds and the likelihood that any infecting organism is located deep within the necrotic tissue and difficult to isolate.

Practice point

Systemic antibiotics may be useful if there are systemic signs of infection, but blood supply to malignant wounds is often poor, so the concentration of antibiotic at the wound site may not be sufficient to have any local effect. Therefore, topical antimicrobials or antiseptics are the preferred choice to treat infection in malignant wounds, for example metronidazole gel, silver-impregnated dressings or medical-grade honey.

Bleeding

The underlying malignancy creates fragile and disorganised blood vessels within the wound. This, along with an abnormal platelet function caused by tumour cell activity, predisposes malignant wounds to bleeding. This usually occurs as light-to-moderate superficial bleeding, but on occasion bleeding can be profuse. Bleeding may occur spontaneously, but is often a result of trauma, particularly during dressing removal and wound cleansing. Ulcerating malignant wounds that overlie superficial blood vessels, for example in the neck, auxilla or groin, may erode a major blood vessel causing profuse spontaneous bleeding, which can be fatal. Although relatively rare, this is obviously extremely distressing for the patient, their family and healthcare staff.

Preventative strategies are vital in the management of malignant wounds with a history of, or potential for, bleeding. Non-adherent dressings that maintain the wound in a moist environment should always be used, and wounds should be cleansed by irrigation or with a sterile gloved hand to prevent wound trauma. Oral or topical antifibrinolytic drugs, such as tranexamic acid, may also help to prevent bleeding (Dean, 1997).

For slow capillary oozing, topical application of sucralfate paste or an alginate dressing may be all that is needed (Emflorgo, 1998; Thomas et al., 1998b), although alginate dressings should be used with care on fragile tumours, as the 'drawing' action may stimulate bleeding (Grocott, 1998).

Moderate-to-heavy bleeding may respond to a haemostatic surgical dressing, which will usually produce rapid haemostasis. Alternatively, an adrenaline soak (adrenaline 1:1000 on sterile gauze) may be effective, as it causes local vasoconstriction. Topical tranexamic acid, made by mixing a crushed tablet with sterile water, can also be effective for moderate bleeding. Both adrenaline and tranexamic acid will require a prescription on a named patient basis, as they are not licensed for this method of application. Continuous heavy bleeding may need referral to a surgeon for cautery or vessel ligation.

> **Practice point**
>
> If massive haemorrhage occurs due to erosion of a major blood vessel, stay with the patient and call for assistance, apply local pressure and packing to the bleeding point (dark green or blue towels are ideal as they mask blood stains) and monitor the patient's pulse. Sedation may be appropriate for distressed patients (usually with morphine IV, IM or SC and/or Midazolam SC). It is important to have a plan in place if haemorrhage is a potential problem, including easy access to necessary equipment and sedation, and relatives should be warned in advance when possible.

Radiation skin damage

Around 60% of cancer patients receive radiation therapy as part of their treatment. External beam radiotherapy (teletherapy) will inevitably deliver some portion of the dose to the skin, as the radiation beam must pass through the skin to reach its target. Consequently, patients develop both acute and chronic skin changes. The degree of skin reaction may be influenced by a number of factors:

- Treatment factors:
  - high total dose of radiation;
  - low-energy radiation or electrons;
  - treatment of the head and neck, breast or pelvic area;
  - large volume of normal tissue included in the treatment field;
  - tangential treatment fields;
  - use of 'bolus' materials.
- Patient factors:
  - older age;
  - immunosuppression;
  - concurrent chemotherapy or steroid therapy;
  - poor nutritional status;
  - tobacco smoking;
  - chronic sun exposure.

Acute skin reactions develop as a result of radiation disrupting cell division in the stratum basale. As cells are lost from the skin surface through everyday wear and tear, they are not replaced. Radiation also induces vascular damage and activation of proinflammatory and coagulation pathways, contributing to a local inflammatory response (Stone et al., 2003). Acute skin reactions only occur within the radiation treatment field, and usually appear within the first 2–3 weeks of treatment and may persist for up to 8 weeks post-treatment.

These reactions are classified according to the appearance of the skin:

- *Erythema*: redness, heat and oedema, accompanied by burning and itching sensations;
- *Dry desquamation*: dry and flaky or peeling skin with associated itching; hair loss may occur within the treatment field;
- *Moist desquamation*: exposure of the dermis with associated exudate production, pain and the risk of infection;
- *Necrosis*: skin necrosis and ulcer formation due to damage to capillaries and connective tissue.

(Campbell and Lane, 1996; Rice, 1997; Boots-Vickers and Eaton, 1999)

Radiation may stimulate melanocytes in the epidermis, resulting in skin pigment changes within the treatment field. The pigmentation may take 6 months or longer to fade.

Radiotherapy-induced late skin changes usually appear around 3 months post-treatment or may present years later, and result from damage to

Table 12.2   Guidelines for managing acute radiotherapy skin reactions

Erythema and dry desquamation	Simple, non-perfumed moisturising cream should be applied two to three times a day to provide symptomatic relief and help maintain skin integrity
	Apply 1% hydrocortisone cream sparingly, two to three times a day to itchy, irritable or burning areas of the skin within the treatment field; do not use on areas of broken or infected skin
Moist desquamation	Hydrogel sheets applied to areas of moist desquamation will reduce discomfort and promote healing; they are also cooling and soothing; amorphous (liquid) hydrogels may be used with a secondary dressing in skin folds or the perineum
	Hydrocolloid sheet dressings can be applied *once radiotherapy treatment is finished*; they provide an aesthetically acceptable dressing that promotes comfort and healing
	Other modern dressing products such as semipermeable films, alginates, hydrofibre or foams may also be used and should be selected based on the presenting characteristics of the wound

Source: Kearney and Richardson (2006).

connective tissue and blood vessels of the skin and underlying tissues. Chronic skin changes may present as:

- atrophy of the skin;
- fibrosis and thickening of skin;
- xerosis (dry skin);
- hypo- or hyperpigmentation;
- telangiectasia (small, dilated red blood vessels within the skin);
- radiation-induced skin cancers;
- necrosis and ulceration following minor trauma to the area of treated skin.

(Pearson and Mortimer, 2004)

Management of radiotherapy skin reactions

The initial aim is to delay onset and reduce the severity of acute skin reactions through preventative measures. During treatment, the patient should be advised to care for skin in the treatment field in the following way:

- Wash area normally using warm water and a mild, non-perfumed soap.
- Pat skin dry with a soft towel.
- Apply a simple moisturising cream two to three times a day.
- Avoid deodorants and perfumed skincare products.
- Avoid the use of flannels, brushes, loofah, etc.

- Wear loose comfortable clothing made of natural fibres, such as cotton.
- Protect the treated skin from extreme cold and sunlight.

Numerous skincare products and regimens have been used and recommended for the management of acute skin reactions, but many have little or no evidence to support their use (Glean et al., 2001). While there is not a great deal of evidence for any particular product as a preventative for acute skin reactions, there is support for some general guidelines on skin reaction management (Table 12.2). There are also a number of products that are not recommended for skincare during radiotherapy, such as petroleum jelly, prophylactic topical antibiotics/antiseptics, talcum powder, corn starch and gentian violet (Naylor and Mallett, 2001). The management of late skin changes following radiotherapy focus on maintaining skin integrity and preventing further skin damage. Surgery may be indicated for chronic radiation-induced skin ulceration.

Wound dressings: special considerations

Malignant wounds present in a wide variety of sizes, shapes and locations, from small, dry necrotic skin lesions to extensive ulceration or large, protruding nodular lesions. Add to this the difficult wound symptoms, and finding a suitable dressing can be problematic. The majority of available dressings are often an inappropriate shape and size, or do not have the required characteristics incorporated in a single product needed to manage a malignant wound.

The wound shape and location can make dressing retention an issue, and it is often necessary to avoid adhesive products due to fragile skin, maceration from exudate and skin stripping from frequent dressing changes. Careful dressing selection is also necessary to avoid pain and bleeding caused by dressings adhering to the wound.

Education and support

Not only are malignant wounds difficult for the patient, they also appear to be particularly challenging for healthcare professionals. Qualitative studies that have involved nurses have found that these wounds have a significant impact on them even many years after the episode of care (Wilkes et al., 2003; Alexander, 2010). Nurses felt that they were the most challenging and complex wounds to deal with. While the nurses identified practical problems, such as malodour and application of dressings to difficult areas, the more difficult aspects of patient management were the struggle with the patient's bodily suffering and disfigurement, a perceived invasion of privacy, feeling personally invaded (particularly by the malodour) and feeling helpless (Lindahl et al., 2008; Alexander, 2010). It is therefore important to consider the support required by healthcare staff when they have to deal with the complexities of caring for a patient with a malignant wound. Nursing staff may also need expert advice and support from a clinician with experience in the care of malignant wounds when assessing and developing a care plan for malignant wound management. Managers will also need to consider workload priorities when a patient with a large and/or complex malignant wound is admitted to their service. Not only will wound care activities be time-consuming, the additional psychological support required may add to nursing time spent with the patient.

A number of strategies aimed at improving or controlling wound-related symptoms will reduce the impact of the wound on the patient. The effective management of wound exudate and odour leads to increased levels of patient confidence and comfort. Appropriate wound management attending to the patient's outward appearance can have a very positive effect on self-esteem and emotional distress. Devising a cosmetically acceptable dressing regime that restores body symmetry is important to allow the patient to continue an active social life, maintain a sense of normality and have confidence in social situations.

Provision of specialist services

As malignant wounds are relatively uncommon when compared to other types of chronic wounds, there are no services specialising in the care of these wounds. However, some wound care specialists, oncology specialist nurses and palliative care specialists do have greater clinical experience and knowledge in the care of malignant wounds. Therefore, advice from a local provider of these services should always be sought if the wound is proving too difficult to manage. It is very challenging to manage a complex malignant wound without support of colleagues; a team approach is always recommended.

Formal or informal counselling will also be helpful, along with spiritual care according to the patient's beliefs. The patient and their family should have appropriate social support, as this will decrease stress and anxiety. A great deal of this supportive care can be provided by a specialist palliative care service, so their involvement should be encouraged if available and the patient agrees.

Criteria for specialist referral

Criteria for specialist referral include the following:

- Any person presenting with a previously undiagnosed malignant wound, or a diagnoses of malignancy in a chronic wound should be referred to a specialist oncologist for evaluation of anticancer therapy.
- Referral to hospice service/specialist palliative care team, if available, may be appropriate, even if anticancer therapy is going to be given. The palliative care team will be able to offer symptom management advice, as well as

psychological and social support for the person and their family.

● Depending on expertise, referral to a specialist wound service/professional may also be appropriate if symptoms are proving difficult to control, and for specific advice on wound care products.

Summary

Not only do malignant wounds present with difficult-to-manage symptoms, they are also distressing to patients, their family and carers, and healthcare staff. Therefore, a holistic approach to patient assessment is a key starting point to effective management. In addition, a multidisciplinary approach is required to address patients' needs across the spectrum of physical, psychological, social and spiritual problems.

Malignant wounds are relatively rare and occur in a population with complex health problems, and therefore they are infrequently the subject of research. Thus, there continues to be a lack of high-quality research-based evidence to guide management of these difficult wounds. To date, research that is available has tended to focus on the psychological and social impact of these wounds, which is vital to inform patient care, but practical care of the wound itself still relies on translating evidence from other chronic wounds; this extends to the development and design of dressing products as well. There is, therefore, a need for ongoing clinical research to establish best practice in the care of malignant wounds and allow for the development of evidence-based guidance.

Useful resources

Scottish Intercollegiate Guidelines Network. *Control of pain in adults with cancer.* Available at: http://www.sign.ac.uk/guidelines/fulltext/106/index.html

NHS Clinical Knowledge Summaries. *Palliative cancer care – Malignant ulcer of the skin – Management.* Available at: http://www.cks.nhs.uk/palliative_cancer_care_malignant_ulcer#

Guidelines for Wound Management in Palliative Care. Available at: http://www.nzwcs.org.nz/images/stories/files/woundmanagementguidelines-text.pdf

CancerNursing.org – Free online courses

Wound Management in Cancer and Palliative Care. Avail-

able at: http://www.cancernursing.org/courses/currentcourses/full.asp?CourseID=42

Introduction to Palliative Care Nursing. Available at: http://www.cancernursing.org/courses/currentcourses/full.asp?CourseID=34

BC Cancer Agency. Nursing Practice Reference – *Care of Malignant Wounds.* Available at: http://www.bccancer.bc.ca/HPI/CancerManagementGuidelines/Supportive Care/ChronicUlceratingMalignantSkinLesions/default.htm

Macmillan Cancer Support. *Fungating cancer wounds.* Available at: http://www.macmillan.org.uk/Cancerinformation/Livingwithandaftercancer/Symptomssideeffects/Othersymptomssideeffects/Fungatingwounds.aspx

References

Adderley, U.J., Smith, R. (2007) Topical agents and dressings for fungating wounds. *Cochrane Database of Systemic Reviews*, Issue 2, Art. No.: CD003948. DOI: 10.1002/14651858.CD003948.pub2

Alexander, S. (2009) Malignant fungating wounds: epidemiology, aetiology, presentation and assessment. *Journal of Wound Care*, 18(7), 273–280.

Alexander, S.J. (2010) An intense and unforgettable experience: the lived experience of malignant wounds from perspectives of patients, caregivers and nurses. *International Wound Journal*, 7(6), 456–465.

Alvarez, O.M., Kalinski, C., Nusbaum, J., et al. (2007) Incorporating wound healing strategies to improve palliation (symptom management) in patients with chronic wounds. *Journal of Palliative Medicine*, 10(5), 1161–1189.

Back, I.N., Finlay, I. (1995) Analgesic effect of topical opioids on painful skin ulcers (letter). *Journal of Pain and Symptom Management*, 10(7), 493.

Bale, S., Tebble, N., Price, P. (2004) A topical metronidazole gel used to treat malodorous wounds. *British Journal of Nursing*, 13(11 Suppl), 4–11.

Boots-Vickers, M., Eaton, K. (1999) Skin care for patients receiving radiotherapy. *Professional Nurse*, 14(10), 706–708.

Bower, M., Stein, R., Evans, T., Hedley, A., Pert, P., Coombes, R. (1992) A double-blind study of the efficacy of metronidazole gel in the treatment of malodorous fungating tumours. *European Journal of Cancer*, 28A(4/5), 888–889.

Campbell, J., Lane, C. (1996) Developing a skin-care protocol in radiotherapy. *Professional Nurse*, 12(2), 105–108.

Davis, V. (1995) Goal-setting aids care. *Nursing Times*, 91(39), 72–75.

Dean, A. (1997) Fibrinolytic inhibitors for cancer-associated bleeding problems. *Journal of Pain and Symptom Management*, 13(1), 20–24.

Dolbeult, S., Flahault, C., Baffie, A., Fromantin, I. (2010) Psychological profile of patients with neglected malignant wounds: a qualitative exploratory study. *Journal of Wound Care*, 19(12), 513–521.

Draper, C. (2005) The management of malodour and exudate in fungating wounds. *British Journal of Nursing*, 14(11), 4–12.

Emflorgo, C. (1998) Controlling bleeding in fungating wounds (letter). *Journal of Wound Care*, 7(5), 235.

Finlay, I., Bowszyc, J., Ramlau, C., Gwiezdzinski, Z. (1996) The effect of topical 0.75% metronidazole gel on malodorous cutaneous wounds. *Journal of Pain and Symptom Management*, 11(3), 158–162.

Flock, P., Gibbs, L., Sykes, N. (2000) Diamorphine-metronidazole gel effective for treatment of painful infected leg ulcers (letter). *Journal of Pain and Symptom Management*, 20(6), 396–397.

Fyrmpas, G., Barbetakis, N., Efstathiou, A., Konstantinidis, I., Tsilikas, C. (2006). Cutaneous metastasis to the face from colon adenocarcinoma. Case report. *International Seminars in Surgical Oncology*, 3(2), DOI:10.1186/1477-7800-3-2. Available at: http://www.issoonline.com/content/pdf/1477-7800-3-2.pdf, retrieved on July 6, 2011.

Glean, E., Edwards, S., Faithfull, S., et al. (2001) Intervention for acute radiotherapy induced skin reactions in cancer patients: the development of a clinical practice guidelines recommended for use by the college of radiographers. *Journal of Radiotherapy in Practice*, 2(2), 75–84.

Grocott, P. (1998) Controlling bleeding in fragile fungating tumours (letter). *Journal of Wound Care*, 7(7), 342.

Grocott, P. (1999) The management of fungating wounds. *Journal of Wound Care*, 8(5), 232–234.

Grocott, P. (2000) Palliative management of fungating malignant wounds. *Journal of Community Nursing*, 14(3), 31–38.

Grocott, P. (2007) Care of patients with fungating malignant wounds. *Nursing Standard*, 21(24), 57–66.

Hack, A. (2003) Malodorous wounds- taking the patient's perspective into account. *Journal of Wound Car*, 12(8), 319–321.

Haisfield-Wolfe, M.E., Rund, C. (1997) Malignant cutaneous wounds: a management protocol. *Ostomy/Wound Management*, 43(1), 56–66.

Hampton, S. (2006) Malodorous fungating wounds: how dressings alleviate symptoms. *Wound Care*, 13(6), S31–S36.

Hoskin, P.J. (2004) Radiotherapy in symptom management. In: *Oxford Textbook of Palliative Medicine*, (eds D. Doyle, G. Hanks, N. Cherny, Calman), 3rd edn, pp. 239–255. Oxford: Oxford University Press.

Ivetić, O., Lyne, P.A. (1990) Fungating and ulcerating malignant lesions: a review of the literature. *Journal of Advanced Nursing*, 15, 83–88.

Jemal, A., Bray, F., Center, M.M., Ferlay, J., Ward, E., Forman, D (2011) Global cancer statistics. *CA: A Cancer Journal for Clinicians*, 61(2), 69–90. Available at: http://onlinelibrary.wiley.com/doi/10.3322/caac.20107/pdf, retrieved on July 26, 2011.

Krajnik, M., Zylicz, A., Finlay, I., Luczak, K., van Sorge, A.A. (1999) Potential uses of topical opioids in palliative care: report of six cases. *Pain*, 80(1-2), 121–125.

Kearney, N., Richardson, A. (eds.) (2006) Skin and wound care. In: *Nursing Patients with Cancer: Principles and Practice*. Edinburgh: Elsevier.

Lazelle-Ali, C. (2007) Psychological and physical care of malodorous fungating wounds. *British Journal of Nursing*, 16(15), 16–24.

LeBon, B., Zeppetella, G., Higginson, I.J. (2009) Effectiveness of topical administration of opioids in palliative care: a systematic review. *Journal of Pain and Symptom Management*, 37(5), 913–917.

Lindahl, E., Norberg, A., Soderberg, A. (2008) The meaning of caring for people with malodorous exuding ulcers. *Journal of Advanced Nursing*, 62(2), 163–171.

Lo, S.F., Hu, W.Y., Hayter, M., Chang, S.C., Shu, M.Y., Wu, L.W. (2008) Experiences of living with a malignant fungating wound: a qualitative study. *Journal of Clinical Nursing*, 17(20), 2699–2708.

Lund-Nielsen, B., Müller, K., Adamsen, L. (2005) Malignant wounds in women with breast cancer: feminine and sexual perspectives. *Journal of Clinical Nursing*, 14(1), 56–64.

Maida, V., Corbo, M., Dolzhykov, M., Ennis, M., Irani, S., Trozzolo, L. (2008) Wounds in advanced illness: a prevalence and incidence study based on a prospective case series. *International Wound Journal*, 5(2), 305–314.

Maida, V., Ennis, M., Kuziemsky, C., Trozzolo, L. (2009) Symptoms associated with malignant wounds: a prospective case series. *Journal of Pain and Symptom Management*, 37(2), 206–211.

Malheiro, E., Pinto, A., Choupina, M., Barroso, L., Reis, J., Amarabte, J. (2001) Marjolin's ulcer of the scalp: case report and literature review. *Annals of Burns and Fire Disasters*, 14(1). Available at: http://www.medbc.com/annals/review/vol_14/num_1/text/vol14n1p39.htm, retrieved on August 1, 2011.

McDonald, A., Lesage, P. (2006) Palliative management of pressure ulcers and malignant wounds in patients with advanced illness. *Journal of Palliative Medicine*, 9(2), 285–295.

Mercier, D., Knevitt, A. (2005) Using topical aromatherapy for the management of fungating wounds in a palliative care unit. *Journal of Wound Care*, 14(10), 497–501.

Mohamed, A., Mohamed, A.E., Afzal-Uddin, M., Emran, F. (2010) Fungating breast cancer, how long we are going to see this stage of the disease. Case report and literature Review. *The Internet Journal of Surgery*, 23(2), DOI: 10.5580/c74. Available at: http://www.ispub.com/journal/the_internet_journal_of_surgery/volume_23_number_2/article/fungating-breast-cancer-how-long-we-are-going-to-see-this-stage-of-the-disease-case-report-and-literature-review.html, retrieved on 17 July 2011.

National Cancer Institute (2011) *Breast Cancer Treatment (PDQ®) Stage IIIB, Inoperable IIIC, IV, Recurrent, and Metastatic Breast Cancer.* Available at: http://www.cancer.gov/cancertopics/pdq/treatment/breast/healthprofessional/page7, retrieved on 19 September 2011.

Naylor, W., Mallett, J. (2001) Management of acute radiotherapy induced skin reactions: a literature review. *European Journal of Oncology Nursing*, 5(4), 221–233.

Naylor, W., Laverty, D., Mallett, J. (2001) *The Royal Marsden Hospital Handbook of Wound Management in Cancer Care.* Oxford: Blackwell Science.

Offer, G., Perks, G., Wilcock, A. (2000) Palliative plastic surgery. *European Journal of Palliative Care*, 7(3), 85–87.

Oxford University Press (2011) *Oxford Dictionaries.* Available at: http://oxforddictionaries.com, retrieved on 1 August 2011.

Pearson, I.C., Mortimer, P. (2004) Skin problems in palliative medicine: medical aspects. In: *Oxford Textbook of Palliative Medicine*, (eds D. Doyle, G. Hanks, N. Cherny, Calman) 3rd edn, pp. 618–628. Oxford: Oxford University Press.

Piggin, C., Jones, J. (2009) Malignant fungating wounds: an analysis of the lived experience. *Journal of Wound Care*, 18(2), 57–64.

Price, P., Fogh, K., Glynn, C., Krasner, D., Osterbrink, J., Sibbald, R. (2007) Managing painful chronic wounds: the Wound pain management model. *International Wound Journal*, 4(Suppl 1), 4–15.

Probst, S., Arber, A., Faithfull, S. (2009) Malignant fungating wounds: a survey of nurses' clinical practice in Switzerland. *European Journal of Oncology Nursing*, 13(4), 295–298.

Rice, A.M. (1997) An introduction to radiotherapy. *Nursing Standard*, 12(3), 49–56.

Saeed, S., Keehn, C.A., Morgan, M.B. (2004) Cutaneous metastasis: a clinical, pathological, and immunohistochemical appraisal. *Journal of Cutaneous Pathology*, 31(6), 419–430.

Stein, C. (1995) The control of pain in peripheral tissue by opioids. *The New England Journal of Medicine*, 332(25), 1685–1690.

Stone, H.B., Coleman, C.N., Anscher, M.S., McBride, W.H. (2003) Effects of radiation on normal tissue: consequences and mechanisms. *The Lancet*, 4, 529–536.

Thomas, S. (1992) *Current Practices in the Management of Fungating Lesions and Radiation Damaged Skin.* Bridgend, UK: The Surgical Materials Testing Laboratory.

Thomas, S., Fischer, B., Fram, P.J., Waring, M.J. (1998a) Odour-absorbing dressings. *Journal of Wound Care*, 7(5), 246–250.

Thomas, S., Vowden, K., Newton, H. (1998b) Controlling bleeding in fragile fungating wounds. *Journal of Wound Care*, 7(3), 154.

Twillman, R.K., Long, T.D., Cathers, T.A., Mueller, D.W. (1999) Treatment of painful skin ulcers with topical opioids. *Journal of Pain and Symptom Management*, 17(4), 288–292.

Van Toller, S. (1994) Invisible wounds: the effects of skin ulcer malodours. *Journal of Wound Care*, 3(2), 103–105.

Wilkes, L., White, K., Smeal, T., Beale, B. (2001) Malignant wound management: what dressings do nurses use? *Journal of Wound Care*, 10(3), 65–70.

Wilkes, L.M., Boxer, E., White, K. (2003) The hidden side of nursing: why caring for patients with malignant malodorous wounds is so difficult. *Journal of Wound Care*, 12(2), 76–80.

World Health Organization (1996) *Cancer Pain Relief: With a Guide to Opioid Availability*, 2nd edn. Geneva: World Health Organization.

World Health Organization (2002) *National Cancer Control Programmes: Policies and Managerial Guidelines*, 2nd edn. Geneva: World Health Organization.

Wu, J.J., Huang, D.B., Pang, K.R., Tyring, S.K. (2006) Cutaneous metastasis to the chest wall from prostate cancer. *International Journal of Dermatology*, 45(8), 946–948.

Young, C.V. (2005) The effects of malodorous fungating malignant wounds on body image and quality of life. *Journal of Wound Care*, 14(8), 359–362.

13 Skin Integrity and Dermatology

Julia Schofield

United Lincolnshire Hospitals NHS Trust, and School of Life and Medical Sciences, University of Hertfordshire, Hertfordshire, UK

Overview

- The skin is an important and highly visible organ. Skin breakdown affects a significant number of people each year and has a major impact on sufferers, relatives and their carers.
- The majority of people with skin conditions will self-care, with only a relatively small proportion opting to seek further advice, usually from a non-specialist doctor or nurse in the community.
- In some geographical areas, there is a lack of publically funded dermatologists. This often means that patients with common inflammatory skin conditions have limited specialist support and may rely on local traditional remedies or over-the-counter treatment.
- There are a range of dermatological conditions that wound care practitioners will come into contact with, such as eczema, allergic dermatitis, cellulitis, 'red legs' and skin cancers. These need to be recognised in order to optimise prevention, assessment and management of a patient with a skin integrity problem.
- The development of combined clinics, where dermatology and wound management teams work closely together to manage patients with chronic wounds such as leg ulcers, is beneficial, particularly in areas where specialist resources are scarce.

Introduction

This is an important chapter for healthcare professionals managing people with wounds and skin integrity problems. Whilst continuity and collaboration among multidisciplinary teams including tissue viability and other specialities such as dermatology, immunology, plastic surgery, lymphovascular medicine and care of the elderly are essential to ensure optimal patient care, each member of the multidisciplinary team should have some basic understanding of related clinical areas. This is particularly relevant in situations where ready access to other specialities is limited. There is evidence in the United Kingdom that the level of training and knowledge of a range of healthcare professionals in skin disease is limited and probably inadequate (Schofield et al., 2009). In particular, neither preregistration nurse training nor undergraduate medical training includes compulsory dermatology and

---

Wound Healing and Skin Integrity: Principles and Practice, First Edition. Edited by Madeleine Flanagan.
© 2013 John Wiley & Sons, Ltd. Published 2013 by John Wiley & Sons, Ltd.

skin integrity education (Davies and Burge, 2009). There are also large numbers of clinicians, who are able to prescribe widely for patients with skin conditions and compromised skin integrity, who receive little or no training in skin disorders. This chapter seeks to raise awareness about the burden of skin disease and the importance of understanding dermatological disease when managing a patient with wounds and skin integrity problems. Chronic skin conditions are considered first as they are commoner in everyday practice; however, it is also important to be able to recognise and manage the more commonly presenting acute skin conditions.

Prevalence and incidence of skin disease

A healthcare needs assessment (HCNA) on skin conditions in the United Kingdom provides good evidence that skin disease is common with studies from unselected populations around the world suggesting that around 23–33% have a skin problem that can benefit from medical care at any one time (Schofield et al., 2009). In the United Kingdom, surveys suggest that around 54% of the population experience a skin condition in a given 12-month period. Most (69%) of these people will self-care, but around 14% will seek further medical advice, usually from a doctor or nurse in the community. In England and Wales, patients are required to attend their primary care general practitioner before being referred for a specialist opinion; there is good data showing that skin conditions are the most frequent reason for people to consult their general practitioner with a new problem. About 24% of the population in England and Wales (12.9 million people) visited their general practitioner with a skin problem in 2006. People die from skin conditions. For example, in the United Kingdom in 2010, there were 4297 deaths due to skin disease, of which nearly half were due to malignant melanoma. Other causes of death from skin disease include cutaneous squamous cell carcinoma (SCC).

Quality of life

The impact of skin disease on quality of life is well documented and it is known that skin diseases such as psoriasis, atopic eczema and acne can have a significant impact on the quality of life and that this impairment can be greater at times than for life-threatening conditions such as cancers (Harlow et al., 2000; Basra and Finlay, 2007). There is strong evidence that many common skin diseases are also associated with significant psychosocial morbidity, which may go unrecognised without the use of appropriate assessment tools (Picardi et al., 2000). Some of this is due to the public's view that skin appearance is as important as, if not more important than, disability and loss of function.

Cost of skin diseases

There are significant costs both to individuals and to healthcare systems in the management of skin disease (Diepgen, 2006). Whilst many of these costs relate to long-term skin conditions such as psoriasis and eczema, there are also significant costs related to the management of patients with skin conditions related to loss of skin integrity both in community settings and in hospital and will be considered later in this chapter. These conditions, and other types of skin disease, such as hand dermatitis, cause disability and loss of earnings (Schofield et al., 2009).

What skin conditions are common?

The spectrum of skin disease seen in different geographical areas and practice settings varies (Lopez and Murray, 1998; Bickers et al., 2006). For example, the common reasons that people present to the general practitioner in England and Wales are for the management of skin infections and eczema but the commonest reasons that people are referred for specialist outpatient dermatology advice is for the diagnosis and management of skin lesions (in particular skin cancer), eczema, psoriasis and acne (Schofield et al., 2009). With regard to hospital admissions in the United Kingdom, cellulitis is the commonest reason for people to be admitted to hospital with a skin condition and these admissions are nearly all emergency admissions. Most patients admitted with cellulitis have a limb affected, and the mean length of hospital stay is approximately 7 days. It is also well recognised that inpatients admitted with other medical problems often have coexisting dermatology problems requiring specialist dermatology input involving the diagnosis and management of a range of conditions. The commonest of these are listed below:

- skin conditions related to venous and gravitational stasis eczema;
- leg ulcers and their management;
- allergic contact dermatitis developing in patients with problems of skin integrity using topical products;
- skin cancer;
- skin changes in the elderly such as asteatotic eczema;
- skin disease related to systemic medical conditions such as cutaneous vasculitis and pyoderma gangrenosum;
- drug reactions, including very rare 'sick skin' conditions such as toxic epidermal necrolysis.

Why is knowing about skin disease important?

First and foremost an understanding of basic good skin care is important in order to optimise healing and maintain skin barrier function. This is particularly important in the elderly. There are also a broad range of dermatological factors that need to be recognised in order to optimise prevention, assessment and management of a patient with a skin integrity problem. This can be demonstrated by the following clinical situations that the healthcare professional may encounter when managing a patient with altered skin integrity:

- **Prevention:** A patient presents with varicose eczema. Management of the varicose eczema may prevent the development of venous ulceration.
- **Assessment:** A patient with inflammatory bowel disease presents with an acute enlarging wound due to pyoderma gangrenosum. The wound will not respond to conventional wound management alone. The key here is to confirm the diagnosis and start oral prednisolone, a treatment that would be contra-indicated in the management of most wounds.
- **Management:** A patient with a chronic venous leg ulcer develops an acute widespread eczema affecting the leg first and then the rest of the body. Recognition and management of a possible allergic contact dermatitis to a topical preparation is key to optimising care.

- **Reassessment:** Objective reassessment of a leg ulcer shows that it has failed to shrink or heal after 12 weeks of optimal therapy. Could this be a SSC rather than a chronic venous ulcer, as initially thought?

Management principles

Assessment considerations

There are some key points relevant to general medical problems and, specifically, dermatological disease that can be established as part of the patient assessment.

Medical history

When taking a patient's medical history it is important to identify the following medical problems:

- *Diabetes mellitus*: This can lead to impaired healing, peripheral neuropathy and vasculopathy.
- *History of hypertension, angina and heart attacks*: These are features of ischaemic heart disease. This can be associated with heart failure and leg oedema. The patient may also have peripheral vascular disease (see below).
- *Peripheral vascular disease*: It can present with leg pain, which may just occur on exercise (intermittent claudication) or at rest when it is usually worse when the foot is elevated.
- Other general medical problems such as anaemia, inflammatory bowel disease, renal impairment or liver disease. These conditions have associated cutaneous manifestations such as pruritus in anaemia, liver and kidney disease. Pyoderma gangrenosum is associated with inflammatory bowel disease.

Skin disease and skin care

Ask about the following:

- *History of eczema or psoriasis or any other skin condition.* If the patient admits to a skin condition, ask how long it has been present, and try to identify aggravating or relieving factors. In particular, ask which treatments are currently being used and whether they help. A history of eczema may mean that the patient has a skin that is more sensitive to irritants. Patients with psoriasis can demonstrate a phenomenon called koebnerisation which is when psoriasis develops in a break in the skin.

- *What is the patient's daily skin care regimen?* This is important because many patients use a range of products that can be irritant to the skin. This includes antiseptic creams, some shower gels and soaps, and alcohol wipes. Some patients may have developed true allergy to a product they are using, although this is more unusual.

What medication is the patient taking?

Understanding a patient's medication is important for two reasons:

- a skin problem may be a reaction to a medication;
- the medication will give clues to general medical conditions which the patient may not have mentioned.

Are there any known allergies?

Understanding a patient's allergies is important for two reasons:

- so that the healthcare professional avoids the use of a medication or topical treatment that may exacerbate or precipitate a problem;
- to clarify whether any of the current problems could be related to an allergic reaction to a product being used.

Patient examination: general considerations

Start your examination by getting an idea of the patient's general condition. For example, ask yourself whether the patient looks generally well or ill. It is useful to take the patient's temperature in a patient with red legs to help assess whether the problem is an infection or dermatitis. In a patient with swollen legs, it will be useful to get an idea of whether the patient has any cardiovascular/respiratory problems.

Skin examination

Wherever possible, and particularly where the patient has an obvious skin problem, the entire skin should be examined as well as hair, nails and mucosal surfaces. Good lighting is important and a magnifying glass is also useful. Without experience in dermatology you cannot be expected to know the correct terminology to use but there are some simple tips that will help you to be able to describe or discuss skin problems with other members of the multidisciplinary team. For example, check all over for dry skin, signs of scratching (excoriations), a widespread rash and any suspicious-looking skin lesions. Get an idea of the distribution, the extent and colour of any skin problem, the sites involved, symmetry, shape and arrangement. It may be helpful to touch the skin, for example if you suspect cellulitis then the abnormal skin will feel warmer than the surrounding normal skin. Examine the hair and nails and have a look at mucosal surfaces such as the conjunctivae, lips, gums, tongue and buccal mucosa. In drug reactions or blistering disorders, oral and genital ulceration may also be present.

Important common skin problems and their management

Long-term skin conditions

Eczema/dermatitis

The clinical features of all types of eczema and dermatitis are similar and include dry skin which is often red and scaly, sometimes with weeping. Typically, eczema is very itchy, and constant scratching can lead to secondary infection or impetiginisation. The management of all types of eczema is similar and is discussed at the end of this section.

Understanding the range of different types of dermatitis and eczema can be confusing for the non-specialist. By and large, the term eczema is used to describe poorly demarcated skin inflammation with surface changes such as scaling or thickening arising from an endogenous (from within) process, as opposed to those caused by external agents, where the term contact dermatitis is often used. Atopic eczema is by far the commonest endogenous eczema and occurs mainly in children and young adults and, although healthcare professionals should be aware of atopic eczema as it is so common, it is more likely that practitioners will encounter other types of endogenous eczema such as asteatotic, gravitational stasis and varicose eczema. By contrast, dermatitis is the term usually used to suggest an external factor, and contact dermatitis describes an inflammatory response occurring as a result of contact with external factors such as irritants or specific allergens.

Endogenous eczema

Asteatotic eczema

Asteatotic eczema is a common type of eczema that occurs typically on the lower legs of the elderly and is due to very dry skin. Asteatosis means 'without oil' and the condition occurs as a result of lack of fatty acids in the skin. Because the skin is dry, it no longer works as an effective barrier and so soaps and other irritant products such as bubble baths or shower gels tend to cause an inflammatory (eczematous response). The condition is also known as eczema craquele because the clinical appearance is 'cracked' (Figure 13.1). Although the condition is most commonly seen on the lower legs, it can be very widespread affecting the trunk and upper limbs. Typically, the skin is itchy and scratching exacerbates the problem.

Varicose and gravitational eczema

These terms are often used interchangeably by clinicians but this is not recommended. The term varicose eczema should be reserved for an eczematous change occurring on the lower legs in association with chronic venous disease. The prerequisite for this diagnosis is therefore an abnormality of venous return in the lower limb leading to venous hypertension and stasis. This may be secondary to a pre-

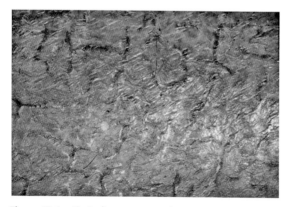

Figure 13.1   Typical appearance of asteatotic eczema in an elderly person. Photo courtesy of Annette Aldridge.

vious deep venous thrombosis and venous eczema can therefore be unilateral.

Gravitational eczema in contrast is usually bilateral and usually occurs secondary to chronic lower limb oedema such as heart failure. The clinical features of the eczematous changes will be similar with either discrete patches of eczema or circumferential changes. The term stasis is added to both of these terms, merely implying a degree of stasis of venous return in both situations. Although the management of the eczema will be the same in both conditions, the management of varicose eczema involves compression stockings whilst gravitational eczema may require modification of diuretic therapy in the first instance. Hence, it is important to be very specific, if possible, when using these terms. Inevitably in some patients both conditions will coexist and a dual approach to management of the underlying pathological process will be required.

Contact dermatitis

There are two types of contact dermatitis that look similar but are differentiated by their history. The distinction is important as investigations and management differ.

Irritant contact dermatitis

Irritant contact dermatitis is much commoner than allergic contact dermatitis and is due to frequent exposure to irritants such as soaps and detergents, for example in hairdressers and healthcare professionals. Anybody exposed to enough irritants is likely to develop irritant contact dermatitis, typically on the hands. However, trapped exudate under bandages or dressings may lead to irritant contact dermatitis and is often seen in patients with exudating venous leg ulcers. The skin damage is usually seen immediately below the wound where fluid leaks or collects under the influence of gravity.

Excessive washing with irritant products, such as soaps and shower gels, in patients with fragile skin such as the elderly, can also cause an irritant contact dermatitis (Figure 13.2). Incontinence-associated dermatitis (IAD) (see Chapter 2) is a type of irritant contact dermatitis that can be associated with pressure damage.

Allergic contact dermatitis

In allergic contact dermatitis, the individual develops a delayed hypersensitivity response to

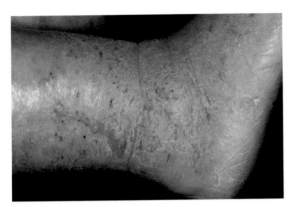

Figure 13.2 Typical appearance of varicose eczema typically associated with venous leg ulceration. Photo courtesy of Julia Schofield.

potential sensitising agents such as metals, perfumes, preservatives or rubber. Common skin sensitising agents can be seen in Table 13.1 and many vary in different geographical locations.

Only those people who are sensitised to that substance will develop a reaction, i.e. it is an idiosyncratic response. Allergic contact dermatitis is common in leg ulcer patients who have been exposed to lots of topical preparations over a long period of time when sensitisation occurs. They may have been using a product for some time before a reaction occurs so it is important to take a good history.

Variations in sensitisation to topical treatments occur in different countries which reflect local practices and availability of topical treatments, for example an increase in sensitivity to Balsam of Peru in leg ulcer patients in France was noted by Machet et al. (2004) in a retrospective review of sensitisation to topical treatments. Although a global decrease in

sensitisation rate with lanolin has been observed during the past 10 years, an increase in sensitisation to glucocorticoids and hydrogels is now being reported. Newer topical treatments and dressing products generally have very low rates of sensitivity with the exception of hydrogels (Machet et al., 2004).

Distinguishing between irritant and allergic contact dermatitis

Making a distinction between the two types of contact dermatitis can be difficult and requires specialist investigation using patch testing. This investigation requires specialist training and is provided by most consultant dermatologists in district general hospitals, with supra-specialist services providing regional patch testing services. A standard battery of allergens at non-irritant concentrations is applied to a patient's back using special chambers within an adherent patch. These are then removed 48 hours later, and a reading of the results is usually done at 96 hours after application.

A wide range of different allergen series is required for different suspected allergies. The skills needed for preparation and interpretation of the results require that this is an investigation that should be performed by dermatology specialists. When allergen positivity is demonstrated, provided it is relevant to the clinical condition, then allergen avoidance is recommended and may lead to cure of the dermatitis. In contrast, the management of irritant contact dermatitis requires attention to skin care and the avoidance of potential external irritants, such as excessive soap and wet work, which can be difficult to achieve in work places that require very frequent hand washing, such as nursing (Saary et al., 2005).

Table 13.1 Potential skin-sensitising agents

Potential allergen	Source
Rubber	Latex gloves, some elastic bandages, hosiery
Fragrances	Bath oils, moisturisers, cosmetics and baby products
Nickel	Jewellery, pens, razors, scissors
Lanolin	Bath additives, moisturisers, emollients, cosmetics and baby products
Topical antibiotics	Creams and ointments, e.g. neomycin, gentamicin
Emulsifier	Most creams/ointments including aqueous cream and steroids
Balsam of Peru	Creams, ointments, perfumes, cosmetics
Colophony	Sap from pine trees used to make medical adhesives, first-aid ointments, cleaning products

Source: Katsarou-Katsari et al. (1998), Diepgen et al. (2007).

Management of eczema

The key principles for the management of eczema are as follows:

- *Avoidance of all irritants*. This includes soaps, bubble baths, alcohol wipes, fabric conditioners and biological washing powders. Aqueous cream, which can be used as a soap substitute, can be an irritant in some patients if left on the skin as it contains sodium lauryl sulphate.
- Avoid the use of a wash-off soap substitutes such as aqueous cream or emulsifying ointment.
- Avoid the regular use of a 'leave-on' emollient to improve barrier function and correct dry skin. Greasier products are more effective than creams. The latter do not form a effective barrier and also contain preservatives which can act as contact sensitisers leading to the development of allergic contact dermatitis. Examples of greasy 'leave-on' emollients include emulsifying ointment and liquid paraffin:white soft paraffin in a ratio of 50:50. There are a range of proprietary products available and these will differ from country to country.
- Topical steroids are an essential part of the management of all types of eczema. In adults, a moderately potent or potent topical steroid is recommended. Short sharp bursts of more potent topical steroids are probably safer than prolonged courses of less-potent topical steroids. Steroid absorption is increased under occlusion which can work to advantage if used under dressings and bandages. Long-term side effects such as steroid atrophy can occur, but usually with prolonged use of potent topical steroids applied to normal skin.

Practice point

Topical steroids are classified by potency (e.g. mild, moderate, potent) of the topical steroid molecules. Potency can be altered by drug concentration and formulation e.g. cream or ointment and is an intrinsic property of the drug and not the same as concentration. Potency ranking is important to predict possible adverse effects.

Product labelling includes drug concentration and not potency which can be confusing. Concentration refers to the amount of steroid in the formulation e.g. clobetasone butyrate 0.05% and does not describe potency of the topical steroid. Clobetasone butyrate 0.05% has moderate potency, whereas, 1% Hydrocortisone has mild potency. It is often incorrectly thought that topical steroid drug concentration relates to potency. In fact, Betamethasone Diproprionate 0.05% is more potent than Hydrocortisone 1% despite the concentration of Betamethasone Dipropionate 0.05% being one-fifth of the concentration of Hydrocortisone 1% (Berth-Jones, 2010)

Topical steroids should *only* be used to control eczema if the above treatment has not been effective, e.g. avoidance of irritants, use of soap substitutes and regular use of emollients. Greasier emollients such as emulsifying ointment are particularly useful to protect the periwound skin surrounding venous leg ulcers. Topical steroids should only be used under the supervision of practitioners who have expertise with their use.

It is essential that even when the skin has recovered and the topical steroid use has discontinued, there is continued avoidance of irritants and use of a soap substitute and leave-on emollient. This should prevent the recurrence of symptoms and a flare of eczema.

Indications for specialist referral

The indications for specialist referral for patients with eczema include the following:

- failure to respond to topical therapy outlined above;
- for the investigation of suspected allergic contact dermatitis using patch testing;
- *diagnostic uncertainty*: if the condition does not respond to the measures above then the diagnosis may be incorrect.

Practice point

You can perform a simple patch test of a dressing or topical preparation yourself. Apply a small amount of the product to the skin under a piece of gauze fixed with tape to the forearm. After 48 hours, remove the dressing and the suspected allergen, marking clearly with a skin marker pen where the suspected allergen was applied. Check the skin after a further 48 hours and if the skin is normal then the patient does not have an allergic contact dermatitis to the product. If the skin reacts by becoming red, itchy and oedematous within the first 48 hours after the potential allergen has been removed this suggests that the patient may have sensitive skin that has become irritated by the product.

Psoriasis

Psoriasis is a common chronic inflammatory disease of the skin arising from a complex interaction between multiple genes, immunological and systemic and environmental factors (Gelfand et al., 2005). It is characterised by well-demarcated scaly plaques which tend to affect the backs of the elbows, knees, lower back, scalp and nails. Psoriasis may also be associated with arthritis (psoriatic arthritis) which can occur in a number of forms. As previously mentioned, patients with psoriasis can demonstrate a phenomenon called koebnerisation which is when psoriasis develops at the site of a break in the skin. Skin injuries caused by shaving, vaccinations, sunburn, surgery, pressure damage or adhesive dressings or tapes can make psoriasis worse.

Management

In addition to the provision of information about long-term management of psoriasis, management involves a range of topical therapies which include vitamin D analogues and tar (Brown et al., 2009). Topical steroids are sometimes used for sensitive areas but are usually to be avoided as they can cause psoriasis to become unstable. Second-line treatments of psoriasis include phototherapy and a range of immunosuppressant agents such as methotrexate, ciclosporin and newer biological therapies for severe recalcitrant disease. Oral retinoids such as acitretin are also used.

Indications for specialist referral

The indications for specialist referral include the following:

- diagnostic uncertainty;
- the need for second-line treatments.

Acute skin conditions

Cellulitis

Cellulitis represents a bacterial skin infection which usually affects a limb. The lower limbs are most commonly involved although any part of the body can develop cellulitis. The features of cellulitis include redness and swelling with increase in temperature of the skin. In more severe cases, blisters and, later, ulceration can occur. Although cellulitis is often localised, it can be extensive and patients can become quite unwell with malaise, fever and rigors. Sometimes there will be lymphangitis, which is manifest by a linear redness from the cellulitic area to the regional lymph nodes which may be swollen and tender. The skin often desquamates as the cellulitis resolves. In severe cases, septicaemia may occur and rarely necrotising fasciitis may occur which can be life-threatening. Any break in the skin can predispose to the development of cellulitis but there are particular systemic and local factors which make cellulitis more likely to occur.

These include the following:

General:

- diabetes mellitus;
- obesity;
- immunosuppression;
- pregnancy.

Local factors:

- peripheral vascular disease and/or oedema;
- previous episodes of cellulitis;
- venous disease +/− venous ulceration;
- lymphoedema including post-radiotherapy;
- recent injury such as trauma or surgical wound;
- tinea pedis/unguium (fungal skin or nail infection) of the affected limb.

Fungal skin infection has been shown to be a significant and easily treated risk factor for lower limb cellulitis (Lewis et al., 2006; Halpern et al., 2008). All patients who develop cellulitis of the lower limb should be examined and if appropriate treated for cutaneous fungal infection.

Management

As cellulitis is caused by a bacterial infection, the treatment is antibiotics. The commonest organism is *Streptococcus pyogenes* and less commonly *Staphylococcus aureus*. Appropriate antibiotics need to be prescribed and penicillin and flucloxacillin represent a sensible choice to cover both organisms. Local antibiotic prescribing policy and advice from the microbiologist should be sought, for example in penicillin-allergic patients. Many patients can be treated with oral antibiotics, but if there are signs of systemic illness then intravenous antibiotics and support may be necessary (Phoenix et al., 2012). In some centres this can be arranged in an outpatient setting or in a dedicated dermatology clinic, but if the patient is very unwell and there is any question of the development of necrotising fasciitis then hospitalisation is required (Wingfield et al., 2012).

Antibiotic therapy should be continued until there is no remaining evidence of infection (redness, pain or swelling) and this may be up to 14 days in some cases. Elevation of the limb to reduce swelling is important. Other general measures such as aspiration of blister fluid and attention to skin care are usually recommended (see Chapter 11).

> **Practice point**
>
> It is essential to identify and manage the underlying cause of the cellulitis to prevent recurrence. In patients with recurrent cellulitis secondary to conditions such as lymphoedema, long-term antibiotics may be necessary to prevent recurrence.

Indications for specialist referral

- patients with cellulitis who are unwell, particularly with fever and rapidly developing cellulitis;
- patients with recurrent cellulitis where further investigation and/or management of the underlying cause is necessary.

> **Practice point**
>
> Remember, that the elderly sometimes do not develop obvious signs of systemic infection such as fever but may have non-specific signs of systemic infection such as confusion, falls and drowsiness.

Pyoderma gangrenosum

Pyoderma gangrenosum is a relatively rare condition that causes painful, rapidly enlarging ulceration usually on the lower limb. This is commoner in people over 50 years of age. There are a range of underlying conditions that may predispose to the development of this condition and the common associations include the following:

- rheumatoid arthritis;
- inflammatory bowel disease (ulcerative colitis and Crohn's disease).

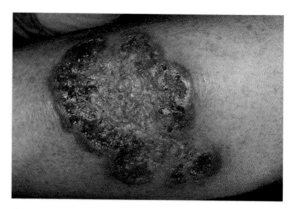

Figure 13.3   Ulceration associated with pyoderma gangrenosum. Photo courtesy of Annette Aldridge.

In a large number of patients no underlying cause is identified. The condition starts suddenly sometimes at the site of minor trauma as a pustule or patch of redness but the ulceration then develops rapidly and the resulting ulcer is deep and painful. The ulcer usually has an obvious purplish surrounding edge as seen in Figure 13.3. Ulcers may be multiple and sometimes coalesce. Even with correct management at an early stage, pyoderma gangrenosum can take a long time to heal and significant scarring is common.

Management

There is no role for surgery in the management of pyoderma gangrenosum; indeed surgical debridement is to be avoided as this can result in enlargement of the ulcer. Management of any underlying relevant systemic disease, such as inflammatory bowel disease, is essential as this may lead to an improvement in the pyoderma gangrenosum. A range of treatments are used depending upon the size and severity of the lesion. These include the following topical treatments:

- For small ulcers, a trial of potent topical steroids may be appropriate for 2–4 weeks. If no improvement is seen, then they should be discontinued.
- Appropriate wound care management should be done, including moist wound management and compression bandaging for a lower limb if there is no contra-indication, for example ischemia.

Systemic treatments that are used to treat pyoderma gangrenosum include the following:

- long-term dapsone and/or minocycline;
- systemic steroids;
- other immunosuppressant agents such as ciclosporin.

If there is surrounding secondary cellulitis then antibiotic therapy may be appropriate, but antibiotic therapy is not helpful for uncomplicated pyoderma gangrenosum.

Indications for specialist referral

- If this diagnosis is suspected then the patient should be referred for specialist assessment and treatment.

'Red legs'

The term 'red legs' is descriptive and not a true pathological diagnoses. Patients are often admitted to hospital with 'red legs' and many are treated empirically as having acute bilateral cellulitis. Bilateral cellulitis is uncommon and the more likely diagnosis in these patients is gravitational or venous eczema with or without secondary infection or allergic contact dermatitis or irritant contact dermatitis (see Figure 13.4). It is important to assess these patients appropriately to avoid unnecessary hospital admissions and intravenous antibiotic therapy (Wingfield et al., 2009).

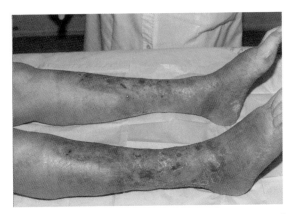

Figure 13.4 Patient with 'red legs'. Photo courtesy of Madeleine Flanagan.

Skin cancer and precancer

Introduction

Skin lesions account for about 50% of a UK dermatologist's workload relating to the diagnosis and management of skin cancer and precancer (Schofield et al., 2009). The incidence of these conditions is increasing year on year and so it is important to have an understanding of the common types of skin cancer and precancer. This section describes the aetiology and clinical features of these lesions.

Precancerous lesions

There are several so-called precancerous skin lesions of which the commonest that may be encountered in the context of skin integrity are solar keratoses and Bowen's disease. Whilst not truly benign, these conditions are not quite malignant. Solar keratoses are common on the sun-damaged skin of the elderly. Their association with the development of squamous cell carcinoma (SCC) is not clear-cut and spontaneous resolution of solar keratoses often occurs. Bowen's disease is less common but has the potential to progress to SCC.

Actinic keratosis

Solar keratoses are common on the light-exposed skin of fair-skinned people who have had a large amount of cumulative sun exposure. The relationship between sunlight and the development of solar keratoses is well documented (Marks et al., 1988). There is debate about the likelihood of malignant

---

Practice point

The key questions to ask when trying to determine the cause of 'red legs' are as follows:

(1) Is the patient ill?
(2) Does the patient have fever?
(3) What are the inflammatory markers? Are they elevated and suggestive of infection?

If the answer to one or more of these questions is yes, it is likely that the patient may have cellulitis or infected eczema (see Figure 13.4). If the answer to all three questions is no, then it is more likely that the patient has a primary dermatological problem which can be managed with topical treatments, probably in an outpatient setting. Some acute providers of dermatology services provide a 'red leg' assessment service which can usefully assess these patients and initiate an appropriate management plan.

change but it is generally accepted that the risk of transformation is very small, except in patients on long-term immunosuppression where this is a very real risk (Alam and Ratner, 2001). The characteristic appearance is that of a pink, scaly, warty, keratotic lesion on the face, scalp, ears and backs of the hands. The diagnosis is often confirmed by gently feeling the surface. Solar keratosis produces a rough, catching surface.

Bowen's disease

Bowen's disease is less common than solar keratosis and represents a skin tumour which has progressed one stage closer to the development of SCC. Also known as intraepidermal carcinoma *in situ* (the equivalent of cervical intraepithelial neoplasia in cervical cytology), it has the capacity to inevitably transform to SCC, although this may take many years. Spontaneous resolution does not occur. Bowen's disease presents as a persistent, well-demarcated, erythematous, scaly plaque on the lower limb of elderly people (Figure 13.5).

The plaque enlarges and may reach several centimetres in diameter. It may be easily confused with skin changes associated with venous ulceration.

Skin cancer

Skin cancer is the commonest type of cancer in human beings (Martinez and Otley, 2001). Skin cancers can be divided into two main types: melanoma and non-melanoma skin cancers (NMSC). NMSCs are principally basal cell carcinoma (BCC) or SCC,

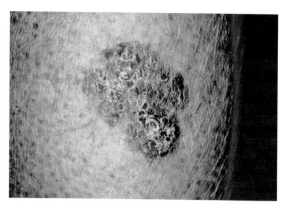

Figure 13.5   A patch of Bowen's disease on the lower leg. Photo courtesy of Julia Schofield.

although there are also other, rarer types such as cutaneous T-cell lymphoma.

Non-melanoma skin cancer

Age, skin type and amount of exposure to ultraviolet radiation are the key risk factors for NMSC. There are a number of other clinical situations that lead to patients having a predisposition to developing NMSC, the most important of these being as follows:

- People with so-called precursor lesions such as Bowen's disease and actinic keratoses: probably about 4–6% of Bowen's disease transforms to SCC (Eedy, 2000) and for actinic keratoses, transformation rates to SCC of 0.025–20% are reported (Alam and Ratner, 2001).
- Patients with a past history of NMSC: the risk of developing a second SCC within 3 years of having one is about 18%, and the risk of developing a second BCC within 3 years of having a BCC (or SCC) is about 44% (Marcil and Stern, 2000).
- Patients with long-term immunosuppression or altered immunity: particularly following renal transplant, where a 500-fold increased risk of NMSC has been reported (Hartevelt et al., 1990).
- BCCs very rarely metastasise but SCCs do, and mortality from NMSC is usually as a result of metastatic spread from SCC.

Basal cell carcinoma

BCC, also known as rodent ulcer, is the commonest type of skin cancer in Caucasian skin. This tumour is much commoner than any of the other malignant or pre-malignant tumours discussed in this chapter. Indeed it is the commonest form of malignant disease (Richmond-Sinclair et al., 2009). BCCs enlarge very slowly but can be highly invasive locally, especially when situated over areas of embryological differentiation. They are said not to metastasise. The commonest sites are the sun-damaged skin of the head and neck, especially in the elderly, who have had long periods of sun exposure over many years. The growing popularity of recreational sun exposure has resulted in an increased incidence of these tumours in younger people who may pick at the lesion causing chronic non-healing ulceration.

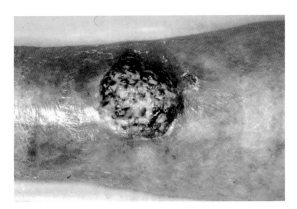

Figure 13.6   Non-healing venous leg ulcer with a large squamous cell carcinoma *in situ*. Photo courtesy of Julia Schofield.

Squamous cell carcinoma

SCC typically arises in the sun-damaged skin of the elderly, typically head, face and lips but can appear on any part of the body including the lower limbs. Figure 13.6 shows an advanced SCC that originally presented as a small 'ulcer' on the lower leg and had been unsuccessfully managed for many years as a venous leg ulcer.

SCCs are much less common than BCCs but incidence increases with age with decreasing latitudes such as the southern United States and Australia. SCC tumours can be aggressive and may arise *de novo*, or there may be a history of a preceding long-standing solar keratosis or a patch of Bowen's disease. They can develop where the skin has been damaged by radiation therapy or may appear in persistent chronic wounds such as venous leg ulcers.

The commonest early clinical presentation is of an indurated crusted keratotic plaque or nodule. The skin changes caused by SCC can be difficult to differentiate from other types of chronic wounds and often looks like a dry scab with thick, adherent scale on a red, inflamed base. The difference is that a SCC does not heal and may intermittently bleed. As the tumour spreads into the dermis, this type of skin cancer can appear like an ulcer with hard, raised edges.

SCCs do metastasise, although tumours arising in solar keratoses are particularly slow to do so. Lesions on the lip spread earlier and have a worse prognosis. The wound care practitioner needs to be vigilant as they may encounter SCC in the context of a non-healing leg ulcer; if suspicious, patients should be immediately referred to an appropriate specialist for assessment.

Malignant melanoma

Despite an overall increase in incidence of malignant melanoma over the past 25 years, melanoma remains a relatively uncommon tumour. However, mortality rates from melanoma are relatively high (Murchie, 2007). The link between sun exposure and melanoma is more complicated than for NMSC. The most significant risk factor is the number of melanocytic naevi (or moles). Red hair, freckles, acute exposure to sunshine in childhood and severe sunburn are all considered relevant risk factors. Incidence is 10–20 times lower in non-whites (Bataille and de Vries, 2008). There are increasing concerns about the use of sun beds in contributing to an increased risk of melanoma (Dale Wilson et al., 2012; Boniol et al., 2012). Although there has been a downturn in the incidence of melanoma in some parts of the world, the link between this and sun avoidance campaigns remains unclear (Bataille and de Vries, 2008; Whiteman et al., 2008) and mortality rates are essentially unchanged.

Malignant melanoma affects young adults, and females are affected more commonly than males. It is generally accepted that the tumour is commoner in those who burn rather than tan in the sun. In about 50% of cases, malignant melanoma presents as a new pigmented lesion, and in the remainder it occurs in a pre-existing lesion (Bataille and de Vries, 2008). Retrospective studies of patients with malignant melanoma have shown that the three most important worrying clinical signs in a pigmented naevus are *change in size, shape* or *colour* (Bataille and de Vries, 2008). Symptoms such as itching are much less important. The commonest type of malignant melanoma is the superficial spreading (80%). This is commonest on the legs of women and the trunk of men. It is a pigmented lesion, usually greater than 7 mm in diameter, and often with an irregular border as seen in Figure 13.7 (Bataille and de Vries, 2008). The pigmentation within the lesion is variable and in some parts may even be absent.

It is important to become familiar with these signs as the wound care practitioner may be the first person to identify a suspicious lesion especially on the lower leg and should immediately refer the patient for specialist assessment.

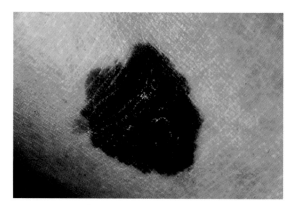

Figure 13.7   Malignant melanoma commonly presents on the lower leg. Photo courtesy of Julia Schofield.

Principles of management of skin cancer and precancer

Although it might be assumed that the management of most skin cancer and precancer is surgical, this is not always the case. In particular, for solar keratoses and Bowen's disease, better cosmetic outcome and low recurrence rates are achieved with medical management using topical treatments such as 5-fluorouracil, imiquimod and photodynamic therapy. Liquid nitrogen cryotherapy, curettage and cautery are treatment options for both conditions and Bowen's disease is sometimes treated with radiotherapy. BCCs and SCCs are usually surgically removed although radiotherapy may sometimes be appropriate. Malignant melanoma is treated by surgical excision, the tumour is not responsive to radiotherapy or current conventional chemotherapy and surgical excision currently provides the best outcome for survival.

> **Practice point**
>
> It may seem like a good idea to take a biopsy of a skin lesion or wound if unsure of the diagnosis, but this invasive procedure should be avoided by non-specialist practitioners for the following reasons:
>
> - The biopsy may be unnecessary as a suitably trained clinician might be able to make the diagnosis.
> - Biopsies only sample localised tissue and may be taken in the wrong area and miss the pathology altogether to give a false negative result (Frost and Adams, 2006).
> - Biopsy wounds may be difficult to heal and can be painful.

> - The pathology report may not be understood or acted upon.
>
> Biopsies should be taken under the guidance of a suitably trained dermatology specialist and should never be taken routinely or as a short cut to diagnosis.

Indications for specialist referral

Suspected skin cancer is best referred for specialist assessment and management. In England, there is very specific guidance about the management of all skin precancer and cancer published by the National Institute of Health and Clinical Excellence (NICE, 2006). The principles in the guidance include the management of precancers and low-risk BCCs by suitably trained primary care healthcare professionals with all other skin cancers managed by skin cancer multidisciplinary teams involving dermatologists, plastic surgeons, histopathologists and radiotherapists. Additionally in England, all suspected malignant melanomas and SCCs are referred and seen by a specialist according the so-called 2-week wait referral process (NICE, 2006). This national guidance sets out clear care pathways and time lines for the management of people with skin cancer in the United Kingdom and has begun to improve outcomes (NICE, 2006).

Provision of dermatology specialist services

Models of service delivery

Specialist dermatology services in some counties such as the United Kingdom and Australia are led by consultant dermatologists working with dermatology specialist nurses to provide a full range of specialist care. However, the availability, interest and enthusiasm of dermatologists in some parts of the world are variable. Where dermatologists are scarce, it is particularly important to identify a local dermatology champion, or if none is available then a physician or surgeon who has developed skills in this area. In some countries, the emphasis on cosmetic dermatology is making this more difficult and patients with skin disease may be suffering.

Wound management, skin integrity and dermatology services are closely linked. It is important for

Table 13.2   Examples of supra-specialist services and the type of conditions treated

Supra-specialist service	Type of conditions seen and services offered
Allergy services	Complex cases of allergic contact dermatitis or urticaria
Genetic dermatology	Rare inherited skin diseases affecting hair and nails, such as epidermolysis bullosa
Photodermatology	Skin disorders related to sunlight, including rare conditions such as porphyria and xeroderma pigmentosum
Lymphovascular services	Diagnosis and management services for patients with skin disease related to lymphovascular disorders
Connective tissue disorders	Joint working with rheumatologists for conditions such as systemic lupus erythematosus and a whole range of other conditions
Paediatric dermatology	Children with birthmarks requiring assessment and treatment
	Diagnosis and management of rare paediatric dermatoses
	Management of complex cases of common paediatric dermatoses, e.g. eczema
Inflammatory skin disorders	Psoriasis and eczema unresponsive to conventional treatment
	Immunobullous disorders
Inpatient services[a]	Severe inflammatory dermatosis, such as eczema, psoriasis, blistering disorders, where outpatient care has proved unsuccessful
	Life-threatening skin conditions, such as toxic epidermal necrolysis or other sick skin conditions
Dermatological surgery and laser unit [a]	Mohs micrographic surgery for skin cancers
	Laser treatment for birthmarks
Skin cancer services	Management of skin tumours; photophoresis services
Genital dermatology[a]	Management of genital dermatoses, including the multidisciplinary management of women with complex vulval disorders
Psychodermatology	The diagnosis and management of skin problems related to mental illness, including a multidisciplinary approach to psychological assessment and support
Specialist laboratory services	Immunohistochemistry, mutation analysis, prenatal diagnostic services, molecular diagnostic services using polymerase chain reaction (PCR)
Research	Recruitment of patients into studies of new therapeutic agents, such as biologic agents. Basic scientific research into the causes of skin disease

[a]Many hospitals offer these services, which should not necessarily be considered supra-specialist services but availability of services varies in different geographical locations.

wound management practitioners to develop links with a range of other specialists such as dermatologists and vascular surgeons and ideally they should have links to supra-specialist services that provide a range of specialist dermatology services. Table 13.2 gives examples of supra-specialist dermatology services and the type of conditions treated.

Summary

There is strong evidence that skin disease is very common and has a significant impact on quality of life and costs to healthcare systems. However, there is a worldwide shortage of suitably trained dermatologists. Even though skin problems are one of the commonest reasons that people present to primary care doctors, very few people are referred for specialist dermatology advice.

An understanding of skin disease is important to maintain skin barrier function and optimise wound healing. A thorough skin assessment that considers a range of dermatological factors will help optimise prevention, assessment and management of patients with impaired skin integrity. This chapter has demonstrated that there is a lot of overlap between wound management and dermatology. Wound management practitioners should improve their knowledge and understanding of dermatology and seek the opinion of local dermatologists where possible so that common and easily managed skin conditions are effectively treated. It is particularly important for patients with skin cancer or inflammatory dermatosis to receive prompt and appropriate management to avoid treatment delays and unnecessary suffering.

Useful resources

Guidelines for Management of Atopic Eczema. *Primary Care Dermatology Society and British Association Dermatologists*: Available at: http://www.bad.org.uk/Portals/_Bad/Guidelines/Clinical%20Guidelines/PCDS-BAD%20Eczema%20reviewed%202010.pdf

The Dermatologist is an electronic journal which shares practical dermatology tips, discusses current issues and summarises research: Available at: http://www.the-dermatologist.com/content/clinical-tips-5

Best Practice Statement. (2012) *Care of the Older Person's Skin*, 2nd edn. London: Wounds UK: Available at: http://www.wounds-uk.com/best-practice-statements/care-of-the-older-persons-skin-best-practice-statement-update

Denyer, J., Pillay. E. (2012) *Best practice guidelines for skin and wound care in epidermolysis bullosa*. International Consensus. DEBRA. Available at: http://www.woundsinternational.com/clinical-guidelines/best-practice-guidelines-for-skin-and-wound-care-in-epidermolysis-bullosa

Clinical Knowledge Summaries: nail and skin. Available at: http://www.cks.nhs.uk/home

Further reading

Penzer, R., Ersser, S. (2010) *Principles of Skin care: A Guide for Nurses and Health Care Practitioners*. Chichester: Wiley Blackwell.

References

Alam, M., Ratner, D. (2001) Cutaneous squamous-cell carcinoma. *New England Journal of Medicine*, 344, 975–983.

Basra, M.K.A., Finlay, A.Y. (2007) The family impact of skin diseases: the Greater Patient concept. *British Journal of Dermatology*, 156, 929–937.

Bataille, V., de Vries, E. (2008) Melanoma – Part 1: epidemiology, risk factors, and prevention. *British Medical Journal*, 337, a2249.

Berth-Jones, J. (2010) Topical treatments used in the management of skin disease. In: *Rook's Textbook of Dermatology* (eds T. Burns, S. Breathnach, N. Cox, C. Griffiths), 8th edn, Vol 4, Chapter 73, pp. 25–30. Oxford: Wiley-Blackwell.

Bickers, D.R., Lim, H.W., Margolis, D. et al. (2006) The burden of skin diseases: 2004 a joint project of the American Academy of Dermatology Association and the Society for Investigative Dermatology. *Journal of the American Academy of Dermatology*, 55(3), 490–500.

Brown, B.C., Warren, R.B., Grindlay, D.J.C., Griffiths, C.E.M. (2009) What's new in psoriasis? Analysis of the clinical significance of systematic reviews on psoriasis published in 2007 and 2008. *Clinical and Experimental Dermatology*, 34, 664–667.

Dale Wilson, B., Moon, S., Armstrong, F. J. (2012) Comprehensive review of ultraviolet radiation and the current status on sunscreens. *The Journal of Clinical and Aesthetic Dermatology*, 5(9), 18–23.

Davies, E., Burge, S. (2009) Audit of dermatological content of U.K. undergraduate curricula. *British Journal of Dermatology*, 160, 999–1005.

Diepgen, T.L. (2006) The costs of skin disease. *European Journal of Dermatology*, 16, 456–460.

Diepgen, T.L., Weisshaar, E. (2007) Contact dermatitis: epidemiology and frequent sensitizers to cosmetics. *Journal of the European Academy of Dermatology & Venereology*, 21(Suppl 2), 9–13.

Eedy, D.J. (2000) Non-melanoma skin cancer and the 'new National Health Service': implications for U.K. dermatology? *British Journal of Dermatology*, 142, 397–399.

Frost, T., Adams, J. (2006) An audit of skin specimens received over a five-year period, 2000–2004 inclusive, at a District General Hospital laboratory. *British Journal of Dermatology*, 155(Suppl 1), 58.

Gelfand, J.M., Weinstein, R., Porter, S.B., Neimann, A.L., Berlin, J.A., Margolis, D.J. (2005) Prevalence and treatment of psoriasis in the United Kingdom: a population-based study. *Archives of Dermatology*, 141, 1537–1541.

Halpern, J., Holder, R., Langford, N.J. Ethnicity and other risk factors for acute lower limb cellulitis: a UK-based prospective control study. *British Journal of Dermatology*, 158(6), 1288–1292.

Harlow, D., Poyner, T., Finlay, A.Y., Dykes, P.J. (2000) Impaired quality of life of adults with skin disease in primary care. *British Journal of Dermatology*, 143, 979–982.

Hartevelt, M.M., Bavinck, J.N., Kootte, A.M., Vermeer, B.J., Vandenbroucke, J.P. (1990) Incidence of skin cancer after renal transplantation in The Netherlands. *Transplantation*, 49, 506–509.

Katsarou-Katsari, A., Armenaka, M., Katsenis, K., Papageorgiou, M., Katsambas, A., Bareltzides, A. (1998) Contact allergens in patients with leg ulcers. *Journal of the European Academy of Dermatology and Venereology*, 11, 9–12.

Lewis, S.D., Peter, G.S., Gomez-Marin, O., Bisno, A.L. (2006) Risk factors for recurrent lower extremity cellulites in a US Veterans medical center population. *The American Journal of the Medical Sciences*, 332(6), 304–307.

Lopez, A.D., Murray, C.C. (1998) The global burden of disease, 1990–2020. *Nature Medicine*, 4, 1241–1243.

Machet, L., Couhé, C., Perrinaud, A., Hoarau, C., Lorette, G., Vaillant, L. (2004) A high prevalence of sensitization still persists in leg ulcer patients: a retrospective series of 106 patients tested between 2001 and 2002 and a meta-analysis of 1975–2003 data. *British Journal of Dermatology*, 150, 929–935.

Marcil, I., Stern, R.S. (2000) Risk of developing a subsequent nonmelanoma skin cancer in patients with a history of nonmelanoma skin cancer: a critical review of the literature and meta-analysis. *Archives of Dermatology*, 136, 1524–1530.

Marks, R., Rennie, G., Selwood, T. (1988) Malignant transformation of solar keratoses to squamous cell carcinoma. *The Lancet*, 331(8589), 795–797.

Martinez, J.C., Otley, C.C. (2001) The management of melanoma and nonmelanoma skin cancer: a review for the primary care physician. *Mayo Clinic Proceedings*, 76, 1253–1265.

Murchie, P. (2007) Treatment delay in cutaneous malignant melanoma: from first contact to definitive treatment. *Quality in Primary Care*, 15, 345--351.

National Institute for Health and Clinical Excellence [NICE] (2006) *Guidance on Cancer Services: Improving Outcomes for People with Skin Tumours Including Melanoma: The Manual*. London: NICE.

Phoenix, G., Das, S., Joshi, M. (2012) Diagnosis and management of cellulitis. *British Medical Journal*, 2012(345), 38–42.

Picardi, A., Abeni, D., Melchi, C.F., Puddu, P., Pasquini, P. (2000) Psychiatric morbidity in dermatological outpatients: an issue to be recognized. *British Journal of Dermatology*, 143, 983–991.

Richmond-Sinclair, N.M., Pandeya, N., Ware, R.S. et al. (2009) Incidence of basal cell carcinoma multiplicity and detailed anatomic distribution: longitudinal study of an Australian population. *Journal of Investigative Dermatology*, 129, 323–328.

Saary, J., Qureshi, R., Palda, V. et al. (2005) A systematic review of contact dermatitis treatment and prevention. *Journal of the American Academy of Dermatology*, 53, 845.

Schofield, J.K., Fleming, D., Williams, H.C. (2009) *Skin Conditions in the UK: a Health Care Needs Assessment*. Centre of Evidence Based Dermatology, University of Nottingham, pp. 1–158. http://www.nottingham.ac.uk/scs/divisions/evidencebaseddermatology/research/publications/index.aspx, last accessed on 19 November 2012.

Wingfield, C. (2009) Lower limb cellulitis: a dermatological perspective. *Wounds UK*, 5(2), 13–19.

Wingfield, C. (2012) Diagnosing and managing lower limb cellulitis. *Nursing Times*, 108(27), 18–21.

14 Surgical Wounds

Alan Widgerow

Laboratory for Tissue Engineering and Regenerative Medicine, Aesthetic and Plastic Surgery Institute, University of California, Irvine, CA, USA

Overview

- An acute surgical wound usually undergoes uncomplicated healing and rapid closure by primary intention.
- Measures used to maximise wound healing in surgical patients include keeping the patient warm, well hydrated, pain free and well oxygenated.
- The predominant complication that impedes wound healing in surgical wounds is surgical site infection (SSI).
- A postsurgical wound that does not close and undergoes further bleeding or exudate production and/or is painful after a 4-week period may be considered to be a chronic surgical wound.
- Patients should be given clear guidelines that relate to daily management of their wound, including dressing regime, bathing, activity restrictions and full description of warning signs indicating potential complications.

Introduction

Until fairly recently, the definition of a surgical procedure was one that creates a wound. With the advent of new technology and techniques, procedures such as those performed by natural orifice translumenal endoscopic surgery (NOTES) result in no external wound and may not quite fulfil the criteria of a surgical wound as defined by traditional terms. However, the vast majority of surgical procedures today still result in external wounds that may be complicated by delayed healing. So whether a surgical procedure is diagnostic or therapeutic, open exposure or minimal access, emergency or elective, incisional or excisional, the resulting wound is subject to the complex process of tissue repair and possible complications and thus requires a treatment plan to effectively manage the wound and subsequent scar.

Classification of surgical wounds

The healing of a surgical wound and its ultimate closure may follow a number of different pathways (Figure 14.1). The commonest surgical wound is one that heals by primary intention. Wound edges are approximated with sutures, clips or skin

---

Wound Healing and Skin Integrity: Principles and Practice, First Edition. Edited by Madeleine Flanagan.
© 2013 John Wiley & Sons, Ltd. Published 2013 by John Wiley & Sons, Ltd.

Mode of healing	Definition	Picture
Primary	Wound edges are brought together in apposition with sutures, clips or skin closure strips. Epithelialisation takes place within 48 hours and most of these wounds are sealed within the first 24–48 hours.	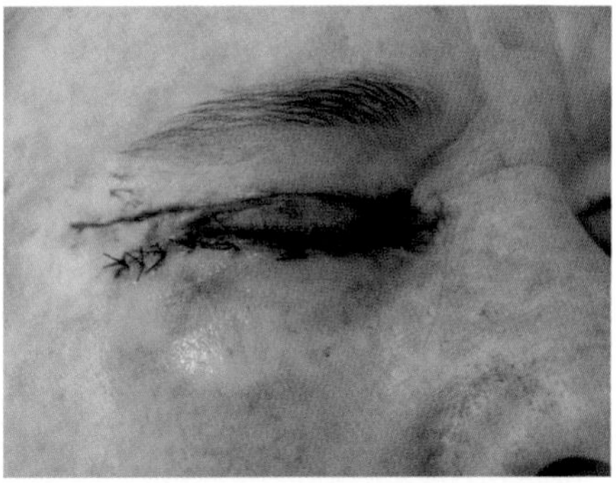
Secondary	A wound that is left open, intentionally or unintentionally, and heals by granulation tissue formation, contraction with or without eventual epithelialisation.	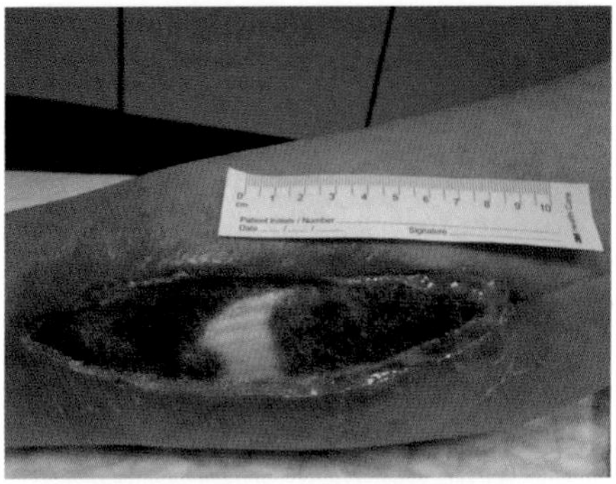
Tertiary	The wound is deliberately left open to allow for drainage, to compensate for major intra-compartment pressure or to control major contamination with the intention of undergoing additional surgery (delayed closure) to close the wound.	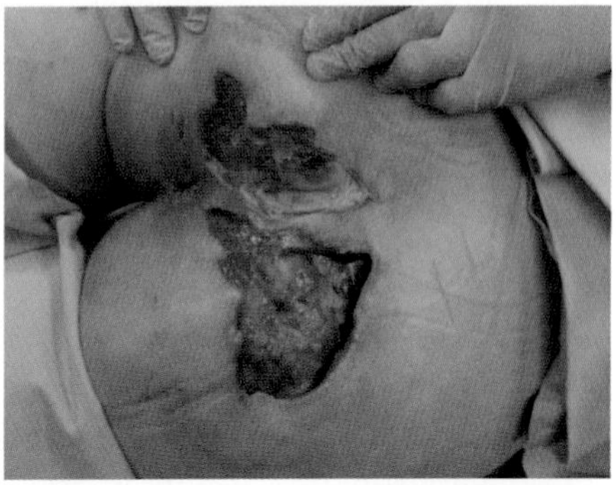 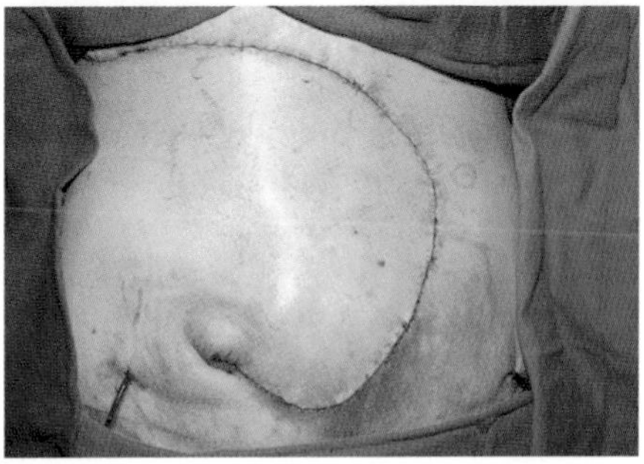

Figure 14.1   Healing pathways. Photos courtesy of Alan Widgerow (eye), Nuno Cunha (leg surgical wound) and Madeleine Flanagan (pressure ulcer and skin flap).

closure strips. Epithelialisation takes place within 48 hours and most of these wounds are sealed within the first 24–48 hours. Full thickness healing (not maturation) usually occurs within 8–10 days. This occurs rapidly as very little 'dead space' exists within the wound, so little new tissue needs to be produced to fill the healing void. The sequential generation of new tissue (repair) takes place from the depths of the wound up until migration of epithelial cells completes the process and forms a protective (although initially vulnerable) barrier for the skin surface. In wounds healing by primary intention, many of the biological processes that result in tissue repair occur simultaneously causing efficient, rapid wound closure. The only evidence of this complex biological sequence is often a small leakage of fluid (caused by the inflammatory process) or a bloody exudate, both of which usually diminish and resolve within the first few days.

A wound that is left open, intentionally or unintentionally, heals by granulation tissue formation from the base of the wound upwards, and contraction with or without eventual epithelialisation, in a process called secondary intention. Healing time depends on the amount of granulation tissue that is needed to fill the 'dead space' of the wound to initiate wound contraction, epithelialisation and closure. The greater the tissue loss in a wound healing by secondary intention, the longer it will take to heal due to the amount of granulation tissue that needs to be produced. Due to this process of protracted healing with significant granulation tissue and contraction, the scarring may be significant and extensive in wounds that heal by secondary intention.

In certain situations, a wound is deliberately left open to allow for drainage, to compensate for major intra-compartment pressure or to control major contamination with the intention of undergoing additional surgery to close the wound. This is sometimes referred to as tertiary intention healing or delayed closure. Once circumstances have improved in relation to the above parameters (controlled exudate, acceptable intra-compartmental pressure, clean wound), the patient is returned to the operating theatre to have their wounds surgically closed.

In addition, surgical wounds are classified according to bioburden and risk of infection (Cruse and Foord, 1980). Clean wounds are non-traumatic wounds created in a background of minimum inflammation where the surgical field is essentially sterile. Clean–contaminated wounds are those where anatomic areas with infective potential (gastrointestinal tract, respiratory tract) are entered but without significant contamination. A contaminated wound is one where trauma or surgery has resulted in significant contamination either from external foreign material exposure, for example, tar, grit from the road surface or internal spillage of contaminated contents from the gastrointestinal tract or similar anatomic areas. Dirty or infected wounds are those where obvious necrotic tissue, pus or potentially infective elements such as denuded bone fragments present within and complicate the wound at the time of surgery (Burns et al., 2003; Uçkay et al., 2010).

The ideal wound that surgeons strive to deal with is the acute surgical wound that undergoes uncomplicated healing and rapid closure. An acute wound by definition is one where skin and underlying tissue has undergone an interruption in integrity but wound closure follows a rapid, uneventful process. However, not all surgical wounds are in healthy tissue and delays in healing may be unavoidable if significant trauma (such as crush injuries) or grossly contaminated wounds present as a background to the surgical wound. In these types of circumstances, healing may be delayed over a longer time period than anticipated and a chronic wound develops. Much discussion has taken place over when an acute wound becomes chronic, and although many attempts have been made to define the chronic wound concept, it is perhaps easiest and most logical to label a wound as being chronic when it does not adhere to a normal healing sequence in terms of symptoms, signs or time to heal. So a surgical wound that exudes, bleeds, is excessively painful or merely takes longer to heal may well be on its way to chronicity and should be recognised as such. A wound that has not matured to its anticipated healing endpoint of closure and undergoes further bleeding or exudate production and is painful after a 4-week period may be considered to be a chronic surgical wound. To a certain extent this chronicity in surgical wounds can be avoided by the surgeon's attention to meticulous surgical technique, gentle tissue handling and good preoperative preparation of the patient. These factors contribute to rapid tissue healing in acute surgical wounds and are important elements that every surgeon should strive to achieve.

Principles of surgical wound management

The principles of surgical wound management are to provide optimal conditions for postoperative wound healing by:

- keeping patients warm, well hydrated, well oxygenated and pain free;
- controlling haemostasis;
- facilitating effective wound drainage;
- protecting the incision site;
- minimising surgical site infections and other postoperative complications;
- optimising scarring;
- providing appropriate postoperative information and aftercare.

Despite a lack of direct clinical evidence to support the provision of specialist wound care services for managing patients with hard-to-heal surgical wounds, clinical guidelines recommend a structured approach to patient management supported by guidance from specialist teams with wound management expertise (NICE, 2008).

Surgical wounds: assessment considerations

A range of factors have the potential to impact on surgical wound healing, wound closure and scarring including preparation of the patient and surgical facility, to the unique nature of the injury or individual disease, to the surgical technique, postoperative management and circumstances. Additional factors influencing surgical wound healing are those intrinsic to the patient, which affect them systemically. These include factors such as the age of the patient, concurrent disease or state of health, nutritional status and medications (Sørensen et al., 2005; Franz et al., 2008).

The process of aging is accompanied by inevitable physiologic changes that may impact on wound healing (Gosain and DiPietro, 2004; Rioux et al., 2006). Skin changes including decreased levels of collagen and elastin, and thinning of the dermo-epidermal junction result in fragility and vulnerability to injury and delayed healing (Gosain and DiPietro, 2004). Neutrophil quantity and function, macrophage phagocytosis, growth factor production and function, keratinocyte migration and epithelialisation may be impeded. Additionally, a decline in the immune system may result in increased susceptibility to postoperative infections. However, although historically healing in the aged was considered defective, there is now consensus that healing in the elderly may be delayed but the final aesthetic appearance of scars looks similar to that of young people (Gosain and DiPietro, 2004). In many cases, patients presenting for surgery have concomitant diseases that may have precipitated or contributed towards the surgical intervention, or could just be a compounding factor. The majority of these diseases or their treatments may slow the wound healing sequence. Diabetes, in particular with its associated microangiopathy, neuropathy and increased circulating glucose renders the patient more susceptible to wound complications which can seriously impact the body's capacity to heal normally. The cellular response to injury in diabetic patients is delayed, immune function is compromised and defects in collagen synthesis and deposition results in weakened strength of the final scar (Gottrup et al., 2005; Kao et al., 2009).

Other conditions that affect surgical wound healing on a circulatory basis include atherosclerosis (impaired perfusion), chronic venous insufficiency (peripheral pooling), anaemia or sickle cell disease (impaired oxygenation) and chronic obstructive pulmonary disease (reduced delivery of oxygen to the tissues) (Gottrup et al., 2005; Franz et al., 2008). Autoimmune diseases such as systemic lupus erythematosus and rheumatoid arthritis affect collagen deposition resulting in defective granulation tissue formation (Burns et al., 2003; Gosain and DiPietro, 2004; Gottrup et al., 2005).

Medications that affect wound healing include steroids, anti-inflammatory and immunosuppressive drugs. Most of these drugs affect various stages in the wound repair sequence including phagocytosis, inflammation, collagen deposition and angiogenesis (Gottrup et al., 2005). Radiation therapy also affects wound repair by disturbing leucocyte production and interfering with fibroblast function (Tibbs, 1997; Franz et al., 2008).

Healthy patients undergoing surgery do not usually have problems with their nutritional status. However, the elderly and medically infirm patients may have concomitant nutritional deficiencies which need to be taken into consideration when assessing patient's preoperatively.

Preoperative management

The ultimate goal as clinicians should be to min- imise the time patients spend in the hospital envi- ronment. The exposure to microorganisms, the inca- pacity or limited capacity of the patient in this envi- ronment and the psychological impact that hospi- talisation has the potential to complicate the wound healing process. Thus, the longer the patient has been in the hospital before surgery, the greater the potential for postoperative complications (WHO, 2009). Patients should have surgery as soon as their general health allows.

The most commonly cited complication of wound healing is that of SSI and much of the patient prepa- ration and 'good surgical practice' is aimed at pre- venting SSI. The most frequently identified risk factors for SSI are diabetes mellitus, age, obesity, incorrect antibiotic usage (or non-usage) (Lübbeke et al., 2008; Trussell et al., 2008; WHO, 2009; Uçkay et al., 2010). In addition, factors such as malnu- trition, steroid use, smoking, radiotherapy, and rheumatoid arthritis increase the likelihood of local infection and/or wound dehiscence. The follow- ing preventative measures are considered as having a high level of evidence (grade IA) in minimising SSI according to evidence-based guidelines (NICE, 2008; WHO, 2009; Uçkay et al., 2010):

- surgical hand preparation and skin preparation using chlorhexidine and alcohol;
- appropriate antibiotic prophylaxis;
- postponing of an elective operation in the case of active, systemic infection.

One of the most important strategies in avoiding SSI is that of surgical hand preparation. This relates to hand-cleansing preparation before undertaking wound procedures in other clinical environments such as hospital wards, outpatient departments as well as in the operating theatre. Semmelweis (1818– 1865) was the first to recognise the importance of hand antisepsis in his obstetric clinic. Using chlori- nated lime, he succeeded in lowering the incidence of postpartum maternal infection (Hugonnet and Pittet, 2000; Uçkay et al., 2010). Since that time, anti- sepsis and skin preparation has remained an impor- tant strategy in avoiding wound complications.

Investigators in the United States randomised skin preparation in 897 adults undergoing clean– contaminated surgery using chlorhexidine glu- conate (CHG) and alcohol or povidone iodine. SSI occurrence within 30 days was compared in the two groups. CHG–alcohol patients presented with a lower rate of SSIs overall (superficial and deep) (Darouiche et al., 2010). In another SSI rele- vant study, researchers in the Netherlands screened 6771 new patients to identify nasal carriers of *Staphylococcus aureus*. Total 1251 carriers were iden- tified and of these 918 were randomly treated with 2% mupirocin twice daily plus CHG soap for 5 days or with placebo treatment. SSIs, par- ticularly deep infections, were significantly lower in the mupirocin–CHG group (Bode et al., 2010). This current recommendation for skin prepara- tion would advise CHG–alcohol in preference to povidine iodine. However, treating carriers of *S. aureus* as described above is less clear, it is possi- ble that preoperative skin preparation or bathing with CHG–alcohol may be as effective in prevent- ing SSIs without extra expense of treating carri- ers, but this still needs proof. Thus, current recom- mendations for treatment for carriers is reserved for high-risk procedure patients such as cardiac surgery, orthopaedic implants, etc. (Bode et al., 2010; Darouiche et al., 2010; Wenzel, 2010).

Preoperative surgical hand preparation was subject to a Cochrane review (Wenzel, 2010). Hand rubbing with an alcohol-based formulation was considered as effective as scrubbing. The minimum duration appears to be 2–3 minutes for both meth- ods. Overall, patient bathing/showering 24 hours prior to surgery using CHG–alcohol preparations and skin preparation with the same combination at the start of surgery appears to be the current favoured method of preoperative skin preparation.

In the majority of surgical procedures performed today, prophylactic antibiotics are administered. However, clean elective short-duration surgery not involving implant insertion, dermatologic surgery and certain smaller foot and ankle procedures do not warrant preoperative antibiotic prophylaxis (NICE, 2008; WHO, 2009; Uçkay et al., 2010). In most cases, first or second-generation cephalosporins administered as a single dose 30–60 minutes prior to the procedure is sufficient as antibiotic prophylaxis (McDonald et al., 1998; Uçkay et al., 2010). Surgi- cal procedures lasting longer than 4 hours or those involving major blood loss may warrant a second dose of antibiotic, although this too is not defini- tive and should be decided according to individual circumstances (Weber et al., 2008). Essentially, very few situations (except significant trauma, exposure of large areas of the body) warrant antibiotic prophylaxis for longer than 24 hours (Prokuski, 2008; WHO, 2009; Uçkay et al., 2010).

As far as preoperative hair removal is concerned, clipping rather than shaving is recommended by consensus guidelines (NICE, 2008; WHO, 2009), although the evidence is of poor quality and still open to scrutiny (Uçkay et al., 2010). Shaving appears to subject the patient to risk because of the potential for skin damage and ingrown hairs. The length of time between shaving and surgery appears to be relevant; the longer the time the greater the risk of damage to the skin barrier. If shaving is essential, it should be performed as close to the time of surgery as possible (Cruse and Foord, 1980). No trials are evident comparing efficacy of clipping with a depilatory cream. However, the evidence found no difference in SSIs among patients who have had hair removed prior to surgery and those who have not (Sax et al., 2007; Uçkay et al., 2010).

Hair clipping before surgery is now considered a matter of debate. It appears to be preferable to recently shaved areas especially if accompanied by traumatic cuts or ingrown hair but may have no advantage over clean unshaven areas (Tanner et al., 2008; Uçkay et al., 2010; Wenzel, 2010).

Other interventions such as avoiding hypothermia, hypoglycaemia, supplementary oxygen, etc., all have important parts to play in a multimodal approach to wound care in a surgical patient but further scientific validation is still needed to demonstrate the clinical efficacy of many of these parameters.

Intraoperative management

Most SSIs are believed to be acquired during surgery (Ayliffe, 1991; Uçkay et al., 2010). Prevention measures in the surgical theatre have contributed to decreased SSIs. However, the actual proportion of SSI acquired in the operating theatre versus postoperative care on hospital wards and the proportion of infections originating from the patient, the environment or from surgical staff is still not known (Uçkay et al., 2010).

The risk of postoperative wound infection is related to the patient's general health and existing comorbidities, the nature of the injury or delayed presentation. However, there is a definite correlation with the events and factors occurring during the surgical period that impact on postsurgical complications as seen in Table 14.1.

To begin with, the duration of surgery is important. In an American study, Procter et al. analysed nearly 300,000 general surgery operations performed at 173 hospitals with the National Surgical Quality Improvement Program (NSQIP) database. They demonstrated that length of hospital stay (LOS) increased as the operative duration increased. LOS increased by about 6% per every 30 minutes of operative duration. The 30-day rate of infectious complications rose by almost 2.5% for every 30 minutes of operative duration (start of incision to closure). That rate increased to 31.4% for cases that took more than 6 hours to complete (Procter et al., 2010). Thus, the expertise of the surgeon has definite impact on healing not only from a tissue handling and surgical technique perspective but also time spent in the operating theatre.

Gentle tissue handling, dissection within tissue planes conserving blood supply, maintaining haemostasis, good judgement in removal of nonviable tissue and foreign material, elimination of dead space and tension-free closure are all important factors that relate directly to surgical experience and expertise and impact on time to healing and scarring (Franz et al., 2008; Aggarwal and Darzi, 2008; Procter et al., 2010). A certain degree of tissue trauma during surgical procedure is inevitable. Furthermore, compromising the blood supply by indiscriminate surgical exploration and tissue manipulation or by promoting haematoma formation will ultimately result in increased complications such as SSIs. Suturing techniques should facilitate tension-free closure and closure of the deeper tissue spaces by subcutaneous buried suturing (WHO, 2009). Wound edges should be everted, and sutures placed equidistant apart with dermal and epidermal approximation. Where possible following subcutaneous closure of tissue, wound-edge approximation should be undertaken with subcuticular sutures hidden beneath the skin. This avoids unsightly scarring produced by large external sutures.

An often overlooked intraoperative factor that may have a major impact on wound healing is temperature control. This relates to ambient theatre temperature and its bearing on patient temperature. Hypothermia is the situation that needs

Table 14.1   Extrinsic factors affecting surgical wound healing

Timing	Factors impacting healing (extrinsic)	Recommendations
Pre-operative	Patient anxiety and stress Skin preparation Preoperative hair removal Antibiotic prophylaxis	Explain surgical procedure and postoperative management of the wound
		CHG and alcohol
		Clipping in preference to shaving; if shaving has to be done, do as close to surgery as possible
		Clean, elective, short surgery – Hair removal not necessary
		Longer surgery, implants, contaminated – Hair removal recommended
Intra-operative	Duration of surgery Surgical technique Temperature control Normoglycaemia Anaesthesia	Minimise length of surgical procedure
		Gentle tissue-handling, good haemostasis, well-judged debridement, careful closure
		Maintain ambient theatre temperature, avoid exposing patient, cold infusion fluids; avoid hypothermia, keep patient warm
		Maintain balanced blood sugar levels, hypoglycaemia may impact on postoperative infection
		Keep the patient well hydrated, well oxygenated and pain free
Postoperative	Dressing regimen Wound drainage Wound cleansing Patient compliance	Tension free; care with circumferential dressings, check ability of dressing to absorb wound fluid
		Encourage free drainage of wound fluid, prevent haematoma formation
		Careful choice of non-toxic cleansing agents
		Good patient education re wound care, dressing change, vigilance for signs of complications and skin care
All	Patient factors: advancing age comorbidities tissue perfusion smoking poor nutritional state obesity	Optimise the patient's preoperative condition to reduce the risk of postoperative complications

Source: Data from NICE (2008), Franz et al. (2008) and WHO (2009).

to be avoided intraoperatively which may result from cold theatres, exposed patients, cold infusion fluids and inadequate patient resuscitation. Controlling temperature requires the co-operation of facility managers (theatre temperatures above 36°C), anaesthesiologist (fluids, resuscitation), theatre scrub nurse (cleaning, exposure) and surgeon (exposure, time, surgical expertise preventing major blood loss, etc.). Several studies have shown the benefit of normothermia to optimise wound outcome and patient recovery (Kumar et al., 2005; Scott and Buckland, 2006; Uçkay et al., 2010). Hypothermia appears to affect cellular function relating to haemostasis, coagulation, immune competence and endocrine systems (Uçkay et al., 2010).

Warming of the patient during surgery should form an integral part of intra- and postoperative care of the surgical patient (Fakhry et al., 2012). Maintenance of normoglycaemia in the intraoperative and immediate postoperative period appears to be important in avoiding postoperative infections, although the evidence for this is less apparent than that for normothermia (Kao et al., 2009; Uçkay et al., 2010).

Postoperative management

In practical terms, measures used to maximise wound healing include keeping the patient warm, well hydrated, pain free and well oxygenated. Surgery itself results in catabolic stress response that may impair wound healing. This response results in a sympathetic nervous system release of catecholamine mediators that can result in vasoconstriction which may be released by hypoxia, hypovolaemia or hypothermia postoperatively (Haridas and Malangoni, 2008; Kao et al., 2009; Uçkay et al., 2010).

Wound drainage

Excessive bleeding may result from inadequate intraoperative haemostasis or background systemic problems such as disseminated intravascular coagulation (DIC). Either way a haematoma constitutes a 'space-occupying lesion' impeding circulation due to direct mechanical pressure and from indirect effects from toxic metabolites secreted by the haematoma itself (Keep et al., 2005). Sutures should be removed, the haematoma adequately evacuated and the wound thoroughly cleansed and allowed to heal by either secondary intention or closed once the risk of infection has diminished.

Wound drainage decisions by the surgeon are important, particularly if excessive drainage, bleeding, dead space or cavities are anticipated. Open or closed drainage systems are appropriate for different clinical situations and also depend on surgeon preference.

Wound closure

Wound strength is weakest at approximately 2–3 weeks postoperatively, often coinciding with removal of external sutures and is weaker in older patients and those with a low serum albumin (Lindstedt and Sandblom, 1975). Sutures should be removed as soon as the wound can withstand external tension forces. Timing varies but generally facial wound sutures are removed earliest (5 days), abdominal and orthopaedic sutures usually later (7–14 days). In areas of less tissue tension such as the face and/or where a layered closure has been performed, sutures may be removed at 5–7 days; high-tension areas may necessitate removal of sutures anywhere from 10 days to 3 weeks. Slow

absorbing (or on occasion non-absorbing) subcuticular sutures buried beneath the skin provide for long-term wound support.

A delicate balance exists between wound dehiscence and scarring caused by leaving sutures in too long or spreading of the surgical scar due to premature removal. Clips and staples should be removed at the earliest possible time to avoid 'cross hatch' scarring (marks caused by the staples crossing the incision line). Of course the surgeons' preference (related to suture technique, materials, etc.) is important in this decision-making process.

The suture used most commonly by plastic surgeons for skin closure is a slowly absorbable monofilament suture placed subcuticularly beneath the skin in the dermis in a continuous fashion. This allows good long-term stability of the skin edges with minimal reaction (monofilament vs. multifilament) and no external skin marks. For smaller areas (face, etc.) interrupted (separate) sutures of non-absorbable material is commonly used as these areas usually are not closed under tension and the sutures are removed early so skin marks are unlikely. Aside from these two common occurrences, a whole host of absorbable sutures is used particularly to close subcutaneous layers. These sutures are seldom used externally on the skin except where removal could be problematic (children) or inaccessible (groin, scalp, axilla, etc.). Skin glue may be used after suture removal to absorb tension or common tapes such as microporous tape may be used for supporting the maturing scar.

Practice point

Is it safe to get wound sutures wet?

Stitches can get wet under most circumstances. The old adage that all stitches must remain dry is no longer true. Sometimes the surgeon dresses the wound with a complex dressing and instructs that sutures are kept dry as a soaked soggy dressing is a focus for infection. However, if the stitches are exposed (small area) and the patient showers in clean running water rather than bathes in dirty water, contact of the area with clean running water will do no harm. However, every circumstance is different and the surgeon's input is clearly a prerequisite before wetting the stitches.

Wound dressings: special considerations

Postoperative wound dressings must absorb wound fluid, allow moisture vapour permeability, be waterproof, act as a bacterial barrier, be atraumatic on removal and non-sensitising to the wound and periwound skin as well as cost-effective.

One of the most practical choices for postoperative dressings is an adhesive polyurethane film incorporating an absorbent pad. There are many variations of this type of dressing which if frequently used following surgery: selection depends on availability, cost-effectiveness and patient preference.

No definitive conclusions can be drawn about the effectiveness of postoperative wound dressings from current studies. A Cochrane review assessed the effectiveness of various dressings and topical agents on surgical wound healing and concluded that the qualities of studies were insufficient to determine any superiority of dressing protocol or topical agent over another (Vermeulen et al., 2004). Although no specific dressing regimen has been shown to be of more value, dressings should be chosen to suit the particular conditions at the incision site and monitored carefully for strike-through or leakage.

Practice point

Are postoperative dressing necessary in smaller sutured wounds?

Although elaborate postoperative dressings are not necessary in smaller surgical wounds, using a small postoperative pad, or microporous tape as a dressing to protect the suture line and provide hydration and prevent drying out of the wound exudate is important. This minimises the inflammatory process needed for the body to remove an eschar and promotes optimal scarring.

Patient postoperative wound care advice should include specific instructions about when dressings need to be changed and abandoned for good. It would be convenient to prescribe a set of rules pertaining to timing of first dressing change, frequency of dressing change and type of dressing recommended for surgical wounds. In reality, most studies to date including a Cochrane review (Vermeulen et al., 2004) have failed to definitively provide an ideal set of principles for a postoperative wound care regimen. Instead the logical approach is to revert to the basic principles described in Table 14.2.

Practice point

When can postoperative dressings be safely removed and not replaced?

Initial wound dressing changes are variable and depend on the direct wound properties (exudate, bleeding, redness, infection), the nature of the reconstruction (simple closure, skin graft, flap) and the circumstances that the patient finds themselves in (hospital, home with expert help, home with inadequate help). This should form part of the discharge instructions that the patient is given prior to discharge. In many cases, the first wound inspection is done by the surgeon before the patient leaves the hospital. Postoperative dressings can be safely permanently removed in two circumstances: first, when full epithelialisation and healing has taken place; and second, once protective coverings are no longer needed which varies depending on the wound type, location and initial size. Although it may appear that the two events are simultaneous, a newly epithelialised skin surface or a freshly healed skin grafted area is still very vulnerable to damage from mechanical trauma such as from scratching or from friction from clothing and may need protection for longer. Therefore, every wound should be assessed on an individual basis depending on the nature of the skin covering and the type of operative closure.

Factors delaying healing in the presurgical, surgical and postsurgical periods involve extrinsic factors, which are those related to the physical environment, the nature of trauma or type of surgical procedure, the expertise of the surgeon and anaesthetist and the postoperative care (Table 14.1). Other extrinsic factors that commonly detrimentally affect wound healing include alcohol abuse and smoking. Both affect the immune system, interfere with healing and may be associated with exaggerated scarring (Wong et al., 2004, Franz et al., 2008).

Surgical wound infection

Wound infection in surgical wounds is characterised by redness, pain, heat, swelling of the wound and periwound area and is essentially the same as in any other type of wound. However, these signs can be confusing as they are similar to the normal inflammatory response seen in wound healing in the first few days postoperatively, but if the

Table 14.2   General principles: post operative management of surgical wounds

Principle	Action	Reference
• Maintain haemostasis; anticipate post operative bleeding or in some cases pre-operative bleeding, e.g. traumatic injuries to facilitate free drainage	Select absorptive dressings to match anticipated wound symptoms and/or suitable drainage system (open or closed) to promote drainage.	Vermeulen et al. (2004)
• Optimise local wound healing environment	Select an appropriate dressing and topical agent for surgical wounds healing by secondary intention.	Vermeulen et al. (2004) NICE (2008)
• Apply dressings without tension, especially circumferential dressings to minimise circulatory problems, e.g. ischaemia, tissue necrosis, skin blisters	During application of circumferential dressings apply a temporary 'spacer' that is removed on completion to release tension.	NICE (2008)
• Provide effective pain control	Prescribe adequate analgesic cover for post-operative period and dressing changes. Use appropriate low adherent dressings.	SIGN (2004) WHO (2009)
• Improve aesthetic appearance of incision by using appropriate wound closure techniques	Consider use of tissue adhesives to close clean surgical incisions excluding areas of high tension. No difference in healing between sutures, tapes and adhesives.	Brolmann et al. (2012)
• Minimise risk of SSI and other related post operative complications	Implement meticulous surgical hand preparation and patient skin preparation using chlorhexidine and alcohol.	NICE (2008) WHO (2009)
	Antibiotic prophylaxis is not necessary for clean, elective, short duration non prosthetic surgery.	NICE (2008) WHO (2009)
	Avoid topical antimicrobial agents for surgical wounds that are healing by primary intention.	NICE (2008) Vermeulen et al. (2004)
	Use sterile saline for wound cleansing up to 48 hours after surgery.	NICE (2008)
• Optimise post operative scar quality	Control inflammation, hydrate & support scar. Support incisional scars prone to vector forces with microporous tape/dressings applied longitudinally along the scar.	Mustoe (2002) Austin et al. (2011)
• Patients require adequate information about post operative wound care and vigilance for signs of complications	Advise patients that they may shower safely 48 hours after surgery.	NICE (2008)
	Clear instructions must be given in relation to getting sutures or other methods of skin closure wet and what signs and symptoms to be aware of relating to complications.	SIGN (2004) NICE (2008) WHO (2009)

signs persist or get worse and a purulent discharge appears or the patient becomes systemically ill, a wound infection is likely. One of the most reliable indicators of wound infection is pain or soreness in and around the wound. Patient reports of discomfort should alert the clinician to the possibility of early wound infection even if there are no obvious clinical signs of infection (Gardner et al., 2001) (Box 14.1).

Immediate management of wound infection may relate directly to surgical technique. If wounds are closed with excessive tension, sutures or clips can cause local vascular compromise and necrosis providing the ideal conditions for wound infection. Sutures (either all or alternate) need to be removed urgently to conserve tissue viability. Foreign materials such as drains should be removed and the wound should be thoroughly cleaned and a dressing regime implemented that can cope with increased exudate. Occasionally, if infective signs are recognised early enough, local topical (in critically colonised wounds) or systemic antimicrobials

Box 14.1   Characteristics of surgical site infection

- Occurs within 30 days of the surgical procedure;
- involves skin or subcutaneous tissue around the incision (superficial) or deeper soft tissues, such as the fascia and muscles (deep).

May involve one or more of the following:

- increasing tenderness/pain around incision area;
- localised oedema, redness, discolouration, heat, cellulites;
- increased wound fluid;
- purulent discharge from incision;
- offensive odour from incision site;
- abscess formation;
- delayed healing of incision;
- spontaneous wound dehiscence;
- evidence of infection from histopathology (organisms isolated from culture of fluid or tissue), or radiology.

(WHO, 2009)

may solve the problem without reopening the wound. These efforts should be tried initially but if a purulent discharge is present, in most cases the surgical wound will require drainage and cleansing. A treatment plan can then be implemented for delayed wound closure once the infection is under control.

Postoperative surveillance of infection rates is an essential component to the prevention of SSI (WHO, 2009). In studies conducted in Brazil, Holland, the United Kingdom and the United States, SSI rates were reduced by 33–88% when feedback was given directly to the surgeon and staff complied to standardised infection control policies (Trussell et al., 2008; Uçkay et al., 2010). As the majority of postoperative superficial SSIs occur within 28 days of surgery, 30 days is now the accepted length of surveillance for infections after operations that do not involve prosthetic implantation (WHO, 2009).

Regular patient follow-up visits should be scheduled after surgery. Patients should be given clear guidelines prior to discharge relating to the daily management of their wound including dressing regime bathing, activity restrictions and a full description of signs and symptoms that may indicate wound infection. It is estimated that without postdischarge wound surveillance, at least 50% of

SSIs may remain undetected and under-reported (Uçkay et al., 2010).

Management of surgical scars

The end result of any surgical procedure or wound healing is scarring. Controlling the process and influencing the outcome of scarring is far more achievable than in previous years (Mustoe et al., 2002). This is because much of the biological sequence and the signalling mechanism occurring at a cellular level is now better understood (Widgerow et al., 2009; Widgerow, 2011a). Inflammation is a necessary sequence in all wound healing mechanisms. However, prolonged or excessive inflammation results in exaggerated scars. A set of principles that appears to minimise scarring has been published which include support, controlled inflammation, adequate hydration and remodelling/maturation of collagen (Mustoe et al., 2002; Widgerow et al., 2009; Widgerow, 2011a, 2011b; Bush et al., 2011). These principles form the basis upon which strategies for scar control can be formulated. Simply put, scar management should satisfy the principles of the acronym SCAR (support, controlled inflammation, adequate hydration, remodelling of collagen).

Supporting a scar, particularly a long surgical scar, in areas where vector forces continually pull on the scar has long been recognised as beneficial to scar outcome (Hugonnet and Pittet, 2000; Burns et al., 2003; Uçkay et al., 2010). Take, for example the presternal chest area where forces are generated on the scar from neck, shoulder and arm movements and additionally from the weight of breasts in some women (Figure 14.2).

The direct response to such vector forces is increased production of collagen in an effort to keep the wound closed. Vitamin E has a collagenase-like effect, which may weaken the scar and lead to stretching of scar tissue (Baumann et al., 1999).

The best and least expensive form of scar support is the microporous tape which is a breathable porous tape (not plastic or fabric) (Widgerow et al., 2000; Atkinson et al., 2005). The tape must be applied longitudinally along the scar path and not at right angles as seen in Figure 14.3.

This ensures that support is consistent and not intermittent in some areas. The tape should not be

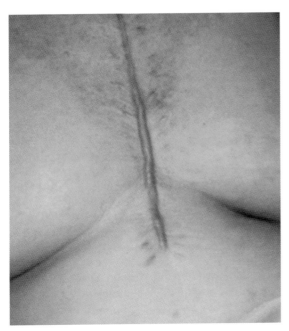

Figure 14.2 Hypertrophic presternal scar in female patient. Photo courtesy of Alan Widgerow.

removed but left in place for as long as possible until it spontaneously separates from the skin or becomes tatty. Premature removal of the tape results in skin stripping which sets up an inflammatory response with negative consequences for the scar. Although small surgical scars may not need support, some

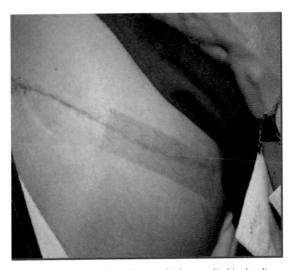

Figure 14.3 Application of tape which is applied in the direction of the scar. Photo courtesy of Alan Widgerow.

small scars heal very well with this simple method of occlusion and support.

Practice point

Cuts on fingers are continually stressed with external forces. Application of a single layer of microporous tape is an ideal method of supporting the scar and avoiding maceration, which is sometimes seen with common plasters as this helps to speed up the maturation process.

Hydration of the scar surface is the basis of action of 90% of scar management treatments currently available (Liu et al., 2011). Most oils, lotions, creams and dressings have beneficial effects on scars purely based on their hydrative capacities (Mustoe et al., 2002; Tandara and Mustoe, 2008). Healthy skin has a mature stratum corneum characterised by minimal transepidermal water loss (TEWL). Damage to the stratum corneum stimulates keratinocytes to produce cytokines, which activate dermal fibroblasts to synthesise collagen. Excessive collagen production is known to cause abnormal scarring (Mustoe et al., 2008).

An effective barrier to TEWL from the stratum corneum is silicone (either in the form of dressing sheets or gels) or plant-derived gels which have been popular for many years for scar management (Mustoe et al., 2008; Tandara and Mustoe, 2008; Widgerow, 2011b). Although silicone is frequently used in the management of larger scars or hypertrophic scars, the evidence of efficacy and mechanism of action are inconclusive (Namazi et al., 2011). A Cochrane review cites 13 trials involving 559 patients and concludes there is weak evidence of benefit of silicone gel sheeting as a prevention for abnormal scarring in high-risk individuals, due to poor-quality studies that are susceptible to bias (O'Brien and Pandit, 2006). Despite the lack of conclusive evidence of its efficacy and mechanism of action, silicone gel will likely continue to be used in scar treatment protocols because it is a non-invasive modality with few adverse effects and is preferred by many patients over invasive procedures such as intralesional steroid injections (Reish and Eriksson, 2008). Interestingly, animal studies comparing silicone dressings to occlusion with microporous tape for small surgical incisions have shown no significant differences in scar quality (O'Shaughnessy et al., 2009; Tollefson et al., 2012) prompting calls for further investigation in humans.

Keloid and hypertrophic scarring arises often as a natural consequence to normal scarring where exaggeration takes place because no scar management has been instituted or where suturing technique is lacking or infection has occurred. The scar steadily increases in its collagen composition and grows according to the placing of the incision (does not overgrow its boundaries). The natural history of a hypertrophic scar is gradual resolution over approximately 1 year with the scar colour changing from pink to white, and the scar flattening and remaining as a broad flat scar (see Chapter 3). Optimal scar management can prevent this occurrence in up to 80% of postsurgical clean incision wounds (Widgerow et al., 2009).

The principles of scar management (support, hydration, scar maturation through collagen modulation and controlled inflammation) are applicable to the prevention of hypertrophic scarring but *do not* relate to keloid scarring which is a completely different mechanism of scarring and important to recognise (Wolfram et al., 2009). Management of keloid scars should be referred to a plastic surgeon with expertise in this area.

Common reconstructive surgical options

A split-thickness skin graft is made up mainly of epidermal components interspersed with occasional dermal remnants as seen in Figure 14.4.

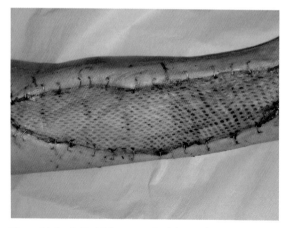

Figure 14.4   Split-thickness meshed skin graft. Photo courtesy of Alan Widgerow.

This technique is frequently used by the reconstructive surgeon to cover defects of dermis but may also be used for deeper wounds. The graft itself survives the first 3 days by plasmatic imbibition, a process whereby nutrients are absorbed from the wound bed to ensure survival of the graft. Almost simultaneously, blood vessels on the edge of the graft line themselves up with capillaries on the wound bed edge and start a primitive early circulation, a process called inosculation. Then new vessels (neovascularisation) begin to form to establish a blood supply to ensure the long-term survival of the skin graft. During this period, the graft needs to be protected from mechanical interference and movement, from contamination and from collections of blood or fluid that could accumulate beneath the skin graft lifting it from its bed and preventing inosculation and vascularisation. Dressings should be carefully chosen to provide stability and absorb exudate during the critical first few days of the process and moist wound dressings such as silicone wound-contact layers have the best outcomes and are well accepted by patients (Wiechula, 2003). The graft site should be assessed daily and redressed every few days depending on the dressing product used. A retentive dressing is placed over the primary dressing, but care must be taken to ensure it is not too tight and does not restrict blood flow.

Most skin grafts do better if covered by an absorbent, low-adherent, compression dressing for the first 7–10 days. In certain situations, however (facial burns, etc.), the surgeon may elect to leave the graft exposed so that excess fluid can be 'milked' from under the graft ensuring a good percentage 'take' of the skin graft. Even after skin grafts have taken (approximately a 10-day period), caution is needed to protect them for the next 3–4 weeks to ensure long-term survival. The patient should be instructed on suitability for bathing, protective dressings, compression according to a treatment plan tailor-made to suit the wound, any coexisting disease and personal circumstances.

Skin grafts may take many months to reach full stability and strength, during which time they are susceptible to mechanical trauma and infection. As time progresses (particularly after 3 weeks) the likelihood of rejection is greatly diminished. The donor area of a split-thick skin graft consists of epithelial cells interspersed in a bed of dermal adnexal structures. It is from these structures that epithelial cells arise, grow, divide and heal the wound; this process requires a stable moist wound environment. The donor site needs to be protected from mechanical abrasion, contamination and fluid collection. In the elderly, where adnexal structures may be limited and the process of epithelialisation is slow, serious consideration must be given to the choice of split skin grafting to avoid the creation of a second chronic wound compounding the initial problem.

Full-thickness skin grafting is undertaken where the wound involves total loss of skin. The graft comprises epidermal and dermal components and on occasion may include other structures such as cartilage in a composite graft. In most cases, these grafts require good compression and techniques such as tie-over dressings may be used to secure the dressing onto the surface of the graft ensuring good compression and contact with the wound bed. 'Tie-over' pressure dressings are often made of sponge or foam and are sutured or stapled on top of the full thickness skin graft. They must stay intact for a minimum of a week and must not be removed. This allows capillary regrowth to re-establish the blood supply and prevents collection of fluid beneath the graft. Tie-over dressings are usually removed after 7–10 days at which time a good assessment of early graft take can be made.

The principles of postoperative management of skin grafts (Table 14.3) need to be carefully followed to ensure success. It is interesting how in recent years, negative-pressure wound therapy (NPWT) has surpassed the use of flaps to treat many complex wounds. Many cases, such as lower limb defects with exposed bone that would previously been selected for free tissue transfer now have NPWT used temporarily to encourage granulation tissue growth over exposed structures and then secondary reconstruction with a much simpler skin graft becomes an option (Levin, 2008). In this way, the 'reconstructive ladder' that was used to choose a reconstruction based on the complexity of the wound, the health status of the patient and the long-term result has been altered by the introduction of this new technology.

Constant vigilance for skin graft or flap failure is important. Signs to observe include oedema, swelling, discolouration (blue venous congestion or black demarcation of a flap denoting circulatory failure particularly in first 48 hours), pain, dehiscence/separation of the flap/graft from surrounding tissue (over first 10 days). The quicker any of these signs are observed and action taken,

the better. The action may involve various medications to stimulate circulation: simple removal of sutures in a tension area; drainage of a haematoma; re-exploration and reanastomosis of vessels in free tissue transfers. With free tissue transfer, the anaesthesiologist has a major responsibility during the procedure and immediately after surgery to ensure constant maintenance of blood pressure to ensure good flow to the flap reconstruction area. Maintenance of general and local body temperature is also important. Various objective flap monitoring devices (oxygen, temperature, circulation) are available to recognise imminent flap failure but simple vigilance and knowing what to look for can prevent major complications with this type of surgery.

Education and support

Patients need to be fully informed about the process of looking after their postoperative wounds especially as they are discharged home early. They need to be taught the early signs of wound infection: increased pain/tenderness, redness and warmth of the surrounding skin, increased exudate, for example, serous fluid, pus and should be told to report these signs and symptoms to a healthcare professional without delay (NICE, 2008).

The instructions that follow are generic as different wounds, types and location of surgery will necessitate variation to these instructions.

Patient education for postoperative wound management should include the following information:

(1) likely frequency of dressing change;
(2) explanation of how to remove wound dressing and tapes;
(3) instructions on how to cleanse the wound and periwound skin;
(4) correct application of new dressing and disposal of soiled dressings;
(5) anticipated date of removal of wound drainage/suture/other skin closure;
(6) where to obtain supplies necessary for dressing change;
(7) what activities to avoid, for example, strenuous exercise;
(8) avoidance of self-prescribed or traditional remedies;
(9) knowing when to seek advice from a healthcare professional;

Table 14.3   General principles: postoperative management of skin grafts

Principle	Action
• Compressive dressing to prevent collection of blood, serum, pus accumulating beneath skin graft or flap	Gently pack defect with a moist dressing and securely bandage in place or use 'tie over dressing' to secure graft in place. For flaps apply low adherent primary dressings making sure not to compromise circulation.
• Constant observation of wound especially in first 48 hours for signs of graft or flap failure	Early identification of signs of infection: increasing redness, oedema, pain, warmth, bleeding or purulent drainage or accumulation of serous fluid at the surgical site. Refer to surgeon immediately.
• Prevent swelling or mechanical damage to flap or graft	Elevate affected limb to prevent oedema. First allow dependent hanging of limb over side of bed, then graded mobilisation over a time period to full weight bearing
• Prevent collection of moisture in wound from exudate, incontinence	Protect incision line from risk of infection with absorbent, low adherent dressings.
• Remove sutures when appropriate (early enough to prevent poor scarring and late enough to prevent dehiscence)	Timing of suture removal depends on individual wound characteristics and location.
• Prevent risk of further trauma	Immobilisation and protection of lower extremity grafts and flaps is necessary for 3–6 weeks. Restrict mobility for patients with grafts/flaps on lower limb for 10 days to 2 weeks depending on size, site and nature of the reconstruction.

(10) how to manage scar;
(11) contact details of whom to contact in case of concern;
(12) when to come back to follow-up appointment.

Criteria for specialist referral

Those caring for patient after surgery need to understand the surgical procedure, its inherent risks and knowledge of the patient's comorbidities to identify postoperative wound complications as early as possible. Complications obviously vary depending on the type of surgical procedure but advice should be sought initially from the surgeon who performed the procedure if any of the following circumstances apply:

- haematoma formation and inadequate drainage;
- wound dehiscence;
- wound infection and sepsis;
- abnormal scarring (hypertrophic/keloid scarring).

Factors known to affect tissue repair like smoking, diabetes, cardiovascular disease, lung disease, blood loss and length and type of surgical proce-

dure are important predictors of wound complications. A study by Sørensen et al. (2005) highlighted the value of identifying patients at high risk of developing wound problems prior to surgery and suggests development of surgical pathways would help to improve patient's preoperative condition with the aim of reducing postoperative wound complications.

Summary

Surgical wounds may present with healing problems in a variety of different ways. If the wound is closed and clean, the primary goal is to keep it this way by reducing risk factors pertaining to the general health of the patient, the avoidance of SSIs and informing the patient on caring for the wound. Various principles are important to follow before, during and after surgery and interventions related to these periods appear to improve chances of uneventful wound healing.

Techniques for closure and reconstruction of surgical wounds differ and necessitate distinct management options for the differing methods of closure. Complications of surgical wounds including dehiscence, infection and bleeding may involve specialised interventions but in most cases, the well-defined principles of wound care are applicable. Wound management does not end with closure, as healing outcome is also impacted by the appearance and sensitivity of the resultant scar. Scar management should therefore be part of all surgical wound management programmes. Patient information, multidisciplinary co-operation, integration of services and psychosocial support are essential to provide the patient with a comprehensive surgical wound care strategy.

Useful resources

NICE (2008) *Clinical Guideline 74 – Surgical Site Infection. Prevention and Treatment of Surgical Site Infection.* Available at: www.nice.org.uk

World Health Organization (2009) *Guidelines for Safe Surgery: Safe Skin Surgery Saves Lives.* Available in Spanish, Chinese, Arabic, French, Russian. Available at: http://www.who.int/patientsafety/safesurgery/en/

References

Aggarwal, R., Darzi, A. (2008) Symposium on surgical simulation for training and certification. *World Journal of Surgery*, 32, 139–140.

Atkinson, J.A., McKenna, K.T., Barnett, A.G., McGrath, D.J., Rudd, M. (2005) A randomized, controlled trial to determine the efficacy of paper tape in preventing hypertrophic scar formation in surgical excisions that traverse Langer's skin tension lines. *Plastic and Reconstructive Surgery*, 116, 1648–1656.

Ayliffe, G.A. (1991) Role of the environment of the operating suite in surgical wound infection. *Reviews of Infectious Diseases*, 13, 800–804.

Baumann, L.S., Spencer, J. (1999) The effects of topical vitamin E on the cosmetic appearance of scars. *Dermatologic Surgery*, 25, 311–315.

Bode, L.G., Kluytmans J.A., Wertheim H.F., et al. (2010) Preventing surgical-site infections in nasal carriers of *Staphylococcus aureus*. *New England Journal of Medicine*, 362, 9–17.

Brölmann, F.E., Ubbink, D.T., Nelson, E.A., Munte, K., van der Horst, C.M., Vermeulen, H. (2012) Evidence-based decisions for local and systemic wound care. *British Journal of Surgery*, 99, 1172–1183.

Burns, J.L., Mancoll, J.S., Philips, L.G. (2003) Impairments to wound healing. *Clinics in Plastic Surgery*, 30(1), 47–56.

Bush, J.A., McGrouther, A., Young, V.L., et al. (2011) Recommendations on clinical proof of efficacy for potential scar prevention and reduction therapies. *Wound Repair and Regeneration*, 19, S32–S37.

Cruse, P.J., Foord, R. (1980) The epidemiology of wound infection. A 10-year prospective study of 62,939 wounds. *Surgical Clinics of North America*, 60(1), 27–40.

Darouiche, R.O., Wall, M.J. Jr., Itani, K.M. (2010) Chlorhexidine-alcohol versus povidone-iodine for surgical-site antisepsis. *New England Journal of Medicine*, 362, 18–26.

Eriksen, N.H., Espersen, F., Rosdahl, V.T., Jensen, K. (1995) Carriage of *Staphylococcus aureus* among 104 healthy persons during a 19-month period. *Epidemiology and Infection*, 115(1), 51–60.

Fakhry, F.M., Montgomery, S.C. (2012) Peri-operative oxygen and the risk of surgical infection. *Surgical Infections*, 13, 228–233.

Franz, M.G., Robson, M.C., Steed, D.L., et al. (2008) Guidelines to aid healing of acute wounds by decreasing impediments of healing. *Wound Repair and Regeneration*, 16, 723–748.

Gardner, S.E., Frantz, R.A., Doebbeling, B. (2001) The validity of the clinical signs and symptoms used to identify localized chronic wound infection. *Wound Repair and Regeneration*, 9, 178–186.

Gosain, A., DiPietro, L.A. (2004) Aging and wound healing. *World Journal of Surgery*, 28(3), 321–326.

Gottrup, F., Melling, A., Hollander, A. (2005) An overview of surgical site infections: aetiology, incidence and risk factors. *EWMA Journal*, 5(2), 11–15.

Haridas, M., Malangoni, M.A. (2008) Predictive factors for surgical site infection in general surgery. *Surgery*, 144, 496–501.

Hugonnet, S., Pittet, D. (2000) Hand hygiene – beliefs or science? *Clinical Microbiology and Infection*, 6, 350–356.

Jenkins, M., Alexander, J.W., Mac Millian, B.G., et al. (1986) Failure of topical steroids and vitamin E to reduce postoperative scar formation following reconstructive surgery. *Journal of Burn Care and Rehabilitation*, 7, 309–312.

Kao, L.S., Meeks, D., Moyer, V.A., Lally, K.P. (2009) Perioperative glycaemic control regimens for preventing surgical site infections in adults. *The Cochrane Database of Systematic Reviews [Computer File]*, 8, CD006806.

Keep, R.F., Xi, G., Hua, Y., Hoff, J.T. (2005) The deleterious or beneficial effects of different agents in intracerebral hemorrhage: think big, think small, or is hematoma size important? *Stroke*, 36, 1594–1596.

Kumar, S., Wong, P.F., Melling, A.C., Leaper, D.J. (2005) Effects of perioperative hypothermia and warming in surgical practice. *International Wound Journal*, 2, 193–204.

Leaper, D.J., Gottrup, F. (1998) Surgical wounds. In: *Wounds: Biology and Management* (eds D. J. Leaper, K. G. Harding), pp. 23–40. Oxford: Oxford University Press.

Levin, L.S. (2008) Principles of definitive soft tissue coverage with flaps. *Journal of Trauma*, 32, S161–S166.

Lindstedt, E., Sandblom, P. (1975) Wound healing in man: tensile strength of healing wounds in some patient groups. *Annals of Surgery*, 181(6), 842–846.

Liu, A., Moy, R.L., Ozog, D.M. (2011) Current methods employed in the prevention and minimization of surgical scars. *Dermatologic Surgery*, 37, 1740–1746.

Lübbeke, A., Moons, K.G., Garavaglia, G., Hoffmeyer, P. (2008) Outcomes of obese and obese patients undergoing revision total hip arthroplasty. *Arthritis and Rheumatism*, 59, 738–745.

Mangram, A.J., Horan, T.C., Pearson, M.L., Silver, L.C., Jarvis, W.R., Hospital Infection Control Practices Advisory Committee. (1999) Guideline for prevention of surgical site infection. *Infection Control and Hospital Epidemiology*, 20, 250–278.

McDonald, M., Grabsch, E., Marshall, C., Forbes, A. (1998) Single-versus multiple-dose antimicrobial prophylaxis for major surgery: a systematic review. *Australian and New Zealand Journal of Surgery*, 68, 388–396.

Mustoe, T.A., Cooter, R.D., Gold, M.H., et al. (2002) International clinical recommendations on scar management. International advisory panel on scar management. *Plastic and Reconstructive Surgery*, 110(2), 560–571.

Namazi, M.R., Fallahzadeh, M.K., Schwartz, R.A. (2011) Strategies for prevention of scars: what can we learn from fetal skin? *International Journal of Dermatology*, 50, 85–93.

NICE. (2008) Clinical guideline 74 – Surgical site infection. Prevention and treatment of surgical site infection. Available at: www.nice.org.uk, last accessed on 19 November 2012.

O'Brien, L., Pandit, A. (2006) Silicon gel sheeting for preventing and treating hypertrophic and keloid scars. *The Cochrane Database of Systematic Reviews [Computer File]*, 1, CD003826.

O'Shaughnessy, K.D., De La Garza, M., Roy, N.K., Mustoe, T.A. (2009) Homeostasis of the epidermal barrier layer: a theory of how occlusion reduces hypertrophic scarring. *Wound Repair and Regeneration*, 17(5), 700–708.

Perrenoud, D., Homberger, H.P., Auderset, P.C., et al. (1994) An epidemic outbreak of papular and follicular contact dermatitis to tocopheryl linoleate in cosmetics. *Dermatology*, 189, 225–33.

Procter, L.D., Davenport, D.L., Bernard, A.C., et al. (2010) General surgical operative duration is associated with increased risk-adjusted infectious complicate rates and length of hospital stay. *Journal of the American College of Surgeons*, 210, 60–65.

Prokuski, L. (2008) Prophylactic antibiotics in orthopaedic surgery. *Journal of the American Academy of Orthopaedic Surgeons*, 16, 283–293.

Reiffel, R.S. (1995) Prevention of hypertrophic scars by long term paper tape application. *Plastic and Reconstructive Surgery*, 96, 1715.

Reish, R.G., Eriksson, E. (2008) Scars: a review of emerging and currently available therapies. *Plastic and Reconstructive Surgery*, 122(4), 1068–1078.

Reus, W.F., Mathes, S.J. (1990) Wound closure. In: *Plastic Surgery: Principles and Practice* (eds M. J. Jurkeiwicz, T.J. Krizek, S. J. Mathes, S. Ariyan), pp. 20–22. St. Louis, MO: Mosby.

Rioux, C., Grandbastien, B., Astagneau P. (2006) The standardized incidence ratio as a reliable tool for surgical site infection surveillance. *Infection Control and Hospital Epidemiology*, 27, 817–824.

Sax, H., Allegranzi, B., Uçkay, I., Larson, E., Boyce, J., Pittet, D. (2007) 'My five moments for hand hygiene': a user-centred design approach to understand, train, monitor and report hand hygiene. *Journal of Hospital Infection*, 67, 9–21.

Scott, E.M., Buckland, R. (2006) A systematic review of intraoperative warming to prevent postoperative complications. *AORN Journal*, 83, 1090–1104.

Sørensen, L.T., Hemmingsen, U., Kallehave, F., et al. (2005) Risk factors for tissue and wound complications in gastrointestinal surgery. *Annals of Surgery*, 241, 654–658.

Tandara, A.A., Mustoe, T.A. J. (2008) The role of the epidermis in the control of scarring: evidence for mechanism of action for silicone gel. *Journal of Plastic, Reconstructive and Aesthetic Surgery*, 61(10), 1219–1225.

Tanner, J., Swarbrook, S., Stuart, J. (2008) Surgical hand antisepsis to reduce surgical site infection. *The Cochrane Database of Systematic Reviews [Computer File]*, 1, CD004288.

Tibbs, M.K. (1997) Wound healing following radiation therapy: a review. *Radiotherapy & Oncology*, 42(2), 99–106.

Tollefson, T.T., Kamangar, F., Aminpour, S., Lee, A., Durbin-Johnson, B., Tinling S. (2012) Comparison of effectiveness of silicone gel sheeting with microporous paper tape in the prevention of hypertrophic scarring in a rabbit model. *Archives of Facial Plastic Surgery*, 14(1), 45–51.

Trussell, J., Gerkin, R., Coates, B., et al. (2008) Impact of a patient care pathway protocol on surgical site infection rates in cardiothoracic surgery patients. *American Journal of Surgery*, 196, 883–889.

Uçkay, I., Harbarth, S., Peter R., Lew, D., Hoffmeyer, P., Pittet, D. (2010) Preventing surgical site infections. *Expert Review of Anti-infective Therapy*, 8(6), 657–670.

Vermeulen, H., Ubbink, D., Goossens, A., de Vos, R., Legemate, D. (2004) Dressings and topical agents for surgical wounds healing by secondary intention. *The Cochrane Database of Systematic Reviews [Computer File]*, 2, CD003554.

Weber, W.P., Marti, W.R., Zwahlen, M., et al. (2008) The timing of surgical antimicrobial prophylaxis. *Annals of Surgery*, 247, 918–926.

Wenzel, R.P. (2010). Minimizing surgical-site infections. *New England Journal of Medicine*, 362, 75.

Widgerow, A.D. (2011a) Cellular extracellular cross talk in scar control. *Wound Repair and Regeneration*, 19, 117–133.

Widgerow, A.D. (2011b) Scar management – the principles and their practical applications. *WCET Journal*, 31(1), 18–21.

Widgerow, A.D., Chait, L.A., Stahls, R., Stahls, P. (2000) New innovations in scar management. *Aesthetic Plastic Surgery*, 24, 227–234.

Widgerow, A.D., Chait, L.A.C., Stals, R., Stals, P., Candy, G. (2009) Multimodality scar management program. *Aesthetic Plastic Surgery*, 33 (4), 533.

Widmer, A.F., Rotter, M., Voss, A., et al. (2009) Surgical hand preparation: state-of-the-art. *Journal of Hospital Infection*, 74(2), 112–122.

Wiechula, R. (2003) The use of moist wound-healing dressings in the management of split-thickness skin graft donor sites: a systematic review. *International Journal of Nursing Practice*, 9, S9–S17.

Wolfram, D., Tzankov, A., Pülzl, P., Piza-katzer, H. (2009) Hypertrophic scars and keloids – a review of their pathophysiology, risk factors, and therapeutic management. *Dermatologic Surgery*, 35(2):171–181.

Wong, L., Green, H.M., Feugate, J.E., Yadav, M., Nothnagel, E., Martins-Green, M. (2004) Effects of "secondhand" smoke on structure and function of fibroblasts, cells that are critical for tissue repair and remodeling. *BMC Cell Biology*, 7, 1.

World Health Organization (2009) *WHO Guidelines for Safe Surgery: Safe Surgery Saves Lives*. WHO/IER/PSP/2008.08-1E

15 Neglected Wounds

Kim Deroo[1], Lesley Robertson-Laxton[1], Sabina Sabo[2] and
Arlene A. Sardo[1,3]

[1]Wound and Chronic Disease Management, Nursing Practice Solutions, Inc., Toronto, Ontario, Canada
[2]Wound Care, Nursing Practice Solutions, Inc., Toronto, Ontario, Canada
[3]Faculty of Health Sciences, School of Nursing, McMaster University, Hamilton, Ontario, Canada

Introduction

Wounds can be difficult to manage for a variety of reasons and at best may cause misery for patients and at worst may be life-threatening. Many wounds do not heal simply due to inappropriate clinical management. There are many reasons for this including a lack of knowledge and understanding by the clinician, inadequate resources, reliance on outdated practices or failure to refer to specialist colleagues.

The aim of this chapter is to provide a concise, practical guide to wounds that may be mismanaged due to lack of clinical experience. These wounds are not seen in everyday clinical practice and as a result there is less shared expertise to help guide best practice. The following types of wounds are discussed:

- body piercings;
- bullous pemphigoid;
- calciphylaxis;
- fistulas;
- necrotising fasciitis;
- pyoderma gangrenosum;
- self-inflicted wounds;
- skin tears.

BODY PIERCINGS

Overview

The trend in body piercings has grown over the past two decades with a prevalence as high as 50% in some populations (Mayers et al., 2002). Piercings are most commonly found in the ears as well as eyebrows, lips, tongue, nose, chin, uvula, navel, nipple and genitals. Metals such as nickel alloy and gold-plated jewellery are most likely to cause allergic reactions. Reasons for piercing range from aesthetics, ritual initiation to sexual stimulation. As many piercings are performed by individuals themselves or by unlicensed personnel, the rates of complications are difficult to ascertain; however, estimates are as high as 30% (Stirn, 2003). Persons experiencing complications may be reluctant to seek care due to embarrassment or fear that the jewellery needs to be removed (Caliendo et al., 2005).

Wound Healing and Skin Integrity: Principles and Practice, First Edition. Edited by Madeleine Flanagan.
© 2013 John Wiley & Sons, Ltd. Published 2013 by John Wiley & Sons, Ltd.

Risk factors (post-piercing infection)

- Anatomic location of piercing;
- Diabetes;
- HIV infection or other immunosuppressive disorders;
- Corticosteroids or other immunosuppressive medicines;
- Clinical expertise of piercer;
- Post-piercing hygiene and aftercare;
- Delay in seeking treatment.

Factors delaying healing

- Anatomic location of piercing;
- Trauma associated with piercing;
- Continued presence of a foreign body;
- Unsterilised or improperly sterilised piercing equipment;
- Allergy to metal jewellery.

Complications

- Uncontrolled bleeding;
- Local infection – abscess, cellulitis (most commonly Group A *Streptococcus*, *Staphylococcus aureus*, *Pseudomonas*, MRSA);
- Sepsis;
- Contact dermatitis;
- Keloid formation, permanent scarring;
- Transmission of hepatitis B, C and D, HIV, leprosy and tuberculosis;
- Risk of tetanus;
- Non-menstrual toxic shock;
- Accidental traumatic tearing;
- Infected breast implants, endocarditis, granulomatous mastitis and minor duct damage – nipple piercings;
- Altered speech, tooth/gum damage, swollen lips, difficulty swallowing, permanent nerve damage and airway obstruction from aspiration of jewellery and post-piercing swelling from tongue and oral piercings;
- Auricular perichondritis, leading to permanent deformity such as 'cauliflower ear', ear piercing;
- Sterility and urethral strictures – genital piercings.

Principles of wound management

The aims of wound management for individuals with body piercings are to:

(1) promote effective self-care to maximise healing;
(2) minimise risk of wound infection, sepsis and development of long-term complications.

Practical management

- Health care professionals should be proactive in educating adolescents and adults about the risks of body piercings and that healing may take time.
- Individuals should have a tetanus vaccination before body piercing if they have not had one in the past 10 years.
- Individuals with a predisposition to hypertrophic or keloid scarring should be advised that body piercing is associated with high risk of recurrence.
- Antibiotic prophylaxis should be considered in those with corrected congenital cardiac conditions who are contemplating piercings.
- Wound management should take into account the specific body part involved. Genital piercings can be especially problematic due to the local environment, which can delay healing for as long as 6–9 months.
- Piercings should be cleaned with clean, warm water. There is no evidence to support the use of salt water or other topical preparations, such as antibiotics, antiseptics and lavender oil, to promote healing.
- Antibacterial mouthwash can be used three to four times a day to promote healing of mouth or tongue piercings.
- Application of topical preparations is more likely to increase the risk of infection due to poor handwashing and contamination of topical treatments and may cause skin sensitivities.
- Antimicrobial therapy should be given early in the course of infection as sepsis is often difficult to treat. Treatment should include broad-spectrum antibiotics (including antipseudomonal coverage), for example with ciprofloxacin when oral antibiotics are appropriate. If infection is severe or slow to respond, more aggressive measures should be

considered, including surgical drainage and intravenous antibiotics.
- If complications occur, management should focus on prevention of endocarditis and development of sepsis.

Practical tips

- Piercing guns should be avoided, especially for cartilaginous piercings as this increases the risk of infection due to tissue damage from blunt trauma (Das, 2002; Keene et al., 2004).
- Stress the importance of handwashing before touching unhealed piercings and touch as infrequently as possible to minimise infection risk.
- Jewellery should not be removed or changed during healing to maintain the piercing and prevent closure.
- If infection is suspected, removal of jewellery may encourage abscess formation, retaining the jewellery at the site may facilitate better drainage.
- If healing is delayed then the jewellery should be removed and referral to a surgeon for drainage should be made.
- Loose clothing should be worn over unhealed piercings as tight clothing can cause friction, irritation and increased moisture, leading to skin maceration, and the risk of bacterial or fungal growth.
- Piercings will usually take several months to heal fully. Advise individuals not to play with or chew on their piercing as this can lead to the formation of scar tissue.

Healing rates

Healing is generally slower in pierced sites due to the factors highlighted above. One of the most com-

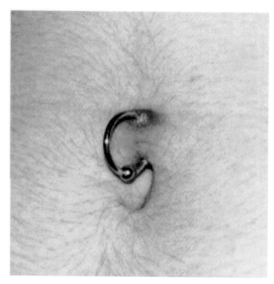

Figure 15.1 Persistent infection associated with navel piercing. Photo courtesy of Dr Peter Molan.

mon reasons for delayed healing is persistent low-grade infection (Figure 15.1).

Healing rates are approximate and are dependent on site and host specific considerations (Table 15.1).

Criteria for specialist referral

- Delayed healing of piercing after considering variations in healing rates;
- Unresolved local infection, spreading cellulitis, sepsis;
- Refer to surgeon for drainage of any abscess formation;
- Unexplained fever, malaise, muscle or joint pain within 4 months of a body piercing (consider infectious endocarditis);
- Signs of cardiac, urology or neurological complications;
- Hypertrophic or keloid scarring, skin tears.

Table 15.1 Healing rates for body piercing

Anatomical location of piercing	Complete healing (typical)	Complete healing (maximum)
Face and mouth	6–8 wk	3 mo
Earlobe	4–6 wk	3 mo
Cartilage and tragus (ear)	4–6 mo	1 yr
Nipple	2–3 mo	6–8 mo
Navel	3–4 mo	9 mo
Genital	3–4 mo	9 mo

Source: Data from Stirn (2003), Mayers et al. (2002) and Antoszewski et al. (2009).

Summary

Most body piercings will eventually heal without significant complication although up to a third may result in superficial localised infection. Individuals contemplating body piercings should be made aware of the risks associated with delayed healing and subsequent scarring so that they can make an informed choice. They should understand the importance of post-piercing aftercare and know when and where to seek professional medical advice if concerned.

Further reading

The Association of Professional Piercers. Available at: http://www.safepiercing.org

References

Antoszewski, B., Szychta, P., Fijalkowska M. (2009) Are we aware of all complications following body piercing procedures? *International Journal of Dermatology*, 48(4), 422–425.

Caliendo, C., Armstrong, M.L., Roberts, A.E. (2005) Self-reported characteristics of women and men with intimate body piercings. *Journal of Advanced Nursing*, 49(5), 474–484.

Das, P. (2002) Piercing the cartilage and not the lobes leads to ear infections. *The Lancet Infectious Diseases*, 2(12), 715.

Keene, W.E., Markum, A.C., Samadpour, M. (2004) Outbreak of *Pseudomonas aeruginosa* infections caused by commercial piercing of upper ear cartilage. *Journal of the American Medical Association*, 291(8), 981–985.

Mayers, L.B., Judelson, D.A., Moriarty, B.W., Rundell, K.W. (2002) Prevalence of body art (body piercing and tattooing) in university undergraduates and incidence of medical complications. *Mayo Clinic Proceedings*, 77, 29–34.

Stirn, A. (2003) Body piercing: medical consequences and psychological motivations. *Lancet*, 361, 1205–1215.

BULLOUS PEMPHIGOID

Overview

Pemphigus vulgaris (PV) and bullous pemphigoid (BP) are rare autoimmune blistering diseases. IgG autoantibodies bind to the skin basement membrane in patients with pemphigoid disorders activating inflammatory mediators.

In BP, autoantibodies attack the basement membrane of the epidermis causing subepidermal bullae (large blisters) which are less fragile than those of PV. Patients with BP usually have lots of intact, tense bullae, rather than ruptured blisters covered with scabs. In contrast, the autoantibodies of patients with PV disrupt the intercellular junctions in the epidermis, causing big, flaccid blisters that burst scab and expose the underlying dermis. Patients with PV often present first with mouth ulcers and later develop bullae on the skin.

BP is more common than pemphigus and most commonly affects persons 70 years of age or older (Langan et al., 2008). BP often requires long-term use of immunosuppressive agents and recurrence is common. Drug-induced BP develops in a small subgroup of patients. Penicillamine and furosemide are most frequently implicated, although cases associated with captopril, penicillin and its derivatives have been reported.

Risk factors

- Associated with other autoimmune diseases, for example, myasthenia gravis;
- Triggered by environmental factors, for example, drugs, stress, pregnancy (removal of the trigger factor does not bring about resolution of the condition.);
- Older age groups;
- Patients taking multiple medications;
- Ultraviolet irradiation, radiotherapy.

Differential diagnosis

Differential diagnosis includes other blistering diseases of the skin and mucous membranes:

- dermatitis herpetiformis;
- bullous drug eruptions;
- epidermolysis bullosa;
- erythema multiforme impetigo, which may be mistaken for the various stages of bullous pemphigoid;
- urticaria;
- bullous eruption of systemic lupus erythematosus.

Clinical features

- Initial presentation varies.
- Pruritus may be initial manifestation (before appearance of lesions).

- A rash may appear before blisters. Skin blisters are widespread appearing on normal or erythematous skin.
- Blisters commonly occur in the flexural areas, groin and axillae.
- Blisters extend rapidly and burst.
- Erosions may be evident after the blisters break.
- Nail lesions may occur (paronychias, nail dystrophies and subungal haematomas).
- The oral cavity is most often affected.
- Bullae in the mouth are painful and heal slowly.
- Other mucous membranes (conjunctivae, oesophagus and genitalia) may be involved.

Factors delaying healing

- Immune suppression;
- Corticosteroid treatment;
- Local infection/secondary infection.

Complications

- Wound/skin infection;
- Secondary infection related to immunosuppressive treatment;
- Glucocorticoid-induced bone loss, heart disease, hypertension, diabetes, gastric ulceration, agranulocytosis;
- Pressure ulceration;
- Death (related to coexisting disease).

Principles of wound management

The aims of wound management for lesions caused by bullous pemphigoid are to:

(1) reduce blister formation and determine the minimal dose of medication necessary to control the disease process;
(2) ensure that all therapeutic regimes are individualised to the patient and any pre-existing conditions;
(3) promote healing of blisters and erosions;
(4) monitor patient's progress until they are in complete remission and treatment can be stopped.

Practical management

- Take a detailed past medical history, as this may reveal triggers associated with bullous pemphigoid (e.g. chronic inflammatory skin conditions) and medications (e.g. antibiotics, furosemide).
- Proper diagnosis is necessary to determine if bullae are related to the disease or are drug-induced, but diagnostic criteria are not clear-cut.
- Treatment of bullous pemphigoid depends on the severity of the disease.
- For localised disease, potent topical steroids plus systemic anti-inflammatory (tetracycline and nicotinamide) may be sufficient.
- Topical steroids are better tolerated than oral steroids in the elderly.
- For more severe cases, systemic steroids along with immunosuppressives may be needed to control the disease.
- Treatment to help prevent osteoporosis: calcium and vitamin D supplements should be commenced to prevent osteoporosis if systemic steroids will be given for more than 1 month.
- Small blisters benefit from application of topical steroids, but large, raw, denuded skin benefits from a moist wound environment. Silicone wound contact layers are useful to cover large areas and minimise further trauma.
- For exudating or bleeding wounds, alginates help control exudate and maintain a moist wound environment.

This section is based on best practice described by Wojnarowska et al. (2002), Kirtschig et al. (2010), and Walling and Sontheimer (2009).

Criteria for specialist referral

- Clinical suspicion of bullous pemphigoid or other blistering diseases;
- Signs of sepsis;
- Rapid deterioration of lesions;
- Uncontrolled pain.

Summary

BP is a chronic inflammatory disease which is usually self-limiting within 2–5 years, if treated appropriately. But it can persist with remissions and exacerbations for many years. During a flare up large areas of the skin can blister and break down incapacitating the patient and have a huge impact on quality of life. Mortality is associated with older patients and those who have existing co-morbidities. The immunosuppressant effects of treatment cause many side-effects including delayed healing and need to be carefully monitored. A multidisciplinary approach and referral to those who have specialist experience of managing these patients are essential.

Further reading

Schmidt, E., della Torre, R., Borradori, L. (2011) Clinical features and practical diagnosis of bullous pemphigoid. *Dermatologic Clinics*, 29(3), 427–438, viii–ix.

Walling, H.W., Sontheimer, R.D. (2009) Cutaneous lupus erythematosus: issues in diagnosis and treatment. *American Journal of Clinical Dermatology*, 10(6), 365–381.

References

Kirtschig, G., Middleton, P., Bennett, C., et al. (2010) Interventions for bullous pemphigoid. *The Cochrane Database of Systematic Reviews [Computer File]*. 6(10), CD002292.

Langan, S.M., Smeeth, L., Hubbard, R., et al. (2008) Bullous pemphigoid and pemphigus vulgaris–incidence and mortality in the UK. *British Medical Association*. 337, a180.

Wojnarowska, F., Kirtschig, G., Highet, A.S., Venning, V.A., Khumalo, N.P. British Association of Dermatologists (2002) Guidelines for the management of bullous pemphigoid. *British Journal of Dermatology*, 147(2), 214–221.

CALCIPHYLAXIS

Overview

Calciphylaxis is a rare, debilitating condition in which calcification of small- and medium-sized arteries (most commonly, cutaneous and subcutaneous arterioles) occur in patients with renal disease. Calciphylaxis causes ischemic necrosis of the dermis, subcutaneous tissue, muscle, fascia (calciphylaxis cutis) and internal organs (visceral calciphylaxis), leading to calcification of the soft tissues. Incidence is estimated at 1% per year in patients undergoing dialysis (Ng and Peng, 2011). Co-morbidities associated with calciphylaxis include chronic renal failure, diabetes, hypercalcaemia, hyperphosphataemia and secondary hyperparathyroidism. These abnormalities are common in patients with end-stage renal disease. Those who develop calciphylaxis have often undergone renal transplant.

Risk factors

- End-stage renal insufficiency;
- Diabetes;
- Hypoalbuminaemia;
- Caucasian race;
- Female gender;
- Obesity;
- Warfarin;
- Corticosteroids or other immunosuppressive medicines.

Differential diagnosis

- necrotising fasciitis;
- Pyoderma gangrenosum;
- Bullous pemphigoid;
- Vasculitis;
- Erythema nodosum;
- Lupus erythematosus.

Clinical features

- Calciphylaxis lesions develop suddenly and progress rapidly, generally on the lower extremities, hands and torso.
- Present as multiple, mottled, erythematous papules, plaques or nodules and develop into stellate, purpuric (star-shaped, purplish) lesions that develop into black, painful, necrotic wounds, resulting in deep, extensive dry gangrene.
- Lesions typically occur in areas with high adipose tissue content, including abdomen, thighs, calves and buttocks, with ischemic necrosis occurring in fingers and toes.
- Pain can be unbearable, burning with intense itching.
- Prognosis is poor with up to 6 months' life expectancy after skin breakdown.
- Diagnosis is confirmed by skin biopsy.

Factors delaying healing

- Elevated levels of serum calcium and phosphate;
- Inadequate blood supply;
- Increased clotting times.

Complications

- Haematoma;
- Tissue necrosis;
- Secondary infection of wounds and sepsis;
- Pressure ulceration;
- Amputation.

Principles of wound management

The aims of wound management for lesions caused by calciphylaxis are

(1) prevention of further calcification occurring in the soft tissues;
(2) prevention of further skin breakdown and stabilisation of any remaining viable tissue;
(3) minimising risk of wound infection and sepsis;
(4) preparation of the wound bed for healing or skin grafting.

Wound treatment should be implemented quickly and monitored carefully.

Practical management

- Judicious antibiotic therapy should be instigated and guided by microbiological wound cultures.
- Aggressive surgical debridement of necrotic tissue is *contraindicated* until perfusion status is established. Arterial Doppler/ABI should be used to determine perfusion to lower leg wounds (Martin, 2008).
- The decision to debride wounds, and to what extent, depends on the patient's overall health and the clinical picture.
- Leave stable eschar intact to maintain skin integrity and minimise infection risk. Remember, surgical debridement may increase risk of sepsis and is likely to worsen wound pain.

- Patients with calciphylaxis may have prolonged bleeding times due to uremia; surgical debridement should be approached cautiously.
- Moist necrotic tissue should be debrided using selective debriding agents such as hydrogels, larvae, chemical debridement using enzymatic agents.
- Vacuum-assisted closure therapy has been successful in several cases of calciphylaxis after surgical debridement and prior to skin grafting.
- Pain management is important especially prior to dressing procedures, and consultation with pain-management specialists may be necessary.
- Pain management is difficult as some analgesics work for some but not all patients. Ketamine 10% combined with hydrogel, opioids, gabapentin, amitriptyline can help control the pain. Over-the-counter analgesia is ineffective.
- Patients with calciphylaxis are at high risk of pressure damage. Implementation of a pressure ulcer prevention programme is essential to minimise further skin breakdown.
- Antimicrobial dressings moistened with hydrogel and covered with a silicone foam dressing can help minimise infection and maintain moisture to promote autolytic debridement.
- Use low-adherent dressings (silicone foam dressings, nonadherent foam, nonadherent layer under cover dressing) to minimise trauma and secondary skin tears.
- Avoid exacerbating ischaemia by checking bandages and dressing tapes such that they are not too tight.

This section is based on best practice described Martin (2004) and Chetan et al. (2012).

Criteria for specialist referral

- Clinical suspicion of calciphylaxis;
- Signs of sepsis;
- Rapid deterioration of necrotic lesions;
- Uncontrolled pain.

Summary

The diagnosis of calciphylaxis should be considered in patients with end-stage renal disease and atypical tissue necrosis or subcutaneous nodules. Early recognition of calciphylaxis and multidisciplinary treatment, including diligent wound care, frequent debridement and appropriate revascularisation, can result in improved wound healing and limb salvage.

Further reading

Hess, C.T. (2002) Calciphylaxis: identification and wound management. *Advances Skin Wound Care*, 15(2), 64.

Arseculeratne, G., Evans, A., Morley, S. (2006), Calciphylaxis–a topical overview. *Journal of the European Academy of Dermatology and Venereology*, 20, 493–502.

Feeser, D.L., Calciphylaxis. *Journal of Wound, Ostomy and Continence Nursing*, 2011, 38(4), 379.

References

Martin, R. (2008) The mysterious calciphylaxis: wounds with eschar – to debride or not to debride? *Ostomy Wound Management*, 50(4), 64–66, 68–70.

Ng, A., Peng, D. (2011) Calciphylaxis. *Dermatologic Therapy*, 24(2), 256–262.

Vedvyas, C., Winterfield, L.S., Vleugels, R.A. (2012) Calciphylaxis: a systematic review of existing and emerging therapies. *Journal of the American Academy of Dermatology*, 67, 6, e253.

FISTULAS

Overview

A fistula is an abnormal opening or tract between two or more organs or spaces. This can involve a communication tract from one body cavity or a hollow organ to another hollow organ or the skin. Fistulas may develop in a dehisced wound or a surgical incision. Simple fistulas have a short direct tract and no organ involvement. Complex fistulas have multiple organ involvement. Fistula with a high output may produce >200 mL of fluid in 24 hours, which is difficult to contain and distressing for patients (Lee 2012). Many patients with fistulae are severely debilitated and immunocompromised, and as a result fistulae development has a significant mortality rate. Fistula management is complex and requires expert clinical knowledge, critical thinking and a high degree of technical skill.

Risk factors

Risk factors are dependent on the type of fistula formation, but in general include

- Co-existing disease: IBD, Crohn's disease, malignancy;
- Emergency surgical procedures;
- Radiation therapy;
- Infection;
- Steroid therapy;
- Malnutrition.

Diagnostic procedures

- Blood to assess electrolyte status;
- Blood cultures if infection suspected;
- Fistulagram indicates location, communicating tracts, abscess;
- Computerised tomography.

Clinical features

The clinical presentation of fistulas varies by type. Symptoms depend on the anatomical location and/or the organs involved but are typically:

- malaise;
- fever;
- failure to recover after abdominal surgery;
- pain and tenderness at fistula site;
- skin/wound breakdown at fistula site;
- odour;
- dehydration;
- electrolyte imbalance;
- sepsis;
- malnutrition.

Factors delaying healing

- Coexisting diseases: IBD, malignancy;
- Inadequate blood supply;
- Distal obstruction;
- Poor surgical technique;
- Abscess formation/sepsis;
- Malnutrition.

Complications

- Multiple organ involvement;
- Dehydration;

- Fluid and electrolyte imbalance;
- Malnutrition;
- Abscess formation;
- Sepsis;
- Perifistula skin excoriation and breakdown;
- Scar tissue;
- High risk of pressure ulceration.

Principles of wound management

The aims of fistula management are

(1) containment of the fistula effluent and odour;
(2) maintenance of fluid, electrolyte balance and nutritional support;
(3) promotion of healing of an open wound with a draining fistula;
(4) prevention and management of peri-fistular skin breakdown;
(5) education of carers and support staff in management of drainage system.

Patients require a complex, individualised plan of care involving a multidisciplinary approach.

Practical management

- Patients with fistula require nutritional support to promote spontaneous closure of fistula and wound healing. Those with low-output fistula will require enteral nutrition whereas those with high-output fistula will require parenteral nutrition.
- Fistula output must be accurately measured so that an appropriate management strategy can be implemented.
- Effluent management, especially when located within a wound, is difficult because the tissue around the fistula does not facilitate adhesion.
- Skin protection may include liquid skin sealants, ostomy paste/strips, hydrocolloids, absorbent dressings, ostomy powder, pouching systems, continuous drainage devices, suction drainage, negative-pressure wound therapy (NPWT).
- Before pouching a fistula, evaluate the patient's abdominal contours when sitting, lying and standing to ensure a good fit.

- Complex pouching methods using adhesive barriers, skin protectants and drainage bags are required to achieve fistula containment and preserve skin integrity while preventing wound contamination.
- A Foley catheter may be carefully inserted into the fistula to direct the flow of effluent into the fistula pouch.
- NPWT may be used to control high-output fistula drainage and odour and accelerate fistula closure by promoting wound healing.
- Prior to discharge ensure the patient/carer know how to change the pouch and protect the skin, when to seek advice and where to get supplies.
- Use a hair dryer to warm the stomahesive or hydrocolloid wafers before applying to the peri-wound skin as this facilitates moulding and adhesion.
- Patients should be encouraged to rest for 15 minutes after application of drainage system to allow body heat to enhance product adherence.

This section is based on best practice described by McNaughton et al. (2010), Datta et al. (2010), and Lee (2012).

Criteria for specialist referral

- Fistulae that have failed to close after 8 weeks of conservative, non-operative management are likely to require surgical repair but should ideally have been free from infection for 6–8 weeks.

Indications for surgical intervention

- Epithelium-lined tract or stoma has formed;
- Distal obstruction;
- Foreign body in fistula tract;
- Formation of large abscess.

Summary

Skin and wound management is an important aspect of the overall medical and surgical management of patients with fistulas and significantly improves patient well-being. When managed correctly, conservative measures help prepare the patient for surgical repair if the fistula does not spontaneously close. Caring for patients with high-output fistula requires teamwork and advanced clinical skills, including familiarity of wound, stoma and skin barrier products and creativity to maximise user wear time and gain patient confidence.

Further reading

Schecter, W.P., Hirshberg, A., Chang, D.S., et al. (2009) Enteric fistulas: principles of management. *Journal of the American College of Surgeons*, 209(4), 484.

References

McNaughton, V., Brown, J., Hoeflok, J., Martins, L., McNaughton, V., Nielsen, E.M. (2010) Canadian Association for Enterostomal Therapy ECF Best Practice Recommendations Panel. Summary of best practice recommendations for management of enterocutaneous fistulae from the Canadian Association for Enterostomal Therapy ECF Best Practice Recommendations Panel. *Journal of Wound, Ostomy and Continence Nursing*, 37, 173–184.

Datta, V., Engledow, A., Chan, S., Forbes, A., Cohen, C.R., Windsor, A. (2010) The management of enterocutaneous fistula in a regional unit in the United Kingdom: a prospective study. *Diseases of the Colon and Rectum*, 53(2), 192–199.

Lee, S.H., (2012) Surgical management of enterocutaneous fistula. *Korean Journal of Radiology*, 13(Suppl 1), S17–S20.

NECROTISING FASCIITIS

Overview

Necrotising fasciitis (NF) is a soft tissue infection that progresses rapidly, threatens limbs, causes toxic shock and if left untreated will cause death (Bucca et al., 2012). It is a necrotising infection involving any layer of the deep soft tissue compartment (dermis, subcutaneous tissue, fascia or muscle). This infection is usually of polymicrobial aetiology and may occur following a minor injury or surgery. Fournier's gangrene is a necrotising infection that involves the genital area (commonly found organisms in patients with NF are *A. streptococcus, Staphylococcus, Pseudomonas, E. coli, Haemophilus apnroilus* that cause toxic shock and haemodynamic instability) (Anaya and Dillinger, 2007; Mullangi and Khardori, 2012). Quick

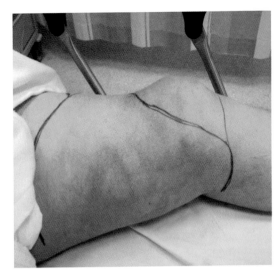

Figure 15.2   Early presentation of necrotizing fasciitis showing typical skin discolouration. Photo courtesy of Gulnaz Tariq.

diagnosis and early aggressive treatment are vital to help prevent serious complications. Misdiagnosis can seriously delay healing. NF is often misdiagnosed for cellulitis (see Figure 15.2), deep tissue thrombosis or abscess (Machado, 2011). Amputation of the affected limb may be necessary to stop the spread of infection. Mortality rates are estimated at 40–76% (Bucca et al., 2012).

Risk factors

- *Comorbidities*: immune suppression, tuberculosis, chronic liver/renal disease, diabetes, malignancy, chronic leg ulceration.
- *Skin trauma*: insect bites, frostbite, surgery, soft tissue contusion.
- *Lifestyle factors*: alcohol abuse, intravenous drug abuse.

Differential diagnosis

- Cellulitis or erysipelas;
- Erythema induratum (nodular vasculitis);
- Pyoderma gangrenosum;
- Limb ischemia, compartment syndrome;
- Deep vein thrombosis or thrombophlebitis;
- Osteomyelitis with soft tissue involvement.

Clinical features

Local

- Erythema, oedema and pain;
- Severe pain out of proportion to physical signs (important feature);
- Pain (not relieved by narcotics);
- Tenderness extends beyond apparent area involvement (unlike cellulitis);
- Dusky blue skin discolouration (cyanosis/mottling);
- Purpura or a haematoma;
- Bullae;
- Necrosis;
- If skin breaks down, probing with a blunt instrument will easily separate the superficial fascial planes.
- Malodorous discharge;
- Crepitus;
- Loss of sensation and pain resolution (late stage).

Systemic

- Patient feels very unwell: flu-like symptoms;
- Low- to high-grade fever;
- Muscle pain;
- Nausea and vomiting;
- Hemodynamic instability;
- Tachycardia;
- Tachypnea;
- Decreased urine output;
- Altered level of consciousness;
- Signs of toxic shock, for example, pyrexia, erythroderma, vomiting, diarrhoea.

Factors delaying healing

- Delayed or misdiagnosis;
- Poor surgical technique;
- Vascular occlusion, ischaemia;
- Tissue and muscle necrosis;
- Septicaemia;
- Co-morbidities.

Complications

- NF carries a significant mortality rate;
- Septic or toxic shock (latter due to streptococcal endotoxin production);
- Soft tissue involvement may lead to vascular occlusion, ischemia and subsequent tissue necrosis, nerve damage and/or muscle necrosis;
- Large area tissue destruction often requires skin grafting, reconstructive surgery or possible amputation.

Principles of wound management

If there is strong clinical suspicion of necrotising fasciitis, exploratory surgery is urgently required, as diagnosis depends on clinical features: lack of bleeding, thrombosed vessels, lack of resistance to finger dissection, grey necrotic tissue and non-contracting muscle.

The immediate aims of surgical wound management are

(1) Extensive surgical debridement of devitalised tissue to remove infected tissue and preserve viable tissue.
(2) Commence intravenous, broad-spectrum antibiotics at high doses. These should cover Streptococci, Staphylococci, Gram-negative rods and anaerobes.
(3) Admission to the intensive care unit for hemodynamic stabilisation which often includes intubation.
(4) Preparation of the wound bed for healing and/or skin grafting.

Practical management

The wound must be observed closely for signs of deterioration. Any concerns should be reported immediately.

- Surgical debridement may be required several times, until the infection is controlled.
- Antibiotic treatment should be discussed with the microbiologist and should be adjusted once culture results are known.
- Extensive surgical debridement creates large open wounds. Closure of the wound is by secondary intention. Vacuum-assisted wound closing devices and skin grafts may promote healing.
- Optimal healing is achieved with the use of advanced wound products that maintain a moist environment, absorb wound exudate and minimise trauma on removal.

- Due to the large size of wounds, dressing changes are complicated and take time to complete. This should be planned for and support asked for from colleagues.
- Nutritional support (parenteral or enteral) is essential due to the high protein and fluid loss from the wound. Patients may need twice their basal calorie requirements.
- Patient and caregiver should be vigilant for signs of infection. Patients should report any signs of infection such as odour, change in exudate, fever, new onset of pain to health care providers immediately.

This section is based on best practice described by Machado (2011), Bucca (2012), and Schuster and Nuñez (2012).

Criteria for specialist referral

- Once NF is suspected or diagnosed, an urgent referral to a multidisciplinary team with experience of managing NF is essential.
- The team should consist of a general surgeon, orthopaedic surgeon (if potential for limb-loss exists), plastic surgeon, infectious disease specialist, microbiologist, urologist (in cases of Fournier's gangrene), intensive care staff and dietician.

Summary

If not promptly diagnosed and treated, NF can progress rapidly to systemic toxicity and death. Once suspected, management should consist of immediate resuscitation, early surgical debridement and administration of broad-spectrum intravenous antibiotics. NF is part of a spectrum of rare necrotising soft tissue infections so diagnosis can be difficult for clinicians unfamiliar with it. This may lead to treatment delays which can result in amputation or fatalities and is made worse by the innocuous clinical signs and symptoms during the early course of the infection as seen in Figure 15.2.

Further reading

Morgan, M.S. (2010) Diagnosis and management of necrotising fasciitis: a multiparametric approach. *Journal of Hospital Infection*, 75(4), 249–257.

Nisbet, M., Ansell, G., Lang, S., Taylor, S., Dzendrowskyj, P., Holland, D. (2011) Necrotizing fasciitis: review of 82 cases in South Auckland. *Internal Medicine Journal*, 41(7), 543–548.

References

Anaya, D.A., Dellinger, E.P. (2007) Necrotizing soft-tissue infection: diagnosis and management. *Clinical Infectious Diseases*, 44(5), 705–710.

Bucca, K., Spencer, R., Orford, N., Cattigan, C., Athan, E., McDonald, A. (2012) Early diagnosis and treatment of necrotizing fasciitis can improve survival: an observational intensive care unit cohort study. *ANZ Journal of Surgery*, doi: 10.1111/j.1445-2197.2012.06251.x

Machado, N.O. (2011) Necrotizing fasciitis: The importance of early diagnosis, prompt surgical debridement and adjuvant therapy. *North American Journal of Medical Sciences*, 3(3), 107–118.

Mullangi, P.K., Khardori, N.M. (2012) Necrotizing soft-tissue infections. *Medical Clinics of North America*, 96(6),1193–1202.

Schuster, L., Nuñez, D.E. (2012) Using clinical pathways to aid in the diagnosis of necrotizing soft tissue infections synthesis of evidence. *Worldviews Evidence Based Nursing*, 9(2), 88–99.

PYODERMA GANGRENOSUM

Overview

Pyoderma gangrenosum (PG) is a rare autoimmune ulcerative skin condition of uncertain aetiology. The name refers to ulcers that develop with a blue-black edge which progressively get worse as seen in Figure 13.4 (see Chapter 13) Approximately half of patients with PG have an underlying systemic disease such as ulcerative colitis, Crohn's disease, chronic active hepatitis and rheumatoid arthritis (Miller et al., 2010). It affects males and females at any age, but is more common over the age of 50 years (Hadi and Lebwohl, 2011).

Risk factors

- IBD;
- Liver disease;
- Leukaemia, myeloma, lymphoma;
- Systemic lupus erythematosus;
- HIV infection;
- Rheumatoid arthritis;
- Trauma, for example, biopsies, surgery.

Differential diagnosis

- Vasculitis, for example, vasculitic rheumatoid arthritis, systemic lupus erythematosus;
- Venous leg ulceration;
- Malignancies, for example, squamous cell carcinoma;
- Infections: bacterial, viral, parasitic, tropical mycoses.

Clinical features

- Presentation is variable:
  - Sudden onset and rapid spread of painful ulcers with systemic illness and fever.
  - Ulceration with spontaneous regression and healing in one area and progression in another.
- Ulceration occurs most frequently on lower legs (pretibial area) and trunk. Lesions initially appear as single or multiple erythematous papules or pustules that may be preceded by trauma.
- Ulcers can progress from nodules to craters within 48 hours.
- Deep ulcerations develop due to dermal necrosis that contains purulent material.
- The classic PG skin lesion usually begins with pustules or fluctuant nodules with an inflammatory, purplish, violet boarder which expands to form an ulcer with raised edges.

Factors delaying healing

- Delayed diagnosis or misdiagnosis;
- Immune suppression;
- Corticosteroid treatment;
- Local infection/secondary infection;
- Co-morbidities, for example, IBD (Crohn's disease, ulcerative colitis).

Complications

- Wound/skin infection;
- Secondary infection related to immunosuppressive treatment;
- Glucocorticoid-induced bone loss, heart disease, hypertension, diabetes, gastric ulceration;
- Uncontrolled pain.

Principles of wound management

The aims of wound management for lesions caused by PG are to

(1) Reduce ulceration and determine the minimal dose of medication necessary to control the disease process.
(2) When associated with systemic disease, the therapeutic approach should also address the underlying disorder, for example, IBD
(3) Ensure that all therapeutic regimens are individualised to the patient and any preexisting conditions.
(4) Promote wound healing using a moist wound environment.
(5) Monitor patient's progress until they respond to treatment.

Treatment of lesions involves systemic treatment, together with local therapies.

Practical management

- PG is a clinical diagnosis made by the characteristic appearance of the ulcer. There is no specific diagnostic test.
- Systemic steroids are effective when delivered in adequate doses, as they prevent formation of new lesions and stop progression of the disease.
- Small ulcers are best managed with potent topical steroids. If wounds are on lower extremities and are minor, compression therapy may be beneficial for oedematous legs.
- More severe disease requires immunosuppressive therapy such as tacrolimus, ciclosporin, methotrexate.
- Analgesia prior to wound care is a high priority.
- Ulcers caused by PG produce copious exudate so calcium alginates and foam dressings are useful.

Wide surgical debridement should be avoided because it may result in enlargement of ulcers (Jackson et al., 2010).

Criteria for specialist referral

- Clinical suspicion of PG;
- Diagnosis or clinical suspicion of IBD;
- Diagnosis or clinical suspicion of arthritic disease.

Summary

Misdiagnosis of PG is not uncommon despite the ulcer being distinctive and should be considered in any non-healing deep ulcer on the lower leg. The prognosis is difficult to predict as patients may spontaneously go into remission or experience flare-ups for no apparent reason. Some studies report that approximately 50% of patients have recurrence (Miller et al., 2010). Long-term follow-up and re-evaluation of the diagnosis (with repeated biopsy, if indicated) are therefore recommended even in those patients who respond to treatment.

Further reading

Nguyen, K.H., Miller, J.J., Helm, K.F. (2003) Case reports and a review of the literature on ulcers mimicking pyoderma gangrenosum. *International Journal of Dermatology*, 42(2), 84–94.

Ruocco, E., Sangiuliano, S., Gravina, A.G., et al. (2009) Pyoderma gangrenosum: an updated review. *Journal of the European Academy of Dermatology And Venereology*, 23(9), 1008–1017.

Weenig, R.H., Davis, M.D., Dahl, P.R. et al. (2002) Skin ulcers misdiagnosed as pyoderma gangrenosum. *New England Journal of Medicine*, 347(18), 1412–1418.

References

Hadi, B.A., Lebwohl, M. (2011) Clinical features of *Pyoderma gangrenosum* and current diagnostic trends. *Journal of the American Academy of Dermatology*, 64, 950–954.

Miller, J., Yentzer, B.A. Clark, A. (2010) Pyoderma gangrenosum: a review and update on new therapies. *Journal of the American Academy of Dermatology*, 62(4), 646–654.

SELF-INFLICTED WOUNDS (SELF-HARM)

Overview

The incidence of deliberate self-harm is on the increase and ranges from minor superficial injuries such as cutting to major trauma such as genital self-mutilation and attempted suicide (Royal College of Psychiatrists, 2010). Individuals who self-harm tend to cause minor physical damage using scissors, razor blades, lit cigarettes, boiling water and bleach, and typically use more than one method over time (Lloyd-Richardson et al., 2007). Self-harm is an expression of emotional distress and can be seen as a distraction that brings relief (Royal College of Psychiatrists, 2010).

Health service staff often have negative attitudes towards those who self-harm, particularly those who do so repeatedly, and individuals may not be treated with compassion or respect. People who present with self-harm injuries frequently experience a significant amount of psychological and emotional distress, which may complicate the ability of the health care provider to care for the injury itself.

Risk factors

- Adolescents and young adults;
- Physical, emotional or sexual abuse in childhood;
- Low self-esteem;
- Poor social support;
- Socio-economic deprivation.

Differential diagnosis

- Dermatitis artefacta (unconscious self-harm);
- Dermatitis para-artefacta or skin-picking syndrome (existing lesions).

Factors delaying healing

- Repeated injury at the same site, for example, picking at scab, reopening of wound;
- Use of dirty objects of harm, for example, needle, razor blade;
- Neglect or delay in seeking help.

Clinical features

- Self-harm behaviours include cutting, hitting, biting oneself, reckless behaviour and bone-breaking.
- Highest prevalence is among young people.
- Self-harm may be life-long, affecting people of all ages.
- Frequent self-harm: typically 2–10 episodes per year.
- History and physical injury may not be consistent.

Complications

- Wound infection;
- Sepsis;
- Post-tourniquet syndrome from the use of string, thread, rubber bands or wire wrapped around a limb or digit resulting in nerve damage and ischemia;
- Permanent damage to tendons and nerves;
- Permanent scarring and disfigurement;
- Self-inflicted fractures are likely to be compound and therefore either are infected or susceptible to infection;
- Increased risk of serious harm or death by suicide.

Principles of wound management

The aims of wound management for individuals who deliberately self-harm are to:

(1) implement appropriate wound management strategies to maximise healing whilst being supportive and non-judgemental.
(2) minimise the risk of wound infection and development of long-term complications, such as scarring.
(3) collaborate with the multidisciplinary team to provide a comprehensive psychiatric, psychological and social assessment of the factors contributing to self-harm.

(National Institute for Health and Clinical Evidence, 2004)

Practical management

- Active listening, being supportive and non-judgemental help to build trust and reduce anxiety. Although it is important to develop a caring therapeutic relationship, it is also important to assess whether self-harming behaviours are being used to manipulate situations and/or staff.
- Individuals who self-harm benefit from continuity of care and are best managed by a limited number of experienced staff so that a rapport can be developed.
- Do not overlook self-harm as a cause of wound in young children or the elderly.

- Treatment is dependent on a detailed assessment of underlying psychological/psychiatric distress. A full account of this should be documented when the individual presents for treatment.
- A thorough skin assessment should be performed, as individuals may self-harm in more than one location. Injuries and wounds are less often seen on the dominant forearm. Areas of the body that are easy to reach are damaged more frequently.
- Self-inflicted wounds require a thorough physical assessment, taking into account the possibility of damage to underlying structures.
- The decision to tell the individual that self-wounding is suspected is a difficult one that should be made on an individual basis with the support of the multidisciplinary team.
- Assessment of the risk of further self-harm or suicide and prompt specialist referral is organised, if necessary.
- Individuals should be fully consulted and given sufficient information to allow an informed choice of treatment options. They must be included in any decision-making to ensure some measure of success.
- Superficial wounds should be managed like any other acute wound.
- Preference should be given to wound treatments that cause the least amount of anxiety (e.g. skin adhesives or skin closure tapes) to avoid further distress.
- Dressing and suture removal must be performed carefully to minimise further anxiety and distress. The patient may have delayed seeking help and may dread the anticipated pain if the dressing has adhered to the wound. Use of a calm approach and soaking the dressing prior to removal is helpful.
- Scarring may be as important as the deliberate act of self-harm. Ensuring that the individual is involved in the treatment plan is important to promote concordance and prevent removal of the dressing and deliberate interference with the wound.
- Evidence is mounting to support the use of cognitive behavioural therapy (CBT) as an effective psychological intervention in decreasing depression and reducing incidents of self-harm (National Institute for Health and Clinical Evidence, 2004 and Slee et al., 2008).

- All persons who have self-harmed should be assessed for further self-harm with particular attention to signs of depression, hopelessness and suicide.

This section is based on best practice described by The Royal Australian and New Zealand College of Psychiatrists (2000, NICE 2004, and the Royal College of Psychiatrists 2010)

Criteria for specialist referral

- A history of repeated injury or non-healing wounds without obvious cause;
- Wounds may be deep and have foreign bodies embedded in them, and may require surgical exploration.
- Referral to mental health services for counselling or CBT should be based on a combined assessment of need and risk of further harm, and must involve the individual concerned.

Information should be communicated with the individual's community doctor and to any relevant mental health services as soon as possible to enable adequate follow-up.

Summary

The development of a therapeutic relationship between the individual who self-harms and health care professionals who focus on self-awareness and an appreciation of the hidden strengths in the individual provides a more considered approach than the traditional medical model of care. A multi-disciplinary approach involving primary care providers, mental health specialists and dermatologists ensures the best chance of success. Intervention needs to focus on reducing the specific issues that contribute to deliberate self-harm and develop alternative skills for positive coping, communication, stress management and strong social support.

Further reading

Guidelines for the Management of Deliberate Self Harm in Young People. Australasian College for Emergency Medicine (ACEM) and The Royal Australian and New Zealand College of Psychiatrists (RANZCP). Available

at: http://www.acem.org.au/media/publications/youthsuicide.pdf.

Australasian College for Emergency Medicine (ACEM) and The Royal Australian and New Zealand College of Psychiatrists (RANZCP) (2000) Available at: http://www.acem.org.au/media/publications/youthsuicide.pdf.

Shepperd, C., McAllister, M. (2003) CARE: A framework for responding therapeutically to the client who self-harms. *Journal of Psychiatric and Mental Health Nursing,* 10(4), 442–447.

References

Lloyd-Richardson, E.E., Perrine, N., Dierke, L., Kelley, M.L. (2007) Characteristics and functions of non-suicidal self-injury in a community sample of adolescents. *Psychological Medicine,* 37, 1183–1192.

National Institute for Health and Clinical Excellence (2004) *Self-Harm. The Short-Term Physical and Psychological Management and Secondary Prevention of Self-Harm in Primary and Secondary Care.* London: NICE.

Royal College of Psychiatrists (2010) *Self-Harm, Suicide and Risk: Helping People who Self-Harm.* Available at: www.rcpsych.ac.uk/files/pdfversion/CR158.pdf.

Slee, N., Garnefski, N., van der Leeden, R., et al. (2008) Cognitive–behavioural intervention for self-harm: randomised controlled trial. *British Journal of Psychiatry,* 192, 202–211.

SKIN TEARS

Overview

Skin tears are traumatic injuries which can result in partial or full separation of the outer layers of the skin as seen in Figure 15.3. These tears occur due to shearing and friction forces or from blunt trauma, and usually occur in either immature skin in neonates or in elderly people (LeBlanc and Baranoski, 2011). Prevalence data is difficult to collect, but there is widespread agreement that skin tears are common (Carville et al., 2007). Pretibial lacerations are one of the most frequently seen skin tears that occur on the lower limb of elderly patients as a result of trauma. Skin tears are often mismanaged and as a result may become chronic wounds.

Risk factors

- Extremes of age – neonates and the elderly;
- *Comorbidities (vascularity):* CVA, chronic heart failure, clotting disorders

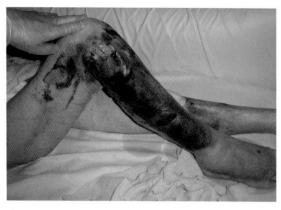

Figure 15.3 Extensive skin tear in an elderly person complicated by a large haematoma. Photo courtesy of Ann Marie Brown.

- History of previous skin tears;
- Dry, fragile skin;
- Medications (e.g. steroids, anticoagulation therapy);
- Echymoses;
- Poor nutrition (including adequate hydration);
- Cognitive or sensory impairment;
- Impaired mobility or vision;
- Predisposition to falls;
- Dependence on others for activities of daily living.

(LeBlanc and Baranoski, 2011)

Differential diagnosis

- Self-inflicted wound;
- Non-accidental injury;
- Cellulitis.

Factors delaying healing

- Significant tissue loss;
- Bleeding and hematomas;
- Infection;
- Oedema;
- Age-related skin changes.

Clinical features

The Skin Tear Audit Research (STAR) is a classification system which describes the appearance of skin tears (Carville et al., 2007).

Category 1a
A skin tear where the edges can be realigned to the normal anatomical position (without undue stretching), and the skin or flap colour is not pale, dusky or darkened.

Category 1b
A skin tear where the edges can be realigned to the normal anatomical position (without undue stretching), and the skin or flap colour is pale, dusky or darkened.

Category 2a
A skin tear where the edges cannot be realigned to the normal anatomical position, and the skin or flap colour is not pale, dusky or darkened.

Category 2b
A skin tear where the edges cannot be realigned to the normal anatomical position, and the skin or flap colour is pale, dusky or darkened.

Category 3
A skin tear where the skin flap is completely absent.

Complications

- Infection: cellulitis, generalised sepsis;
- Necrosis with loss of tissue;
- Pain;
- Delayed wound healing.

Principles of wound management

The aims of wound management for individuals with skin tears are to:

- assess the skin trauma using a recognised classification system, for example, STAR;
- approximate the skin flap if possible without causing traction or further damage;
- secure the skin flap using a non-adherent dressing and apply without tension;
- minimise the risk of wound infection and development of complications;
- reduce the risk of recurrence by educating patient and carers about the risk of further trauma.

Practical management

- Control bleeding: apply pressure and elevate limb, if required.
- Clean wound with normal saline or sterile water to remove any blood clots and pat area dry.
- Approximate the skin flap: use a gloved finger, cotton tip swab or tweezers as appropriate.
  - If flap is difficult to realign, consider moistening with normal saline for 5–10 minutes to rehydrate the flap.
  - Wound closure strips should allow drainage of wound fluid from the flap and may be made from strips of silicone sheet dressings to avoid use of adhesive strips.
  - Sutures and staples are not recommended, but skin adhesive can be useful.
- Apply a skin barrier product to the peri-wound area for protection.
- Apply a low-adherent primary dressing to maintain a moist wound environment, for example, soft silicone or foam dressings.
- Mark dressing with an arrow to indicate the preferred direction of removal and take care when removing dressing so as not to damage the flap.
- Leave dressing *in situ* for as long as possible to avoid disturbing the flap.
- Monitor wound pain as this may be one of the earliest signs of infection and treat promptly.
- Apply a light compression bandage or tubular bandage to the limb if tolerated but check circulation first.
- Adopt good manual handling techniques to avoid further skin trauma.

Criteria for specialist referral

Referral to a surgeon is indicated when the skin tear is extensive or when there is an associated full thickness skin injury, significant and uncontrolled bleeding or large hematoma formation.

Summary

Prevention of skin tears is a vital part of daily skin care practice, especially in the elderly, infants or patients who require assistance with daily care. The skin should be kept hydrated by applying emollients twice a day, and attention should be paid to reduction of pressure, shear and friction by use of appropriate repositioning techniques or pressure-relieving devices. People who experience repeated skin tears should be encouraged to wear long sleeves and socks for protection. The care environment should be evaluated to maintain a safe environment, as any management plan should include strategies to prevent skin tears from occurring.

Further reading

Ayello, E., Sibbald, R.G. (2008) National Guideline C. Preventing pressure ulcers and skin tears. In: *Evidence-Based Geriatric Nursing Protocols for Best Practice* (eds E. Capezuti, D. Zwicker, M. Mezey, T. Fulmer), 3rd edn, pp. 403–429. New York: Springer Publishing Company.

Stephen-Haynes, J., Carville K. (2011) Skin tears made easy. *Wounds International*, 2(4). Available at: http://www.woundsinternational.com.

References

Carville, K., Lewin, G., Newall, N., et al. (2007) STAR: a consensus for skin tear classification. *Primary Intention*, 15(1): 18–28.

LeBlanc, K., Baranoski S. (2011) Skin tears: state of the science: consensus statements for the prevention, prediction, assessment and treatment of skin tears. *Advances in Skin and Wound Care*, 24(9), 2–15.

Section 3

Improving Skin Integrity Services

16 Reducing Wound Care Costs and Improving Quality: A Clinician's Perspective

Theresa Hurd

Wound and Chronic Disease Management, Nursing Practice Solutions, Inc., Toronto, Ontario, Canada

Overview

- Chronic wounds represent a large and growing burden for both patients and healthcare organisations. However, despite the significance of chronic wound care as a health issue, the total costs are often underestimated and poorly understood.
- As cost consciousness becomes increasingly widespread throughout healthcare, there is a greater need for clinicians as well as administrators and policymakers to understand how services can be delivered more efficiently and effectively.
- There is a close relationship between the quality/safety of care and the efficiency/effectiveness of healthcare resource utilisation: A lack of safe, quality care leads to overall increases in healthcare costs. Conversely, the consistent delivery of quality care supports efficient resource allocation, which ultimately makes more resources available for clinical priorities.
- Best-practice wound prevention and care programmes are, in effect, quality programmes. They are designed to put in place evidence-based clinical best practices on a consistent, sustainable basis and involve major organisational change.
- Many of the barriers to best-practice wound prevention and care relate to the fact that wounds can be complex chronic conditions that involve all stages of the continuum and numerous clinical disciplines, while the systems needed to support multi-disciplinary, collaborative care are often absent or underdeveloped.
- Evidence to date shows that best-practice wound prevention and care programmes result in reduced wound healing times and significant cost reductions. As best practices are implemented, errors are reduced and clinical outcomes improve and become more predictable. Appropriate clinical resources are matched with clinical needs. Waste is reduced and cost efficiencies are realised.

Introduction

Chronic wounds represent a large and growing burden for both patients and healthcare organisations. Despite the significance of chronic wounds as a health issue, the impact on health economics is often underestimated. Wounds remain a relatively low-profile concern for many administrators and clinicians. Wound care is often viewed simply as a routine component of basic nursing practice, rather than a complex and multifaceted healthcare challenge with implications that extend across organisations and disciplines. In many cases, the cost of wound care is simplistically and inaccurately

Wound Healing and Skin Integrity: Principles and Practice, First Edition. Edited by Madeleine Flanagan.
© 2013 John Wiley & Sons, Ltd. Published 2013 by John Wiley & Sons, Ltd.

based on the number of dressings used, rather than the total care requirements for all patients across the continuum. Key indicators such as wound prevalence, healing times and infection rates are not always measured and the size and nature of the chronic wound problem may not be fully understood.

In recent years, however, a growing body of research has been contributing to a better appreciation of the high cost of chronic wounds. Further, and most importantly, the testing, development and implementation of best-practice wound prevention and care programmes has been demonstrating how these costs can be reduced, while simultaneously improving the health and well-being of patients. This chapter provides an overview of best-practice wound prevention and care programmes, focusing on economic as well as patient outcomes.

Health economics: a clinician's perspective

In the healthcare sector, health economics aims to provide a set of analytical techniques to assist decision-making, to promote efficiency and equity. Ultimately, health economics is about issues related to scarcity in the allocation of health and healthcare (Shiell et al., 2002). For organisations involved in the delivery of health services, this increasingly important discipline encompasses all of the decisions about how limited healthcare resources – including everything from skilled clinicians and hospital beds to operating funds and emerging new technologies – are used most efficiently to deliver the best possible healthcare.

Health economics is currently receiving considerable attention for most health systems around the world because the available resources are increasingly limited or under strain. Healthcare organisations face growing demands from aging populations with an increasing prevalence of chronic disease and complex co-morbidities. At the same time, there are government funding constraints, shortages of trained professionals and constant pressures to adopt new and often very expensive technologies. The ability to allocate scarce resources is becoming increasingly difficult and challenging.

Health economics and financial issues have been viewed traditionally as a concern primarily for administrators and policymakers. Clinicians, who must focus foremost on the health of their patients, have often approached issues of cost and efficiency as a lower priority, or have confronted these issues only when advocating for a particular treatment on a patient's behalf. Discussions about costs have been avoided or approached sceptically by many clinicians, because they are seen as potentially limiting care options or clinical choice. Financial concerns have often been viewed as separate from or even in opposition to the ultimate goal of providing optimal patient care.

'Cost consciousness' is now much more widespread than in the past, particularly where limited resources must meet growing healthcare demands. There is a need across all care settings to provide cost-effective care in a clinically responsible manner (Britt et al., 1999). A greater focus on costs affects clinicians, although the first and most common response often involves simply tracking specific cost items such as the wound dressings noted above. Within clinical circles, a broader view that encompasses the relationships between the management of healthcare resources and the delivery of care across organisations or health systems is less common.

This broader perspective reveals that health economics and clinical care are, in fact, integrally related. Better clinical care can lead to improved health economics; efficient resource allocation can lead to better outcomes for patients. It is important for clinicians to develop an understanding of health economics and financial issues as they pursue clinical practice and assume leadership roles. This understanding should include a *micro* perspective related to the financing of individual healthcare organisations, and extend to encompass a *macro* perspective of the entire health system, including who pays for healthcare, how these payments are made and how reimbursement affects healthcare services.

The linkages between health economics and clinical practice can be examined through an analysis of quality in the delivery of healthcare services. Quality care has become a high-priority concern for healthcare providers globally, and it is closely interrelated to patient safety, another high-profile concern. Evidence of the growing prominence of quality and safety issues is found in media reports and in the attempts by insurance providers, administrators and legislators to improve standards and link healthcare funding to quality/safety indicators. Wound care is one of the key clinical functions at the centre of these issues. Pressure ulcers and wound infections, in particular, are often linked to patient complications and litigation risk (Baranoski and Ayello, 2008).

The literature demonstrates that a lack of safe, quality care has a direct impact on a variety of cost categories, leading to an overall increase in costs to the healthcare system (Finkelman, 2006). Conversely, the consistent delivery of quality care supports efficient resource allocation, which ultimately makes more resources available for clinical priorities. These relationships can be readily illustrated by wound care, and are further explored below.

Barriers to best-practice wound care and prevention

As a growing body of research confirms that the cost of chronic wounds to both patients and healthcare organisations is already very high and can be expected to grow, the case for improving wound care, both as a quality measure and as a value measure, is compelling. However, a variety of long-standing clinical and institutional barriers must be overcome.

Most of these barriers relate to the fact that wound care is a complex and widespread healthcare challenge that cuts across healthcare sectors (acute, long-term and community care) and clinical disciplines (nurses, physicians, nutritionists, physiotherapists, etc.). Wound care cannot be easily defined as a distinct clinical issue, and there are often no clear lines of responsibility or accountability. Specific barriers that have been identified include

- *Inadequate or poorly maintained measurement and reporting systems*: There may be limited or inconsistent wound care metrics, a lack of data on key indicators (such as wound prevalence, age of wounds, infection rates and healing times) and/or a lack of information on wound care costs.
- *Inconsistent wound assessment*: There may be an absence of consistent head-to-toe assessment protocols applied organisation-wide and recorded systematically for all wound patients

or patients who may be at risk of acquiring wounds.
- *Gaps in evidence-based practice*: Some practices may be outdated or not backed by evidence. There may be no clear predictability for healing times/outcomes for specific wound types and patient populations.
- *Inconsistent application of clinical best practices*: In some cases, there are no clear clinical pathways or protocols applied by clinicians across the organisation. Clinical approaches to wound care may be fragmented or uncoordinated across sectors, departments or clinical disciplines.
- *Inconsistent purchasing practices*: Formularies for the selection, purchasing and use of wound care products may not be in place or followed consistently. There may be waste, duplication and inappropriate/inefficient use of products. Access to products and equipment may be uneven across the organisation.
- *Inadequate training and education*: Training and education specific to wound care may be inadequate and/or not sufficiently competency-based. There may be significant gaps and inconsistencies in nursing skills and knowledge.
- *Lack of interdisciplinary cooperation and coordination*: Clinical disciplines can be highly competitive and protective of certain defined areas of practice, while wound care demands an interdisciplinary, holistic approach.
- *Lack of clear leadership*: There may be little or no leadership or responsibility for wound care at the senior clinical or administrative level, and a general lack of organisational awareness and understanding of wounds as a clinical priority.
- *Communication deficiencies*: Tools and programmes to inform patients and families about wound care and the risks of acquiring wounds may not be in place.

(Flanagan, 2005)

These barriers reflect characteristics of health systems that have been identified in the literature as barriers to the management of chronic diseases in general. A complex, fragmented and disorganised system can be poorly equipped to care for patients with complex chronic conditions that require a collaborative, long-term approach to care (Wagner et al., 1996; Board on Population Health and Public Health Practice 2012). Mannion et al. (2005) recommends that healthcare organisations to support patients with long-term conditions such as chronic wounds:

(1) need for evidence-based care;
(2) reorganisation of practices to meet the needs of patients who require more time, a broad array of resources and closer follow-up;
(3) systematic attention to patients, need for information, self-management and behavioural change;
(4) readiness to access appropriate expertise;
(5) supportive information system.

The costs of wound care

Many of the costs associated with wound care are poorly documented or hidden within other general cost categories such as hospital bed-days or community nursing visits. This is due in part to the relatively low profile of chronic wounds and the complexity of many wound cases, as noted above.

In practice, wound care places a significant burden on the time of nurses and other clinicians, and complex or mismanaged wound cases place heavy and often preventable demands on acute care resources. Health economics research is beginning to confirm that most wound care costs are, in fact, hidden. One UK study suggests the following breakdown:

- *Wound dressings and materials*: These highly visible cost categories typically account for just 17–22% of total wound care costs.
- *Nursing hours*: Nurses perform the bulk of frontline wound care, and nursing hours typically make up as much as 33–41% of the total costs.
- *Hospitalisation*: Hospital admissions and extended hospital stays typically consume more than 37–49% of the total cost of wound care.

Some recent research has attempted to estimate the total cost of wound care across a patient population. For example, a 2-year study completed in the United States followed 9822 patients from 13 states. The total cost to treat 19,047 wounds during 92,668 visits (including physicians, clinics, home nursing, dressings and laboratory services) was US$ 54.3 million, for an average cost per patient of more than US$ 5500. The cost per patient exceeded US$ 100,000 in few cases (Walker, 2009).

Other studies have focused on particular categories of chronic wounds. For example, Canadian data indicate that:

- *Surgical site infections* affect 30–40 patients per 1000 operations. Attributable mortality was estimated at 5%. The excess length of stay (LOS) in hospital was 10.2 days per case (Hurd and Posnett, 2009).
- A 4-week costing study (Friedberg et al., 2002) estimated that 192 people receiving care would annually consume $1 million in nursing care services and $260,000 in wound care supplies. Comparing patients newly admitted during the past 6 months of either study period revealed the median number of nursing visits to have declined from 37 (interquartile range [IQR] 24–42) to 25 (IQR 15–35) over the period ($p = 0.041$). The median number of visits to each patient declined from 3 (IQR 2–4.8) to 2.1 (IQR 1.6–2.4) per week ($p = 0.005$). The median supply cost per case decreased from $1923 (IQR $395–1931) to $406 (IQR $219–920; $p = 0.005$).
- Stage III *pressure ulcers* result in an average LOS in hospital of 18.8 days, at an average cost of C$19,213. Stage IV pressure ulcers require an average LOS of 27.7 days at an average cost of C$29,208, and Stage X pressure ulcers with bone and necrotic tissue involvement result in an average LOS of 73.1 days at an average cost of C$85,436 (Hurd and Posnett, 2009).

Health economists are also attempting to quantify wound care costs across healthcare institutions and systems. The annual cost to a typical hospital in Europe has been estimated at 4000 excess bed-days and €3.3 million (Drew et al. 2007). In the United Kingdom, it is estimated that there are 200,000 people with a chronic wound, costing the National Health Service £2–3 billion annually, or about 3% of the total NHS budget (Posnett and Franks, 2007). The Wound Ostomy and Continence Nursing Society (2010) has estimated that between US$ 2.2 and US$ 3.6 billion is spent yearly for the management of pressure ulcers in the United States. The cost to care for all chronic wounds has been estimated at US$ 10 billion annually throughout North America (Swanson 1999). A study in Australia looked at the number and economic value of bed-days lost to pressure ulcers and concluded that the opportunity cost to Australian hospitals for pressure ulcers alone was A$ 285 million (Graves et al., 2005).

Best-practice wound prevention and care programmes

Best-practice wound prevention and care programmes offer particularly prominent illustrations of the relationships between quality care and health economics (Hurd et al., 2008). These programmes are designed to put in place evidence-based clinical practices across healthcare organisations on a sustainable basis. As such, they are comprehensive processes of organisational change. Specific best-practice protocols for all aspects of wound prevention and care are defined and implemented, along with all of the necessary organisational supports (i.e. information systems, training and education programmes, programme formularies, etc.). Clinical results are measured and monitored to provide continuous feedback and to identify opportunities for improvement. Best practices, in effect, become standardised, predictable and continuously monitored for all patients and all practitioners. These programmes are multi-disciplinary and work across the healthcare continuum, including acute care, long-term care and home care sectors.

The basic relationships between programme implementation, clinical outcomes and resource utilisation are summarised in Figure 16.1.

Key steps in the process are

- The implementation of a best-practice wound prevention and care programme is a starting point. It initiates a comprehensive change process across the organisation, designed to integrate best-practice wound care protocols permanently into regular clinical practices. All levels of the organisation are involved.
- If implemented consistently and rigorously across the organisation, best-practice wound care leads inevitably to improved clinical outcomes for patients. Examples include faster healing times, reduced infection rates, improved comfort, increased mobility and a better quality of life.
- As the programme is established and outcomes improve, the more efficient and effective utilisation of limited healthcare resources is, for example, fewer complications, reduction in length of hospital stays, less admissions and readmissions. Clinicians spend less time on business processes (tracking patient records, sourc-

ing wound care products and equipment, etc.) because clear protocols and formularies are in place.
- More efficient resource utilisation enables continuous programme improvement. Clinicians are able to spend more time directly on patient care and focus on patients with the most serious clinical needs. Information systems enable better coordination of a multi-disciplinary clinical team. The organisation improves its capacity to manage the most high-risk patients and the most complex wounds.
- The benefits of improved efficiency and resource allocation extend beyond wound care as resources become available to meet other healthcare priorities. For example, hospital beds become available for other acute care needs. Since wound care is a multi-disciplinary function that is closely related to common chronic diseases, best-practice programmes are well-positioned within most healthcare settings to generate spin-off benefits and serve as a model for similar quality care initiatives.

Best-practice wound prevention and care programmes differ from many health-care innovations that are focused primarily on new products, new technologies or new clinical approaches. These programmes cannot be viewed as 'add-ons' to existing systems. Rather, they are processes of systemic organisational change. The technology of wound care is well-established and readily available; the challenge is to have it adopted rigorously, consistently and in a disciplined manner by all clinicians and administrative staff.

This fundamental emphasis on organisational change and improvement means that the entire healthcare organisation, from senior leadership to front-line clinical staff, must be involved. The comprehensive nature of this approach creates many challenges. However, it also creates opportunities, in that the basic process demonstrated by wound care can foster broader organisational improvement and be applied to other clinical challenges.

A best-practice wound prevention and care programme is comprehensive and multi-faceted. Table 16.1 highlights the critical programme components and has been adapted and expanded for wound care and prevention from Board on Population Health and Public Health Practice (2012).

The introduction of a best-practice wound prevention and care programme (1) leads to improved clinical outcomes (2) which, in turn, produce a number of cost efficiency and resource utilisation benefits (3). These feed back to allow continuous improvement of the programme (1) while also generating spin-off economic benefits (4).

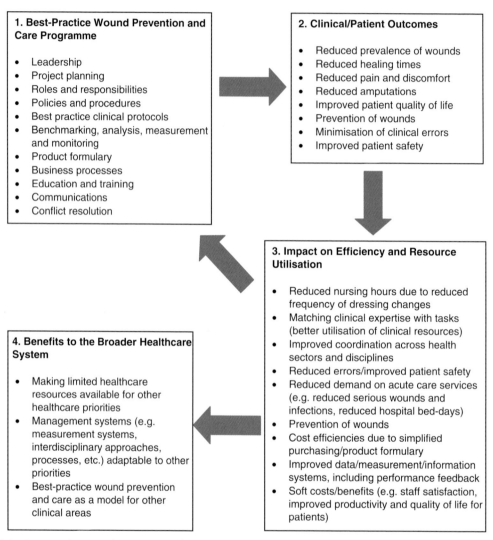

Figure 16.1   Best-practice wound prevention and care.

Clinical results

Best-practice wound care and prevention programmes have been shown to produce a range of positive clinical outcomes from reduced healing times and infection rates to improved comfort, mobility and quality of life for patients. Data from a growing number of programmes in jurisdictions throughout the world indicate that these results can be achieved consistently and predictably in a variety of healthcare settings.

Best-practice programmes place each patient on a predictable clinical pathway towards the optimal healing of their wound(s), or in cases where healing is not an achievable goal, the optimal maintenance of their wound(s). Clinical pathways are part of best-practice standards/guidelines for wound care. There are typical pathways for different types of

Table 16.1   Table summary of key components of a wound care programme

Leadership	• Senior management identified as the driver for change and the face of the project, and committed to support all aspects of the programme from launch to sustainability • Focus on patients and improved clinical outcomes • Identify more effective organisational support to ensure change of care possible • Consistency and discipline: all policies, procedures, protocols and processes enforced evenly, with no exceptions; fair and consistent treatment for all parties • Clear mandate and support for any external experts/resource people to work effectively • Support from leaders in ensuring that all care is equitable and does not vary in quality because of geographic location, gender, ethnicity, etc.
Defined roles, responsibilities	• Clear definition of all roles (e.g. nurses, care providers, physicians, wound care specialists, other clinicians, such as nutritionists and physiotherapists, clinical managers, administrators, senior managers, vendors and suppliers, outside experts, patients, families, etc.) • All have a shared agenda to improve overall quality of care and a safe environment for patients
Project planning	• Planning group consisting of senior management, clinicians, consultants and other experts, representatives of outside agencies, etc. • Detailed project plan with subsidiary plans for training and education, communications, conflict resolution, etc.; timelines, planning tools and process maps included as appropriate
Policies and procedures	• Clear policies and procedures, established across the health-care organisation to guide clinical practices based on evidence-based, best-practice standards of care
Measurement and monitoring (Berendt et al., 2001)	• Comprehensive benchmark analysis of current wound prevalence and wound care practices to identify gaps and areas for improvement • Key metrics and measurement/data collection systems in place prior to programme launch • Regular auditing and reporting • Utilisation review of appropriateness and efficiency of services specific to wound patients
Best-practice, Evidence-based clinical protocols/pathways	• Assembled and developed by the planning group, using available resource and guidelines (standard of care) where appropriate, adapted to suit local requirements and producing new protocols as needed • Patient-centred care; providing care that is respectful and responsible • Provision of care and services based on scientific knowledge to all who benefit and not likely to benefit; avoiding overuse and underuse • Practice changes (e.g. compression of venous leg ulcers, use of advanced dressings)
Process mapping	• Detailed process maps, based on clinical evidence and best practices, provided to case managers, care providers and other clinicians; consistent and disciplined application • Ensure that processes and their implementation is efficient avoiding waste – this includes waste of equipment, wound care products, ideas and energy • Timely ensuring reduction in waste and harmful delays for those who receive and give care
Business processes and product formulary	• Clear business processes to guide all accounting practices, data recording, record keeping, etc. related to wound care, standardised throughout the organisation • Detailed product formulary, linked to clinical protocols, listing all products and equipment • Clear systems for ordering, storing, accessing wound care products and equipment
Documentation	• Documentation tools to support process maps, interreliability of tools • Protocols, pathways and assessment tools to ensure consistent and clear documentation that drives practice
Education and training	• Identification of who needs to be educated and the required content Comprehensive, competency-based training/education programme and resources for all clinicians, using adult learning principles and linked to clinical protocols; rigorous training for administrative staff and other staff to support programme • Team-building, sharing and exchange of ideas; capacity building for long-term sustainability

(Continued)

Table 16.1   (*Continued*)

Communications	• Detailed communication plan guiding regular communication to all groups involved
	• Communications staff involved early in the process and integrated into programme planning
	• All messaging to staff and service providers focused on best practices and the commitment to providing quality care to patients
	• Successes celebrated and communicated to all involved groups
Conflict resolution	• Anticipation of potential conflict areas
	• Emphasise common goal of improved quality of care
	• Process mapping to guide interactions between groups, with tools to assist in conflict resolution (e.g. scripted letter to aid in communication between staff and physicians)
	• Reduce interprofessional competition and rivalry

wounds and different types of patients. Evidence-based guidelines are also available to identify outcomes, assess progress towards these outcomes and support best practices for various types of chronic wounds. These pathways and guidelines are useful in determining both the quality and cost of wound care. The promotion of the appropriate use of resources in a timely manner is an important component of each pathway and thereby promotes cost-effectiveness. These guidelines serve as benchmarks for clinicians and patients, as well as family members and caregivers.

Ongoing measurement and monitoring of clinical outcomes is an integral part of the overall change process. Benchmarks are established, progress is monitored and results are reported regularly across the healthcare organisation. This process allows organisations to compare their performance both within the organisation and with other organisations (Berendt et al., 2001). It also helps to motivate staff, to encourage continuous improvement and, ultimately, to support the sustainability of wound management programmes. The organisation can focus on key performance gaps, identify new opportunities in both quality and cost improvement (Karpiel, 2000).

Improved wound healing

Results from best-practice wound prevention and care programmes have demonstrated significant, and in some cases, dramatic reductions in average healing times. A recent study followed 263 clients with leg ulcers and found significant differences in the healing of lower extremity ulcers was seen between a best-practice-based approach and standard community care (Bolton et al., 2004). Improved

wound healing rates lead, in turn, to a number of associated clinical outcomes. These include

• reduced risk of infection;
• reduced amputations;
• reduced pain and improved comfort for patients;
• improved quality of life;
• improved patient safety.

From a health economics perspective, a key benefit of more rapid, predictable and consistent healing times is reduced time spent by wound patients in acute care. As noted, this is the aspect of care that is most costly to healthcare organisations and, in most cases, it is preventable.

Wound prevention

Prevention measures are integral to any best-practice wound programme. These measures encompass the prevention of avoidable wounds such as pressure ulcers, as well as any complications, deteriorations or infections associated with existing wounds. Screening upon admission and as part of routine clinical assessments is required to identify patients who are at risk of developing a wound such as a pressure ulcer. The level and type of risk should inform prevention decisions. Custom protocols should be designed to reflect these risks, with clinical practice guidelines used as starting points (Baranoski and Ayello, 2008).

A wound that is prevented is, by definition, a 'non-event'. The cost savings attributed directly to prevention measures are therefore difficult to estimate. It can be assumed, however, that for most best-practice programmes, prevention is a major contributor to reduce overall wound prevalence rates (see later). Also, prevention is widely considered to be a low-cost intervention that is far less costly than any of the remedial measures required to correct a preventable problem, and of course is far less consequential for patients. A review of various studies confirms that the costs associated with prevention are limited (Waters, 2005). Finally, wound prevention is integral to the patient safety imperative of healthcare institutions. Increasingly, wounds are being recognised as a major patient safety risk and a reliable indicator of quality of care, including the associated legal liabilities.

Reduced prevalence of chronic wounds

Wound prevalence and incidence rates are perhaps one of the best indicators of the overall effectiveness of best-practice wound prevention and care programmes (Sussman and Bates-Jensen, 2007). Data from programmes in various jurisdictions around the world show that significant reductions in wound prevalence can be achieved in a wide range of healthcare settings.

A comparison of similar programmes implemented in two different acute care institutions, one in Canada and the other in Australia, illustrates the potential to reduce wound prevalence. The first institution is a multi-site teaching hospital serving a large urban community in Ontario, Canada, with two hospital sites and residential aged care services providing care for about 29,000 inpatients annually; the second is an integrated healthcare organisation in Victoria, Australia, that includes a major regional hospital, as well as residential aged care services, with an annual inpatient volume of about 35,000.

Pressure ulcers were identified as a specific clinical issue in both cases. Nurse specialists with expertise in wound care were available, but no broad organisation-wide programmes or capabilities were in place. Wound care efforts at both institutions were characterised by a general lack of awareness and data on wounds, as well as inconsistencies in clinical practice, documentation, purchasing, training and education.

Best-practice programmes were launched first at the Canadian facility in 2007, and then at the Australian organisation in 2009. Key results are summarised in Table 16.2. It is noteworthy that

Table 16.2   Best-practice wound prevention and care programmes: summary of pressure ulcer prevalence and related indicators before and after programme implementation[a]

	Canadian healthcare organisation (Hurd et al., 2012)		Australian facility (Hurd and Trueman, 2012)	
	Pre-implementation (2007)	Post-implementation (2009)	Pre-implementation (2009)	Post-implementation (2011)
Total number of patients	309	301	630	635
Pressure ulcer prevalence (% of patients with pressure ulcers)	21	2.9	15	3.7
Hospital acquired pressure ulcers (% of total pressure ulcers)	89	12	88	25
Daily dressing changes (% of patients receiving daily dressing changes)	40	0	28	1
Use of advanced wound dressings where appropriate	29	100	35	88
Infection rate (% of pressure ulcer patients with infected wound)	7	0	9	0

[a]Note: The Canadian programme was launched in 2007, and was established within approximately 1 year. The post-implementation survey was completed in 2009, following 12 months of operation. The Australian programme was launched in 2009, and was also established within 1 year. The post-implementation survey was completed in 2011, following 6 months' operation.

these reductions in pressure ulcer prevalence were achieved quickly, after about 1 year of programme operation in Canada and 6 months in Australia. Continuous improvement is underway at both institutions, and it is anticipated that pressure ulcer prevalence rates will drop further to a sustainable rate well under 10%.

The impact of best-practice wound prevention and care on health economics

Best-practice wound prevention and care programmes are aimed at producing evidence-based clinical outcomes. However, because they establish robust measurement and monitoring systems and apply clear, consistent protocols and business processes, they are also efficient programmes. They are designed to ensure that the correct combination of clinical resources (e.g. clinician expertise, products, technologies, etc.) reaches each patient as quickly as possible. As such, they eliminate confusion, errors, waste and duplication, all of which can lead to suboptimal clinical outcomes, as well as unnecessarily high costs. These programmes have also been shown to address a major opportunity cost that is attributable to the preventable utilisation of hospital beds and other acute care resources by wound patients (Graves et al., 2005). As these programmes take effect and clinical outcomes are established, they have been shown to produce significant cost savings and major improvements in the allocation of healthcare resources.

The economic impact of best-practice wound prevention and care programmes extend across the entire continuum of care. Ensuring the delivery of best-practice care in the most appropriate setting

from the most appropriate provider is a primary driver in the improvement of cost-effectiveness and efficiency.

Cost-efficiencies and improved utilisation of clinical resources

Wound care is labour intensive, and most of the workload is carried out by nurses. Nursing hours make up roughly one-third of all wound care costs (Drew et al., 2007). The implementation of best-practice wound care can reduce this workload significantly, making nursing hours available for other clinical priorities. It is also noteworthy that, across healthcare, nurses are responsible for using more resources than any other categories of healthcare providers (Finkelman, 2006).

The case profiled in Table 16.3 shows how a shift to best-practice care in Canada produced significant savings, driven in particular by reduced nursing labour. This case (Teague and Mahoney, 2004) involves a 21-year-old man with type 1 diabetes, who was admitted to the medical unit of a major hospital with diabetic ketoacidosis. This patient had three traumatic wounds on his left leg. Prior to the launch of a best-practice programme, he was being treated with a regimen of gauze bandages and topical antimicrobial. Although this treatment was simple and inexpensive in terms of products and materials, this approach required excessive nursing hours and did not heal the wound. The new treatment involved a thorough wound assessment, the introduction of a comprehensive care pathway including multidisciplinary components such as nutrition, advanced dressings based on moist-wound healing principles and far fewer nursing

Table 16.3   Case cost comparison: wound patient before and after implementation of best-practice wound care

Previous care	Cost	Best practice	Cost
Nursing labour $40 × 240 visits	$9600.00	Nursing labour $40 × 6 visits	$240.00
Fucidin acid cream	$240.00	Duplex scan	$161.30
Gauze bandages	$360.00	Multi-layer bandage ×4	$100.00
Gloves	$48.00	Nanocrystalline silver 4 × 4 (×2)	$26.00
		Dressing trays	$6.00
		Gloves	$1.20
Total	$10,248.00	Total	$534.50
Outcome	Not healed	Outcome	HEALED
Difference in cost: $9,713.50			

Table 16.4   Implementation of best-practice wound care in a community-care setting: selected clinical indicators

| | Intervention group | | Control group | |
	Pre-audit	Post-audit	Pre-audit	Post-audit
Mean wound duration (weeks)	60	13	43	46
Advanced dressing and pathway use	41%	88%	47%	46%
Daily dressing changes	38%	13%	44%	49%
Leg ulcers compressed	50%	89%	24%	26%

hours. The result was a healed wound and a total cost savings of close to C$ 10,000.

Across healthcare organisations, reduced dressing changes as a result of best-practice care lead to one of the most immediate cost-efficiency benefits. Table 16.2 shows that the percentage of wound patients receiving daily or more frequent dressing changes in the Australian case introduced above was reduced from 38% to 6% during the first 6 months of programme operation. This is a direct result of substituting dry gauze dressings for advanced wound dressings based on moist wound healing principles. A total of 91 wound dressings within the survey population were being changed at least once per day, for a total of at least 1364 dressing changes per week. Assuming an average of 10 minutes per dressing change (Drew et al., 2007), this represents approximately six full-time equivalent (FTE) nursing staff. The number of wounds changed daily or more frequently was reduced to 11, translating to 77 changes per week, or less than 13 hours of staff time.

The other major cost category for wound care is hospitalisation, which is estimated to consume about one-half of all wound care costs (Drew et al., 2007). Best-practice programmes have been demonstrated to reduce or virtually eliminate extended hospital stays and hospital admissions due to chronic wounds. Table 16.2 shows that infected pressure ulcers were eliminated in both of the cases profiled and that use of daily dressing changes were significantly reduced.

Best-practice wound prevention and care programmes have been particularly effective in reducing costs and improving efficiencies in home/community care organisations. A shift to advanced wound dressings can be particularly significant, for example since as many as one-half of all home visits involve wound care (Hurd et al., 2008). Potential programme results for home/community care are illustrated by a study conducted in another

Canadian healthcare organisation. This organisation serves population of approximately 1.6 million and is responsible for the delivery of in-home nursing visits to 28,000–32,000 patients each day. Forty-seven percent of all nursing visits require some form of wound care.

Programme implementation was preceded by a detailed trial that compared a control group (no change to existing wound care practices) with a similar group for which best-practice protocols were implemented. After 1 year, the implementation group showed significant changes in both wound care practices and wound healing results, as indicated by the average age of wounds (Table 16.4). The average total cost of wound treatment per wound was C$ 3,491 in the intervention group, compared to C$ 15,996 for the control group (Table 16.5). Subsequent roll-out of the programme across the organisation resulted in a total annual savings of C$ 11.8 million, or roughly 5% of the total annual operating budget (Hurd and Posnett, 2009).

Two common themes emerge from the cost data from best-practice wound prevention and care programmes. First, the time spent by nurses and other clinicians on routine tasks such as dressing changes

Table 16.5   Implementation of best-practice wound care in a community-care setting: selected cost indicators

	Intervention group	Control group
Mean dressing changes per week	2.78	5.82
Nurse cost per change	$57	$57
Mean materials cost per change	$39.59	$2.75
Treatment cost to date:		
Nurse cost	$2060	$15,260
Materials cost	$1431	$736
Total treatment cost	$3491	$15,996

is reduced, thereby making more time available for treating the most serious wound cases and managing other clinical priorities. Second, extended hospital stays, admissions and readmissions due to wound deterioration and complication are avoided, thereby making limited acute care resources available for other priorities and removing a major barrier to efficient bed management within acute care institutions. These resource-utilisation outcomes are measured and monitored and become more predictable as best-practice clinical pathways are established, thereby supporting the overall budgeting and resource management functions of healthcare organisations.

Redesigning clinical care, business and information processes

Best-practice wound prevention and care programmes involve comprehensive processes of organisational change that extend well beyond simple introductions of new clinical methods or technologies. Central to the change that occurs within organisations is the simplification and standardisation of decision-making and information-sharing systems:

- Clinical care protocols and process maps are used to define clear decision-making pathways for all staff. These tools help to eliminate confusion and reduce the time required to make patient care decisions and to initiate therapies.
- Measurement and monitoring systems generate regular feedback on clinical outcomes and performance, so that problems are identified and solved, progress is monitored, costs are tracked and areas for improvement are identified.
- Consistent and comprehensive documentation supports the efficient integration of care services delivered by a multidisciplinary clinical team.
- Pathways and documentation systems enable the smooth transition of patients across the continuum of care (e.g. from acute care to a home-care setting). Records and pathways go with the patient, so that care can be continued with minimal re-assessments, delays, questions or confusion.
- Detailed product formularies specify wound care products which are, in turn, linked back to clinical pathways. These formularies eliminate duplication and waste, and create opportunities to reduce costs through bulk purchasing.
- Formularies and clinical pathways also control the acquisition, allocation and use of capital equipment such as pressure-reducing surfaces, to ensure that high-cost devices are carefully monitored and used only where appropriate.
- Clinical training and education programmes are focused on pathways and protocols for consistency and efficiency. They are competency based to support the development of permanent, sustainable clinical capacities and reduce reliance on external expertise.
- The combination of best-practice clinical pathways that are consistently applied and information systems that generate regular performance data creates an organisational environment that supports patient safety. The risk of clinical errors that are costly to patients, healthcare workers and organisations is reduced.

Wound care becomes a fundamental part of clinical practice that is integrally related to the broader chronic disease management, patient safety and quality care agendas of health-care organisations. The systems and processes associated with best-practice wound prevention and care programmes are therefore well-positioned to serve as models for other clinical functions, or to be linked to broader organisational reforms.

Indirect economic benefits

Best-practice wound prevention and care programmes can contribute to a positive and productive workplace environment. Although the launch of a programme can be challenging, clinicians typically respond positively when an evidence-based framework of care is applied consistently and predictably across the entire organisation. Clinicians also appreciate regular feedback on performance. Wound care often represents one of the best available opportunities in healthcare to produce rapid results, leading to improved staff morale, with potential benefits across the organisation.

These programmes also generate economic benefits that extend beyond healthcare into the general society. Each wound that is prevented or healed represents an opportunity for someone to enjoy improved comfort and perhaps, restored mobility or the capacity to continue working. Effective wound care can mean the ability to maintain independent living arrangements or reduce dependencies on family members and other support services. All of these outcomes translate into benefits to individuals and the broader society that may be difficult to measure, but in many ways represent the most important result of best-practice wound prevention and care programmes.

Summary

Experience to date with the development and implementation of best-practice wound prevention and care programmes illustrates the close relationship between quality care and health economics. As quality and safety initiatives are implemented across healthcare organisations, errors are reduced and clinical outcomes are improved and become more predictable. The appropriate clinical resources are matched with clinical needs. Waste is reduced and cost efficiencies are realised. Over time, measurement and monitoring systems enable the continuous improvement of quality and safety, and ultimately patient outcomes and resource utilisation. The prevention and care of chronic wounds is particularly effective in demonstrating these relationships due to the widespread occurrence of these conditions across the healthcare continuum, the close association with a number of common chronic diseases and the multi-disciplinary nature of care and treatment.

In this context of increasingly strained healthcare resources, it is important for clinicians to develop an understanding of the relationships between quality and health economics. This includes an appreciation for the total cost of care and treatment. Clinicians must learn the critical processes involved and understand the importance of safe, quality care, delivered in the most appropriate setting by the most appropriate provider. A broader perspective that encompasses the organisation and the healthcare system as a whole will ultimately support both quality and value.

Best-practice wound prevention and care programmes also illustrate how significant improvements can be achieved through the implementation of protocols, methodologies and technologies that are well-established, evidence-based and readily available. Most of the interventions required are based on the consistent, disciplined application of effective and appropriate nursing practice, rather than any specific new medical technologies or innovations. In this regard these programmes offer valuable lessons: they provide processes and methodologies that can potentially be expanded and adapted to address other healthcare priorities, particularly related to the management of common chronic diseases.

Useful resources

Wound organisations

American Academy of Wound Management (USA). Available at: http://www.aawm.org

Association for the Advancement of Wound Care. Available at: http://aawconline.org

Australian Wound Management Association, Inc. Available at: http://www.awma.com.au

Canada Association of Wound Care. Available at: http://www.cawc.net

European Wound Management Association. Available at: http://www.ewma.org

European Pressure Ulcer Advisory Panel. Available at: http://www.epuap.org

Icelandic Wound Healing Society. Available at: http://www.sums-is.org/english.aspx

National Alliance of Wound Care. Available at: http://www.nawccb.org

National Pressure Ulcer Advisory Panel. Available at: http://www.npuap.org

New Zealand Wound Care Society. Available at: http://www.nzwcs.org.nz

Registered Nurses Association of Ontario: Wound Care. Available at: http://rnao.ca/

South Australia Wound Management Association. Available at: http://www.awma.com.au/sa/

Tasmanian Wound Care Association. Available at: http://www.twca.com.au

Tissue Viability Nurses Association. Available at: http://www.tvna.org

UK Tissue Viability Society. Available at: http://www.tvs.org.uk

Wound Care Information Network. Available at: http://www.medicaledu.com

Wound Care Society. Available at: http://www.woundcaresociety.com

Wound, Ostomy and Continence Nurses Society. Available at: http://www.wocn.org

Wound Management Association of Ireland. Available at: http://www.wmaoi.org

World Union of Wound Healing Societies. Available at: http://www.wuwhs.org

Journals

Advances in Skin & Wound Care. Available at: http://www.aswcjournal.com

Journal of Wound Care. Available at: http://www.journalofwoundcare.com

Ostomy/Wound Management. Available at: http://www.o-wm.com

Wound Repair and Regeneration. Available at: http://www.blackwellpublishing.com

World Wide Wounds. Available at: http://www.worldwidewounds.com

Wounds UK. Available at: http://www.wounds-uk.com

International Wound Journal. Available at: http://www.internationalwoundjournal.com

Educational resources

Institute of Health Economics: Albert, Canada. Available at: http://www.ihe.ca/sitemap

WoundPedia. Available at: http://www.woundpedia.com

Wounds International. Available at: http://www.woundsinternational.com

References

Baranoski, S., Ayello, A.E. (2008) *Wound Care Essentials-Practice Principles.* 2nd edn. Philadelphia, PA: Lippincott Williams & Wilkins.

Berendt, M., Schaefer, B., Heglund, M.J., Barden, C. (2001) Telehealth for effective disease state management. *Home Care Provider*, 6(2), 67–72.

Bolton, L., McNees, P., van Rijswijk, L., et al. (2004) Wound-healing outcomes using standardized assessment and care in clinical practice. *Journal of Wound, Ostomy and Continence Nursing*, 31(2), 65–71.

Britt, H., Sayer, G.P., Miller, G.C., et al. (1999) *General Practice Activity in Australia 1998–99.* Canberra, Australia: Australian Institute of Health and Welfare.

Drew, P., Possnett, J., Rusling, L. (2007) The cost of wound care for a local population in England. *International Wound Journal*, 4(2), 149–155.

Finkelman, A. (2006) *Leadership and Management in Nursing.* 2nd edn. Upper Saddle River, NJ: Prentice Hall.

Flanagan, M. (2005) Barriers to the implementation of best practice in wound care. *Wounds UK*, 1(3), 74–82.

Friedberg, E., Harrison, M.B., Graham, I.D. (2002) Current home care expenditures for persons with leg ulcers. *Journal of Wound, Ostomy and Continence Nursing*, 29(4), 186–192.

Graves, N., Burrell, F., Whitby, M. (2005) Modelling the economic losses from pressure ulcers among hospitalised patients in Australia. *Wound Repair and Regeneration*, 13(4), 462–467.

Hurd, T. (2011) Ballarat Health Services. *Improving Wound Care Outcomes.*

Hurd, T., Posnett, J. (2009) Point prevalence of wounds in a sample of acute hospitals in Canada. *International Wound Journal*, 6(4), 287–293.

Hurd, T., Popovich, K., Antoni, T. (2012) Comparative Analysis of the Implementation of Improved Pressure Ulcer Prevention Programs in Healthcare Organizations in Canada and Australia. Poster presented at: 4th Congress of the Worlds Union of Wound Healing Societies. September 6, 2012; Tokohama, Japan.

Hurd, T., Trueman, P. (2012) Evaluating the costs and benefits of innovations in chronic wound care products and practices. *Wound Ostomy.*

Hurd, T., Zuliani, N., Posnett, J. (2008) Evaluation of the impact of restricting wound management practices in a community care provider in Niagara, Canada. *International Wound Journal*, 5(2), 296–303.

Karpiel, M.S. (2000) APCs challenge hospital EDs and outpatient clinics. *Healthcare Finance Management*, 54(7), 62–66.

Board on Population Health and Public Health Practice (2012) *Living Well with Chronic Illness: A Call for Public Health Action.* National Academies Press, Available at: http://www.nap.edu/openbook.php?record_id= 13272&page=163. Retrieved on January 31, 2012.

Mannion, R., Davies, H.T.O., Marshall, M.N. (2005) Cultural characteristics of "high" and "low" performing hospitals. *Journal of Health Organization and Management*, 19(6), 431–439.

Popovich, K., Tohm, P., Hurd, T. (2010) Skin and wound care excellence integrating best practice evidence. *Healthcare Quarterly*, 13(5), 42–46.

Posnett, J., Franks, P. (2007) The costs of skin breakdown and ulceration in the UK. In: *Skin Breakdown: The Silent Epidemic* (ed. M. Pownall). Hull, UK: Smith and Nephew Foundation.

Shiell, A., Donaldson, C., Mitton, C., Currie, G. (2002) Health economic evaluation. *Journal of Epidemiology and Community Health*, 56(2) 85–88.

Sussman, C., Bates-Jensen, B. (2007) *Wound Care: A Collaborative Practice Manual for Health Professionals.* Baltimore, MD: Lippincott Williams & Wilkins.

Swanson, L. (1999) Solving stubborn wound problem could save millions team says. *Canadian Medical Association Journal*, 160(4), 556.

Teague, L.M., Mahoney, J.L. (2004) Cost effective wound care: how the advanced practice nursing role can positively affect outcomes in an acute care setting. *Wound Care Canada*, 2(1), 32–33.

Wagner, E.H., Austin, B.T., Von Korff, M. (1996) Organizing care for patients with chronic illness. *Milbank Quarterly*, 74(4), 511–544.

Walker, D. (2009) The cost of outpatient wound care. *Today's Wound Clinic*. Available at: http://www.todays woundclinic.com/the-cost-outpatient-wound-care? page=3. Last accessed 19 November 2012.

Waters, N. (2005) The challenges of providing cost effective quality wound care in Canada. *Wound Care Canada*, 3(1), 22–52.

Wound Ostomy and Continence Nurses Society (2010) *Guidelines for Prevention and Management of Pressure Ulcers. Clinical Practice Guidelines Series,* Mount Laurel, NJ. Available at: https://wocn.site-ym.com/store/ view_product.asp?id=692610&hhSearchTerms= Guidelines+and+pressure+and+ulcers, Retrieved on March 2012. Last accessed 19 November 2012

17 Dressings: The Healing Revolution

Douglas Queen[1] and Keith Harding[2]

[1] Wound Healing Research Unit, Medical School, Cardiff University, Cardiff, UK
[2] Research Unit, TIME Institute, Medical School, Cardiff University, Cardiff, UK

Overview

- Wound management originates from humble beginnings as innovative technologies have stimulated advances in new treatments. Wound care has now developed into the global arena with most countries having some advanced wound products available.
- Technological advances mean that dressings now have specific functions, such as the ability to reduce bacterial burden, and need to be selected carefully. This makes dressing choice complicated resulting in a large number of inappropriate dressings being used today.
- Although 50 years old, the principle of moist wound healing and adoption of advanced products is not universal. It is generally accepted that today less than 50% of chronic wounds receive appropriate modern moist wound dressings.
- Advanced wound technologies require key evidence to support their use. But the effectiveness of these products is hindered by the difficulty of choosing the 'right' product for the 'right' wounds at the 'right' time.
- There is a danger today that cost-cutting measures may restrict the development of wound management as a clinical specialty. To survive, data urgently need to be collected to provide information to convince those who determine health policy that wound care is a serious concern.
- Significant funding challenges for healthcare services globally is likely in the future to result in the emergence of specialised, multidisciplinary clinical service delivery in the public and private sectors for patients with wound and skin integrity problems.

Introduction

Over the past 40 years, clinicians have been exposed to a plethora of new advanced wound dressings. Many reviews have been written concerning the development of dressing technology and individual products often updating from the last to reflect the evolution of wound dressings over time (James and Watson, 1975; Eaglstein and Mertz, 1978; Harding et al., 2002; Thomas and O'Donnell, 2006). These publications often present a regional perspective of the development of modern wound care and may not be evidenced based.

However, the development of the modern wound care concept and adoption of advanced products is not universal even today. Healthcare markets in

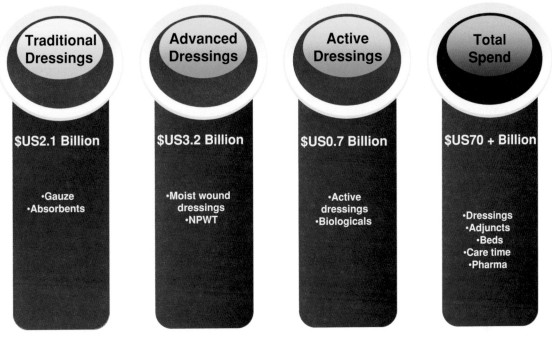

Traditional Dressings

$US2.1 Billion

•Gauze
•Absorbents

Advanced Dressings

$US3.2 Billion

•Moist wound dressings
•NPWT

Active Dressings

$US0.7 Billion

•Active dressings
•Biologicals

Total Spend

$US70 + Billion

•Dressings
•Adjuncts
•Beds
•Care time
•Pharma

Figure 17.1   Estimated size of the global wound dressing market.

different countries develop at different times and evolve at different rates. Expert opinion can vary in different countries and between discrete professional groups resulting in conflicting advice and different practice recommendations. This means that implementation of change in clinical practice can be frustratingly slow and may differ by geographical region and culture.

Today, wound care is a global arena with most countries having some elements of technology and dressing product available. Although traditional wound dressings still account for a significant number of dressing products used even today, there has been an explosion of interactive and advanced dressing products over the past 30 years making wound healing a multibillion dollar industry (Figure 17.1).

However, the efficacy of many wound dressing products has not been empirically and rigorously tested and clinicians may not have the critical appraisal skills to differentiate between good- and poor-quality research evidence. In recent years, the Internet has helped to share best practice and provides a good source of clinical guidelines developed by specialist consensus groups to support clinical decision-making. But this is an area that requires

further improvement if wound management is to mature into a true clinical specialty.

This chapter will review the historical development of advanced wound technologies, highlighting major advances in our understanding of wound healing. It will discuss implications for practice development and the future of wound care as a clinical specialty.

Evolution of new wound dressing technologies

The management of wounds began in Egyptian times (Sipos et al., 2004) with grease-soaked gauze bandages. Over the centuries, a variety of materials such as leaves, mud and marine sponges have been used to cover wounds and although wound contact materials have become more sophisticated, their function to promote healing has remained the same. Up until the 1980s, traditional dressings such as gauze were non-occlusive and dried out adhering to the wound bed. This led to wound trauma and bleeding at dressing removal, causing pain and delayed healing (Rogers et al., 1999).

In the 1960s and 1970s, the pioneering work of a group of researchers into the effects of occlusive dressings stimulated a interest in the development of a new generation of dressing materials which has transformed and challenged traditionally accepted approaches to wound management and improved the management of patients with chronic wounds (Winter, 1962; Hinman and Maibach, 1963; James and Watson, 1975). Others went on to study this phenomenon in humans and demonstrated not only faster healing but also better tissue quality (less scarring) (Alvarez et al., 1983; Foertsch et al., 1998; Eaglstein, 2001) and reduced pain (Nemeth et al., 1991).

During the 1980s, wound care took a new direction with the widespread introduction of products that promoted moist wound healing (Eaglstein and Mertz, 1978; Alvarez et al., 1983; Alvarez, 1988). As the principle of moist wound healing gained acceptance, dressings that were capable of providing conditions that promoted healing became available for the first time. Today, there is a better understanding of local factors that delay wound healing such as the need to control the wound bioburden and absorb chronic wound fluid (Schultz et al., 2003). So wound dressings are now designed to function in specific circumstances and therefore, the choice of product for optimal wound management is not straightforward. Dressing choice should not be made for a single wound factor or indeed one specific function. The wound, the patient and their multiple needs should also be considered.

Optimal wound-care wisdom understands and promotes the need for a moist interactive dressing in chronic wounds with an improved ability to heal (Keast and Orsted, 1998). Unfortunately, best practice does not necessarily follow and a large number of inappropriate dressings are still used today. Any treatment choice should consider other patient-centred factors involved in the quality of their life in addition to healing.

Moist interactive wound care has been in existence for the past three decades in countries such as the United Kingdom and the United States and the concept of moist wound healing is not new. But, even today, the use of dressings promoting moist wound healing in regular wound care practice is too low and it is generally accepted that less than 50% of chronic wounds receive modern moist wound dressings even when they are appropriate (Eaglstein, 2001). The main justification for the continued use of traditional dressings is budget constraints (cost and unavailability) and lack of knowledge, particularly in routine healthcare settings. These are mainly gauze-based dressings, which do little to promote healing or patient comfort.

Dressing manufacturers have been aware of the benefits of moist wound healing for some time, and as a result an evolutionary development process, through innovation, has provided the comprehensive range of moist interactive dressings available today. These products are based on the same principles defined by Winter in 1962 by creating a moist environment to enhance healing, reduce pain and improve scar quality, allowing healing to progress more naturally.

During the evolutionary development of modern dressing materials, manufacturers have become aware of product shortcomings and have designed better product variants. The modern wound care revolution truly began in the late 1980s and early 1990s with an explosion of products and significant scientific and clinical research around the area of moist healing. It is now routinely accepted among key opinion leaders that moist wound healing has been shown to be superior with respect to wound management, when compared with dry dressings (Eaglstein, 1985; Eisenberg, 1986; Eaglstein et al., 1987; Nemeth et al., 1991; Harding et al., 2000). The wound bed preparation paradigm introduced by Sibbald et al. (2000) involved treating the cause, local wound care and patient-centred concerns and began to give some structure to the clinical thought process around dressing choice and a patient-centred approach to care. Treating the cause revolves around the correct diagnosis of the wound aetiology and patient-centred concerns focus on what the patient sees as the primary reasons for receiving treatment for his/her wound.

The healing revolution

One of the earliest moist interactive dressings were polyurethane films which were used in Winter's classic study in 1962 widely acknowledged as being responsible for the concept of moist wound healing. This type of film dressing simply adhered to the surrounding skin trapping moisture at the wound bed. Film dressings provided some pain relief by preventing dehydration of the wound surface and bathing exposed nerve endings in wound fluid. The strong adhesives used to secure the dressing film could cause trauma on removal (Campbell et al., 2000), although today improved adhesive technology and careful removal techniques help to minimise skin damage (Burge, 2004). Strong adhesive bonds in this type of dressing may lead to skin tears unless the adhesive bond is weakened by stretching the dressing laterally and parallel to the wound surface before trying to remove the dressing by gently lifting at a 90° angle above the wound surface. Polyurethane film dressings are not designed to absorb fluid as exudate accumulation may break the seal to the external environment and risk bacterial contamination.

Following the limitations of the film dressings, a number of more absorbent moist wound care dressing categories were developed and a plethora of products became available in the 1980s and 1990s:

- *Hydrocolloid dressings* (Friedman and Su, 1984; Heffernan and Martin, 1994; Chang et al., 1998) were shown to produce a moist environment by gelling on contact with wound fluid. The outer layer of hydrocolloids is protected by a semi-occlusive film covering;
- *Foam dressings* (Thomas et al., 1997; Martini et al., 1999; Ashford et al., 2001; Kammerlander and Eberlein, 2003; Viamontes et al., 2003) provided an easy-to-remove, absorbent, non-adhesive contact surface (some newer products contain adhesive surfaces);
- *Alginates* (Piacquadio and Nelson, 1992; Bale et al., 2001) transform from a fibre to a soft gel on contact with wound fluid and provide a low-adherent wound contact surface that provides a moist wound environment;
- *Hydrogels* (Mandy, 1983; Yates and Hadfield, 1984; Kickhofen et al., 1986; Misterka, 1991; Sdlarik et al., 1995; Whittle et al., 1996; Agren, 1998; Eisenbud et al., 2003) provide high water content in a gel lattice that makes them non-adherent and soothing. This type of dressing rehydrates the wound and facilitates autolysis.

All of these new products were designed with moist wound healing in mind, to promote faster healing. Some products were designed to provide security with regard to adhesion, while maintaining a moist environment. Other products provided moisture balance by absorbing and/or retaining wound exudate. Many modern dressings minimise wound pain by being low adherent and creating a moist environment which soothes exposed nerve endings, e.g. hydrogels, or are biodegradable and easily rinsed from the wound surface, e.g. alginates. Over the years, widespread use of these dressing products on a wide range of different wounds has provided insight into their advantages as well as their limitations.

However, the reality is that there is still not one ideal dressing that can manage all of the different local conditions found in different types of wound.

Film and hydrocolloid dressings have aggressive adhesives which can result in skin stripping around wound margins (Dykes et al., 2001; Finnie, 2002). Foam dressings can also adhere to the wound bed if wound exudation is low and should be used with caution on low-exudating wounds under compression bandages (Malone, 1987). Some products rely heavily on secondary coverings for retention, e.g. amorphous hydrogels, but some dressing combinations can be detrimental to wound healing. For example, an absorptive secondary dressing may remove the moisture from an amorphous hydrogel and dehydrate the wound bed. On the other hand, if an adhesive film is used over an amorphous hydrogel, the excess moisture trapped at the wound margin can cause maceration and cause wounds to deteriorate. Alginates absorb wound fluid but if they become supersaturated, the resultant gel may cause maceration of the surrounding skin or allow strikethrough of excess exudate through the secondary dressing. If a wound is too dry to transform the alginate fibres into a hydrogel-like material, then the wound surface remains dry and the undissolved dressing fibres do not provide moist interactive healing. These are some specific examples of limitations of wound dressings, the skill of dressing selection is to understand which dressing is appropriate for the wound at that specific time as this may change as the wound heals or deteriorates, e.g. becomes infected.

These issues led manufacturers to develop second-, third- and even fourth-generation products of existing dressings to improve their performance so that today clinicians are able to use more absorbent hydrocolloids or foams (Daniels et al., 2002; Goodhead, 2002). Classification of dressings is evolving as variants of modern dressing become available. Technological advances are providing wound contact materials with surfaces to reduce adhesion that are more absorbent (Martinez et al., 1998), e.g. hydrofibres (Legarra et al., 1997a; Bowler et al., 1999; Russell and Carr, 2000; Vloemans et al., 2001; Garcia et al., 2002) and next-generation hydrocolloid dressings (Legarra et al., 1997b).

Dressing evolution led by technology: an example

As the use of film dressings increased, clinicians began to see limitations which created an opening for development of alternative interactive dressings. At the same time, clinicians treating stoma patients noticed that the skin surrounding stomas began to heal under hydrocolloid stoma wafers. This led to the development of hydrocolloid dressings for wound management and the moist wound healing revolution really began. The introduction of hydrocolloids for the treatment of wounds drove both the clinical and technological adoption of the findings of Winter's work some 20 years after his discovery of the importance of moist wound healing (Mollard, 1984). This revolution was also spurred on in the 1980s by a more aggressive approach to the marketing of hydrocolloids than that of previous dressings.

Hydrocolloids comprise an adhesive rubber matrix containing a gel-forming colloidal suspension such as sodium carboxymethylcellulose or gelatin, containing fluid-absorbing particles (Thomas, 2008). Hydrocolloid dressings were modified from stoma products to be more appropriate for wound care. The adhesive wafers were backed by polyurethane films to make them easier to handle and to provide moisture-retentive properties previously offered only by film dressings. Hydrocolloid dressings overcame one of the limitations of film dressings by being able to absorb wound fluid.

Hydrocolloid dressings have been subject to a great deal of research. Much of this has centred around their mechanism of action and has by default led to the expansion of scientific knowledge about wound healing processes. Hydrocolloid dressings have been shown to not only provide a moist environment but to influence healing by creating an environment where the biological process of healing occurs in a more ordered fashion (Chen et al., 1992).

The first hydrocolloid dressing was launched in the United Kingdom in 1982, and was introduced into the United States a year later. This first formulation produced a viscous gel in the presence of exudate. By the 1990s, new formulations were introduced to provide greater absorption and today many companies produce generic versions of hydrocolloids (Thomas, 2008). All of these products are broadly similar in appearance and are used for the same range of clinical indications, despite some differences in their structure and composition. The continued development of hydrocolloid technology has provided a number of new technologies and dressings in other formats such as gels, foams and fibres. In addition, there are a number of combination dressing products available which contain hydrocolloid particles.

Hydrocolloids are not ideally suited for all clinical situations and do not absorb high levels of exudate. This lead to the development of newer technologies in the 1990s when hydrofibre dressings were introduced. Hydrofibre dressings are soft, non-woven pads or ribbons composed of sodium carboxymethylcellulose which absorb wound fluid, transforming it into a soft gel to maintain a moist environment to support healing and promote autolytic debridement (Armstrong and Ruckley, 1997).

This new technology created a new category of dressings that were neither hydrocolloid nor alginate but a hybrid of both and so the term hydrofibre was born. As this name was trademarked, similar dressings cannot refer to themselves as hydrofibres and this dressing category is likely to be renamed as 'gelling fibres' with different sub-categories, which may include alginates as it expands.

Patient-centred dressing evolution: an example

Specialised wound contact materials have been developed to improve the management of wound pain by producing dressings that release easily from the wound surface to minimise trauma. This was a more patient-centred, rather than material-focused, evolutionary approach. The significance of this development was that the approach used changed from material development, e.g. dressing performance, to patient symptom management. Dressing materials were specifically redesigned to have low-adherent coatings such as silicone that did not dry out and adhere.

Silicones are not new to wound care; indeed, they have been used in burns for over 30 years (Brossy, 1981; Bugmann et al., 1998). The most popular dressings were low-adherent silicone gel sheets for the management of burns (Perkins et al., 1983) and hypertrophic scars (Bail et al., 1998). Silicone dressings help minimise pain during dressing removal and have now progressed beyond simple gels and coatings, recently being redeveloped as soft silicone dressing technology.

Soft silicone dressings rely on a hydrophobic silicone layer that prevents the dressing from adhering to the wound surface. They do so by maintaining contact without causing friction and shear, thereby reducing the tear force on removal.

The soft silicones are among the first dressing products to be specifically designed for atraumatic removal from the wound bed and surrounding skin, with a focus on pain management. A variety of product variants now exist, providing a versatile technology for a number of clinical situations (Schwope et al., 1977). There are many patient testimonials supporting the use of these products which have become extremely popular for wounds associated with fragile skin such as skin tears and blistering diseases (Waring et al., 2009) and use for those with delicate skin such as children and the elderly (Cutting, 2008).

Advanced wound technologies

More sophisticated biological approaches to wound management have been around for the 40 years in which advanced wound modalities have evolved. Such an approach began in the burns arena with the use of artificial skin substitutes (Phillips and Gilchrest, 1990), which have become significantly more advanced (Hansbrough et al., 1994; Gentzkow et al., 1996; Barret et al., 2000) with the development of technologies such as Dermagraft (Curran and Plosker, 2002), Apligraf and similar modalities.

Biologically active dressings, based on collagen (Bou et al., 2002; Ishihara et al., 2002), chitosan (Doillon and Silver, 1986), hyaluronic acid (Davidson et al., 1991; Hashimoto et al., 2004), peptides (Skokan and Davis, 1993) and growth factors (Drisdelle, 2003; Henderson et al., 2003) have been developed and evaluated, but most still require evidence to substantiate widespread use beyond complex wounds that are slow to heal. Biologically active dressings have a comparatively high unit cost and there is a general lack of good-quality, cost-effective data to support their use. It is also difficult to accurately predict which wounds would benefit from such technologies and, as such, the overall effectiveness is diluted in clinical trials.

The reintroduction of larvae therapy (maggots) into clinical practice is a novel biological approach to wound debridement and cleansing which has gained popularity in recent years and a number of commercial organisations now farm sterile maggots, increasing their availability (Dowsett, 2003).

Developments in the antimicrobial dressing's category (Cullen et al., 2002; Lansdown, 2003) and regenerated cellulose–collagen dressings (Evans and Land, 2001) have given significant focus to metalloproteases and other pro-inflammatory mediators in wound healing. Current research into these products is greatly adding to our understanding of the role of the inflammatory response in wound healing. However, the true effectiveness of these advanced wound products is hindered by the difficulty of choosing the 'right' product for the 'right' wounds at the 'right' time. The development and evolution of these wound healing products has focused on a more scientific and patient-focused approach rather than based on the properties of the materials or their limitations in the physical wound environment. This has become the preferred approach to product design in the 2000s where the development of wound management products has become more mature.

Some non-dressing approaches to wound healing exist. These generally centre on negative pressure therapy (WUWHS, 2008), hyperbaric oxygen (Wang et al., 2003; Roeckl-Wiedmann et al., 2005), topical oxygen delivery (Quirinia, 2000) and warm-up therapies (Hess and Kirsner, 2003). Other approaches including transcutaneous electrical nerve stimulation, ultrasound and various skin grafting techniques, for example, pinch grafts, have also been tried. Some attempts have been made using systemic drugs to treat recalcitrant wounds but with little success.

Some of the more advanced wound technologies have been successful and in some cases clinical evidence exists, but due to their generally higher perceived costs they are not often part of routine clinical practice and have some further evolutionary steps to make. However, negative pressure therapy remains the most significant therapy category in wound care globally.

However, most of these advanced technologies still require key data to support their use. In recent years, the development of these advanced modalities has focused around a more scientific, clinical and patient-focused approach and is producing evidence that is more applicable to everyday clinical practice. The European Wound Management Association (EWMA) set up a Patient Outcome Group in 2010 to identify recommendations to improve clinical research in wound management which included the following:

- An objective evaluation of dressing performance may not require a comparative study as the relevant data could be assessed using a cohort study with a validated protocol.
- Decisions to adopt a new technology or procedure should not be made on the basis of clinical outcomes alone. Rational choice requires evidence of the costs and benefits of alternatives.
- Studies should be designed to address the relative cost-effectiveness of alternative treatments from the outset, in addition to safety and efficacy data.
- The choice of study duration must consider the type and size of the wound and its natural outcome.

(Gottrup et al., 2010)

The future: wound care as a clinical specialty

Historically, the development of wound care as a clinical specialty has primarily been the remit of clinicians with a special interest. But in reality, the growth of wound care as a clinical specialty has been led by industry through the development and marketing of new wound products and technologies (Queen, 2006).

The introduction of these technological advances has required significant education for clinicians, patients and their carers and has led the way to the development of the clinical specialty of wound management. As clinicians and health service providers have become involved, the demand for evidence of treatment efficacy has increased, resulting in diversion of industry resources previously involved in innovation (e.g. development of diagnostic tools), which has limited the continued development of wound care as a specialty.

Whilst it is important to demonstrate treatment efficacy, there is growing concern about the value and relevance of the RCT in wound care considering the varied and multiple co-morbidities that exist in patients with non-healing wounds as this will affect trial outcome data despite use of specific inclusion/exclusion criteria. In addition, the competitive nature of the industry supporting the wound care market has also impacted the continued evolution of the specialty (Harding, 2008; Queen, 2010).

If the development and adoption of the principle of moist wound healing or the implementation of a multidisciplinary approach are taken as the biggest indicators of specialty development, then some progress has been made but on a limited basis. Today, at best 50% of wound carers use moist wound healing and even less work as part of an integrated multidisciplinary team, so the evolution of wound management still has some ways to catch up with other clinical specialties.

One of the biggest barriers to the evolution of wound care, as a clinical specialty, is awareness and burden of proof, e.g. efficacy data. Both of these barriers could be minimised by policy-driven changes. But this is difficult to achieve as governments, who face significant financial challenges in the delivery of healthcare, are not only ignorant to the costs related to the treatment and prevention of wounds but are focused on what they believe are more important healthcare challenges. Indeed in some countries government agencies are implementing drastic cost-saving steps that are driving the evolution of wound management backwards such as the elimination of specialist wound care nurses. There is a significant danger that cost elimination programmes, if not implemented carefully, will restrict the future development of wound care services and compromise patient care at a time when the burden of chronic wound conditions are growing due to an aging population.

To address these issues, data need to be collected and pooled to provide the information necessary to convince those who drive health policy. Governments learn from governments, so incremental differences regionally can ultimately have an international impact. Politicians need to be lobbied, as do other government decision-makers, to firmly establish wound care as part of their focus and agenda. This will help with the realisation that management of skin integrity and wounds is a huge issue for

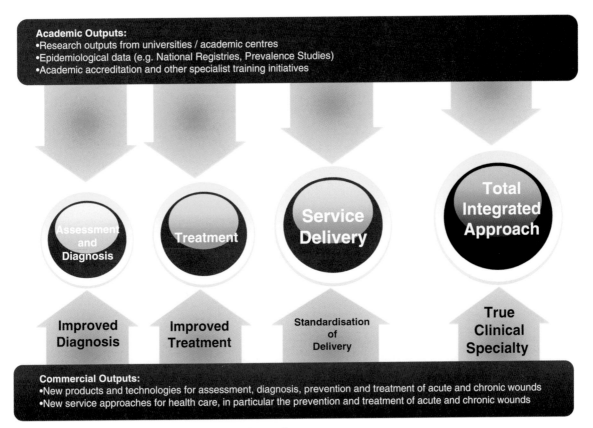

Figure 17.2   Evolution of wound healing as a clinical speciality.

society, which is growing exponentially as people live longer.

Ironically clinicians, academia and industry have a shared agenda which is concerned with raising awareness and development of an educated, more sophisticated marketplace to enhance wound healing as a specialty (Figure 17.2).

Together they need to lead government and policymakers to understand the complexity of wound care and tailor government initiatives and spending to suit the needs the patients with compromised skin integrity. Clinicians have an ethical and clinical responsibility to patients, government has a moral and fiscal responsibility to patients and industry has an ethical responsibility to provide effective treatment options for patients.

A recent publication noted that a key driver of the standardisation of practice is accurate assessment and diagnosis (Queen, 2010). As such, any diagnostic tool will play a pivotal role in the emergence of wound care as a clinical specialty. Figure 17.3

demonstrates the importance that diagnosis has in the evolution and adoption of standardised practice, which will include advanced therapeutics as this evolution occurs.

So the past 50 years has delivered change within practice, but clearly not enough as there still remains significant development to reach the degree of specialisation of other diseases.

Looking to the next 50 years of wound management we would predict

- continued commoditisation of current so-called advanced therapies, with little development of new materials, certainly in the short term (e.g. 10 years);
- some existing therapies (e.g. protease modulation) finding their place within the wound treatment spectrum, with appropriate evidence to support and direct their use;
- the true emergence of biological or pharmaceutical approaches with a better understanding

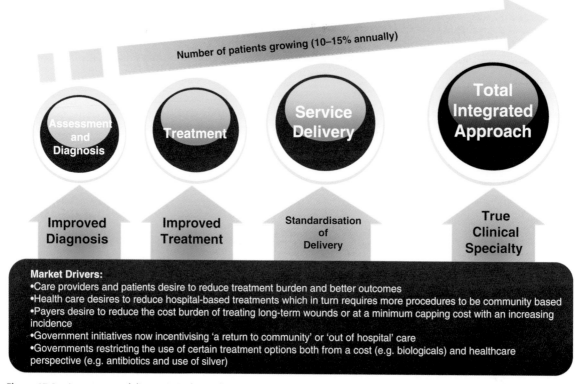

Figure 17.3 Importance of diagnosis in the evolution of wound healing as a clinical speciality (from Queen, 2010).

of where and when to use them, e.g. theranostics;

- the evidence debate being agreed upon with a clearer understanding of the type and level of evidence required for wound care and a wide range of evidence considered appropriate to support the process of clinical decision-making;
- assessment and diagnosis will become as sophisticated as in other clinical areas, including genetic signatures used to identify a patient's 'healability';
- as data are collected and presented, policymakers and funders will have a clearer understanding of the challenges both patients and carers alike face in the management of wounds and associated skin integrity problems;
- due to the significant funding challenges for healthcare services across the world, specialised, multidisciplinary clinical service delivery, both public and private, will emerge for patients with wound and skin integrity problems;

- preventative strategies will become a reality, as governments and payers better understand both the clinical specialty of wound care and also the economics of prevention rather than treatment in this clinical arena;
- as patient care becomes more self-care focused, there will be an emergence of patient educational materials, without the fear of litigation, which provides accurate guidance to self- or family-driven wound care.

Perhaps a stronger focus on the development of better wound assessment and diagnostic tools and more specialised clinical service delivery, rather than the development of more therapies, would help achieve the specialty status of 'woundology' which would have equal recognition to other clinical specialties such as oncology and cardiology. As care becomes more self-driven, either by self-treatment or choice of service provider, the patient's voice will surely lead to more significant changes over the next 50 years. To date, healthcare providers have, to a degree, failed to acknowledge patient concerns as part of the multidisciplinary approach to the prevention or treatment of wounds. Perhaps in future, however, those with the most significant vested interest will finally be heard.

Summary

Wound therapies have evolved significantly over the past four decades, providing more effective and more user-friendly dressings. Technology and product proliferation, however, varies by geography, usually as a function of economics and healthcare policy. From the banana-leaf and potato-peel approaches of the Third World to the sophisticated interactive dressings and growth factors of the developed world, much has advanced in relation to wound contact materials in recent years. However, one could argue that too much dressing choice exists, and the selection of a particular product without sufficient robust trial data to support its use remains, at best, an expensive guessing game.

The increase in clinical knowledge that new technologies and products bring to the wound care arena means that caregivers are better equipped than ever before to make the right treatment choices. Implementation of local wound management protocols based on best practice by an integrated multidisciplinary team using an appropriate treatment that is patient-, wound- and disease-specific will vastly improve healing outcomes compared to those available four decades ago.

Where can technology lead the evolution of wound management in the future? The creativity of clinicians, scientists and technologists has, to date, produced a range of sophisticated dressing materials for a variety of clinical situations. One thing is certain, the future of wound treatment and prevention will continue to evolve to meet new clinical challenges and improve quality of life for patients with compromised skin integrity.

Useful resources

Jones, V., Grey, J.E., Harding, K.G. (2006) ABC of Wound Healing. *British Medical Journal*, 332, 777–780. Available at: www.bmj.com

Stephen, T. (2010). *Surgical Dressings and Wound Management*. England: Medetec Publications.

This book provides a comprehensive review of wound dressing materials including: dressing development, mode of action of generic dressing groups and indications for clinical use. It is available as a printed book or as an e-book at: www.medetec.co.uk

The Surgical Materials Testing Laboratory provides dressing and medical device testing and produces technical reports to assist evidence-based purchasing. Available at: www.smtl.co.uk

References

Agren, M.S. (1998) An amorphous hydrogel enhances epithelialisation of wounds. *Acta Dermato-Venereologica*, 78(2), 119–122.

Alvarez, O. (1988) Moist environment for healing: matching the dressing to the wound. *Ostomy Wound Management*, 21, 64–83.

Alvarez, O.M., Mertz, P.M., Eaglstein, W.H. (1983) The effect of occlusive dressings on collagen synthesis and re-epithelialization in superficial wounds. *Journal of Surgical Research*, 35(2), 142–148.

Armstrong, S.H., Ruckley, C.V. (1997) Use of a fibrous dressing in exuding leg ulcers. *Journal of Wound Care*, 6(7), 322–324.

Ashford, R.L., Freear, N.D., Shippen, J.M. (2001) An in-vitro study of the pressure-relieving properties of four wound dressings for foot ulcers. *Journal of Wound Care*, 10(2), 34–38.

Bail, D.H., Schneider, W., Khalighi, K. Seboldt, H. (1998) Temporary wound covering with a silicon sheet for the soft tissue defect following open fasciotomy. Technical note. *Journal of Cardiovascular Surgery*, 39(5), 587–591.

Bale, S., Baker, N., Crook, H., Rayman, A., Rayman, G., Harding, K.G. (2001) Exploring the use of an alginate dressing for diabetic foot ulcers. *Journal of Wound Care*, 10(3), 81–84.

Barret, J.P., Dziewulski, P., Ramzy, P.I., Wolf, S.E., Desai, M.H., Herndon, D.N. (2000) Biobrane versus 1% silver sulfadiazine in second-degree pediatric burns. *Plastic and Reconstructive Surgery*, 105(1), 62–65.

Bou Torra, J.E., Soldevilla Agreda, J.J., Martinez, C.F., Rueda, L.J. (2002) Collagen powder dressing in the treatment of pressure ulcer. Multicenter comparative study assessing effectiveness and cost. *Revista De Enfermeria*, 25(9), 50–57.

Bowler, P.G., Jones, S.A., Davies, B.J. Coyle, E. (1999) Infection control properties of some wound dressings. *Journal of Wound Care*, 8 (10), 499–502.

Brossy, J.J. (1981) Foam elastomer dressings in surgery. *South African Medical Journal*, 59(16), 559–560.

Bugmann, P., Taylor, S., Gyger, D., et al. (1998) A silicone-coated nylon dressing reduces healing time in burned paediatric patients in comparison with standard sulfadiazine treatment: a prospective randomized trial. *Burns*, 24(7), 609–612.

Burge, T.S. (2004) Removing adhesive retention dressings. *British Journal of Plastic Surgery*, 57(1), 93.

Campbell, K., Woodbury, M.G., Whittle, H., Labate, T., Hoskin, A. (2000) A clinical evaluation of 3M no sting barrier film. *Ostomy/Wound Management*, 46(1), 24–30.

Chang, K.W., Alsagoff, S., Ong, K.T., Sim, P.H. (1998) Pressure ulcers – randomised controlled trial comparing hydrocolloid and saline gauze dressings. *Medical Journal of Malaysia*, 53(4), 428–431.

Chen, W.Y.J., Rogers, A.A., Lydon, M.J. (1992) Characterization of biologic properties of wound fluid collected during early stages of wound healing. *Journal of Investigative Dermatology*, 99(5), 559–564.

Cullen, B., Smith, R., McCulloch, E., Silcock, D., Morrison, L. (2002) Mechanism of action of PROMOGRAN, a protease modulating matrix, for the treatment of diabetic foot ulcers. *Wound Repair and Regeneration*, 10(1), 16–25.

Curran, M.P., Plosker, G.L. (2002) Bilayered bioengineered skin substitute (Apligraf): a review of its use in the treatment of venous leg ulcers and diabetic foot ulcers. *Biodrugs*, 16(6), 439–455.

Cutting, K.F. (2008) Impact of adhesive surgical tape and wound dressings on the skin, with reference to skin stripping. *Journal of Wound Care*, 17(4), 157–162.

Daniels, S., Sibbald, R.G., Ennis, W., Eager, C.A. (2002) Evaluation of a new composite dressing for the management of chronic leg ulcer wounds. *Journal of Wound Care*, 11(8), 290–294.

Davidson, J.M., Nanney, L.B., Broadley, K.N., et al. (1991) Hyaluronate derivatives and their application to wound healing: preliminary observations. *Clinical Materials*, 8(1–2), 171–177.

Doillon, C.J., Silver, F.H. (1986) Collagen-based wound dressing: effects of hyaluronic acid and fibronectin on wound healing. *Biomaterials*, 7(1), 3–8.

Dowsett, C. (2003) An overview of Acticoat dressing in wound management. *British Journal of Nursing*, 12(Suppl. 19), S44–S49.

Drisdelle, R. (2003) Maggot debridement therapy: a living cure. *Nursing*, 33(6), 17.

Dykes, P.J., Heggie, R., Hill, S.A. (2001) Effects of adhesive dressings on the stratum corneum of the skin. *Journal of Wound Care*, 10(2), 7–10.

Eaglstein, W.H. (1985) Experiences with biosynthetic dressings. *Journal of the American Academy of Dermatology*, 12(2 pt. 2), 434–440.

Eaglstein, W.H. (2001) Moist wound healing with occlusive dressings: a clinical focus. *Dermatologic Surgery*, 27(2), 175–181.

Eaglstein, W.H., Mertz, P.M. (1978) New methods for assessing epidermal wound healing: the effects of triamcinolone acetonide and polyethylene film occlusion. *Journal of Investigative Dermatology*, 71(6), 382–384.

Eaglstein, W.H., Mertz, P.M., Falanga, V. (1987) Occlusive dressings. *American Family Physician*, 35(3), 211–216.

Eisenberg, M. (1986) The effect of occlusive dressings on re-epithelializations of wounds in children with epidermolysis bullosa. *Journal of Pediatric Surgery*, 21(10), 892–894.

Eisenbud, D., Hunter, H., Kessler, L., Zulkowski, K. (2003) Hydrogel wound dressings: where do we stand in 2003? *Ostomy/Wound Management*, 49(10), 52–57.

Evans, D., Land, L. (2001) Topical negative pressure for treating chronic wounds: a systematic review. *British Journal of Plastic Surgery*, 54(3), 238–242.

Finnie, A. (2002) Hydrocolloids in wound management: pros and cons. *British Journal of Community Nursing*, 7(7), 338, 340, 342.

Foertsch, C.E., O'Hara, M.W., Stoddard, F.J., Kealy, G.P. (1998) Treatment-resistant pain and distress during pediatric burn-dressing changes. *Journal of Burn Care and Rehabilitation*, 19(3), 219–224.

Friedman, S.J., Su, W.P. (1984) Management of leg ulcers with hydrocolloid occlusive dressings. *Archives of Dermatology*, 120(10), 1329–1336.

Garcia, C.F., Salvador Moran, M.J., Roman Garcia, M.J. (2002) Treatment of skin lesions combining hydrofiber and extra-fine hydrochloride dressings. *Revista De Enfermeria*, 25(2), 50–54.

Gentzkow, G.D., Iwasaki, S.D., Hershon, K.S., et al. (1996) Use of Dermagraft, a cultured human dermis, to treat diabetic foot ulcers. *Diabetes Care*, 19(4), 350–354.

Goodhead, A. (2002) Clinical efficacy of Comfeel Plus transparent dressing. *British Journal of Nursing*, 11(4), 284, 286–287.

Gottrup, F., Apelqvist, J. Price, P. (2010) Outcomes in controlled and comparative studies on non-healing wounds: recommendations to improve the quality of evidence in wound management. *Journal of Wound Care*, 19(6), 239–268.

Hansbrough, J.F., Morgan, J., Greenleaf, G. Underwood, J. (1994) Development of a temporary living skin replacement composed of human neonatal fibroblasts cultured in Biobrane, a synthetic dressing material. *Surgery*, 115(5), 633–644.

Harding, K. (2008) 'Woundology'– an emerging clinical specialty. *International Wound Journal*, 5, 597.

Harding, K.G., Jones, V., Price, P. (2000) Topical treatment: which dressing to choose. *Diabetes/Metabolism Research and Reviews*, 16(Suppl. 1), S47–S50.

Harding, K.G., Morris, H.L., Patel, G.K. (2002) Science, medicine and the future: healing chronic wounds. *BMJ: British Medical Association*, 324(7330), 160–163.

Hashimoto, T., Suzuki, Y., Tanihara, M., Kakimaru, Y., Suzuki, K. (2004) Development of alginate wound dressings linked with hybrid peptides derived from laminin and elastin. *Biomaterials*, 25(7–8), 1407–1414.

Heffernan, A., Martin, A.J. (1994) A comparison of a modified form of Granuflex (Granuflex Extra Thin) and a conventional dressing in the management of lacerations, abrasions and minor operation wounds in an accident and emergency department. *Journal of Accident and Emergency Medicine*, 11(4), 227–230.

Henderson, J.L., Cupp, C.L., Ross, E.V., et al. (2003) The effects of autologous platelet gel on wound healing. *Ear, Nose, and Throat Journal*, 82(8), 598–602.

Hess, C.T., Kirsner, R.S. (2003) Orchestrating wound healing: assessing and preparing the wound bed. *Advances in Skin & Wound Care*, 16(5), 246–257.

Hinman, C.D., Maibach, H. (1963) Effect of air exposure and occlusion on experimental human skin wounds. *Nature*, 200, 377–378.

Ishihara, M., Nakanishi, K., Ono, K., et al. (2002) Photocrosslinkable chitosan as a dressing for wound occlusion and accelerator in healing process. *Biomaterials*, 23(3), 833–840.

James, J.H. Watson, A.C. (1975) The use of Opsite, a vapour permeable dressing, on skin graft donor sites. *British Journal of Plastic Surgery*, 28(2), 107–110.

Kammerlander, G. Eberlein, T. (2003) Use of Allevyn heel in the management of heel ulcers. *Journal of Wound Care*, 12(8), 313–315.

Keast, D.H., Orsted, H. (1998) The basic principles of wound care. *Ostomy/Wound Management*, 44(8), 24–28, 30–31.

Kickhofen, B., Wokalek, H., Scheel, D., Ruh, H. (1986) Chemical and physical properties of a hydrogel wound dressing. *Biomaterials*, 7(1), 67–72.

Lansdown, A.B. (2003) Silver-containing dressings: have we got the full picture? *Journal of Wound Care*, 12(8), 317–318.

Legarra, M.S., Vidallach Ribes, M.S., Esteban, G.M. (1997a) Non-comparative evaluation of a new hydrofiber dressing in the treatment of vascular ulcers. *Revista De Enfermeria*, 20(231), 59–63.

Legarra, M. S., Vidallach Ribes, M.S., Estanban, G.M. (1997b) Non-comparative evaluation of a new hydrofiber dressing in the treatment of vascular ulcers. *Revista De Enfermeria*, 20(231), 59–63.

Malone, W.D. (1987) Wound dressing adherence: a clinical comparative study. *Archives of Emergency Medicine*, 4(2), 101–105.

Mandy, S.H. (1983) A new primary wound dressing made of polyethylene oxide gel. *Journal of Dermatologic Surgery and Oncology*, 9(2), 153–155.

Martinez Cuervo, F., Franco Gutiez, T., Lopez Rebordinos, M.T., Menendez, S., Rodriguez, B. (1998) Treatment of chronic skin ulcers in the elderly. Descriptive study on the use of hydrocellular dressing. *Revista De Enfermeria*, 21(244), 51–60.

Martini, L., Reali, U.M., Borgognoni, L., Brandani, P., Andriessen, A. (1999) Comparison of two dressings in the management of partial-thickness donor sites. *Journal of Wound Care*, 8(9), 457–460.

Misterka, S. (1991) Clinical evaluation of a hydrogel type dressing materials after their 8 years use. *Polimery w Medycynie*, 21(1–2), 23–30.

Mollard, P. (1984) Penile dressings of CMH silicone elastomer foam. *Chirurgie Pediatrique*, 25(2), 117–119.

Nemeth, A.J., Eaglstein, W.H., Taylor, J.R., Peerson, L.J., Falanga, V. (1991) Faster healing and less pain in skin biopsy sites treated with an occlusive dressing. *Archives of Dermatology*, 127(11), 1679–1683.

O'Donnell, T.F. Jr., Lau, J. (2006) A systematic review of randomized controlled trials of wound dressings for chronic venous ulcer. *Journal of Vascular Surgery*, 44(5), 1118–1125.

Perkins, K., Davey, R.B., Wallis, K.A. (1983) Silicone gel: a new treatment for burn scars and contractures. *Burns, Including Thermal Injury*, 9(3), 201–204.

Phillips, T.J., Gilchrest, B.A. (1990) Cultured epidermal grafts in the treatment of leg ulcers. *Advances in Dermatology*, 5, 33–48.

Piacquadio, D., Nelson, D.B. (1992) Alginates. A "new" dressing alternative. *Journal of Dermatologic Surgery and Oncology*, 18(11), 992–995.

Queen, D. (2006) Trends in wound care – our changing environment. *International Wound Journal*, 3, 149.

Queen, D. (2010) The emergence of a clinical specialty in wound care. *International Wound Journal*, 7, 3–4.

Quirinia, A. (2000) Ischemic wound healing and possible treatments. *Drugs Today (Barc)*, 36(1), 41–53.

Roeckl-Wiedmann, I., Bennett, M., Kranke, P. (2005) Systematic review of hyperbaric oxygen in the management of chronic wounds. *British Journal of Surgery*, 92, 24–32.

Rogers, A.A., Walmsley, R.S., Rippon, M.G., Bowler, P.G. (1999) Adsorption of serum-derived proteins by primary dressings: implications for dressing adhesion to wounds. *Journal of Wound Care*, 8(8), 403–406.

Russell, L., Carr, J. (2000) New hydrofibre and hydrocolloid dressings for chronic wounds. *Journal of Wound Care*, 9(4), 169–172.

Schultz, G.S., Sibbald, R.G., Falanga, V., et al. (2003) Wound bed preparation: a systematic approach to wound management. *Wound Repair and Regeneration*, 11(2), S1–S28.

Schwope, A.D., Wise, D.L., Sell, K.W., Dressler, D.P., Skornick, W.A. (1977) Evaluation of wound-covering materials. *Journal of Biomedical Materials Research*, 11(4), 489–502.

Sdlarik, K.M., Vacik, J., Wichterle, O., Hajek, M. (1995) Modern dressings. Hydrogels. *Rozhledy v chirurgii*, 74(1), 3–7.

Sipos, P., Gyory, H., Hagymasi, K., Ondrejka, P., Blazovics, A. (2004) Special wound healing methods used in ancient Egypt and the mythological background. *World Journal of Surgery*, 28(2), 211–216.

Skokan, S.J., Davis, R.H. (1993) Principles of wound healing and growth factor considerations. *Journal of the American Podiatric Medical Association*, 83(4), 223–227.

Sibbald, R.G., Williamson, D., Orsted, H.L., et al. (2010) Preparing the wound bed—debridement, bacterial balance, and moisture balance. *Ostomy Wound Manage*, 46(11), 14–22, 24–28, 30–35.

Thomas, S. (2008) Hydrocolloid dressings in the management of acute wounds: a review of the literature. *International Wound Journal*, 5(5), 02–13.

Thomas, S., Banks, V., Bale, S., et al. (1997) A comparison of two dressings in the management of chronic wounds. *Journal of Wound Care*, 6(8), 383–386.

Viamontes, L., Temple, D., Wytall, D., Walker, A. (2003) An evaluation of an adhesive hydrocellular foam dressing and a self-adherent soft silicone foam dressing in a nursing home setting. *Ostomy/Wound Management*, 49(8), 48–52, 54–56, 58.

Vloemans, A.F., Soesman, A.M., Kreis, R.W., Middelkoop, E. (2001) A newly developed hydrofibre dressing, in the treatment of partial-thickness burns. *Burns*, 27(2), 167–173.

Wang, C., Schwaitzberg, S., Berliner, E., Zarin, D.A., Lau, J. (2003) Hyperbaric oxygen for treating wounds: a systematic review of the literature. *Archives of Surgery*, 138(3), 272–279.

Waring, M., Bielfeldt, S. Brandt, M. (2009) Skin adhesion properties of three dressings used for acute wounds. *Wounds UK*, 5(3), 22–31.

Whittle, H., Fletcher, C., Hoskin, A., Campbell, K. (1996) Nursing management of pressure ulcers using a hydrogel dressing protocol: four case studies. *Rehabilitation Nursing*, 21(5), 239–242.

Winter, G.D. (1962) Formation of the scab and the rate of epithelization of superficial wounds in the skin of the young domestic pig. *Nature*, 193, 293–294.

World Union of Wound Healing Societies (WUWHS) (2008) *Principles of Best Practice: Vacuum Assisted Closure: Recommendations for Use. A Consensus Document.* London: MEP Ltd.

Yates, D.W., Hadfield, J.M. (1984) Clinical experience with a new hydrogel wound dressing. *Injury*, 16(1), 23–24.

Index

Note: page numbers in *italics* refer to figures and tables.